Handbook of Pulmonary Drug Therapy

Handbook of Pulmonary Drug Therapy

Edited by
Samuel V. Spagnolo, M.D.

Professor, Department of Medicine, George Washington University School of Medicine and Health Sciences; Director, Division of Pulmonary Diseases and Allergy, and Attending Physician, George Washington University Medical Center; Chief, Pulmonary Disease Section and Attending Physician, Veterans Affairs Medical Center, Washington

Richard A. Nicklas, M.D.

Clinical Professor of Medicine, Division of Pulmonary Diseases and Allergy, George Washington University School of Medicine and Health Sciences; Attending Physician, George Washington University Medical Center, Washington

Philip Witorsch, M.D.

Clinical Professor of Medicine, Division of Pulmonary Diseases and Allergy, George Washington University School of Medicine and Health Sciences, and Adjunct Professor, Department of Pharmacology, Georgetown University School of Medicine; Attending Physician, George Washington University Medical Center, and Medical Director, Center for Environmental Health and Human Toxicology, Washington

Little, Brown and Company
Boston/New York/Toronto/London

First Edition

Library of Congress Cataloging-in-Publication Data

Handbook of pulmonary drug therapy / edited by Samuel V. Spagnolo, Richard A. Nicklas, Philip Witorsch.
p. cm.
Includes bibliographical references and index.
ISBN 0–316–80474–6
1. Pulmonary pharmacology — Handbooks, manuals, etc. I. Spagnolo, Samuel V. II. Nicklas, Richard A. III. Witorsch, Philip.
[DNLM: 1. Respiratory Tract Diseases — drug therapy — handbooks. WF 39 H2366 1993]
RM388.H36 1993
616.2′4061 — dc20
DNLM/DLC
for Library of Congress 93–26273
CIP

Printed in the United States of America

RRD-VA

Editorial: Laurie Anello
Production Editor: Kellie Cardone
Copyeditor: Beverly Miller
Indexer: Nancy Newman
Production Supervisor: Madeline Belliveau
Cover Designer: Vince Bitel

Contents

Contributing Authors

Aram A. Arabian, M.D.
Assistant Professor, Department of Medicine, George Washington University School of Medicine and Health Sciences; Attending Physician and Associate Chief, Medical Intensive Care Unit, Veterans Affairs Medical Center, Washington

Richard Carl Bernstein, M.D.
Pulmonary Fellow, George Washington University School of Medicine and Health Sciences, Washington

Jonathan G. W. Evans, M.D.
Pulmonary Fellow, George Washington University School of Medicine and Health Sciences, Washington

Cynthia L. Gibert, M.D.
Assistant Professor, Department of Medicine, Georgetown University School of Medicine; Assistant Chief, Infectious Diseases Section, Veterans Affairs Medical Center, Washington

Fred M. Gordin, M.D.
Associate Professor, Department of Medicine, Georgetown University School of Medicine; Chief, Infectious Diseases Section, Veterans Affairs Medical Center, Washington

Peter C. Hill, M.D.
Assistant Clinical Professor, Department of Medicine, George Washington University School of Medicine and Health Sciences, Washington

Steven H. Krasnow, M.D.
Associate Professor, Department of Medicine, George Washington University School of Medicine and Health Sciences; Chief, Oncology Section, Veterans Affairs Medical Center, Washington

Truvor V. Kuzmowych, M.D.
Associate Professor, Department of Medicine, George Washington University School of Medicine and Health Sciences; Chief, Pulmonary Clinic and Pulmonary Diseases Section, Veterans Affairs Medical Center, Washington

Shakun Malik, M.D.
Fellow, Oncology Section, Veterans Affairs Medical Center, Washington

Ann E. Medinger, M.D.
Assistant Professor, Department of Medicine, George Washington University School of Medicine and Health Sciences; Attending Physician and Director, Pulmonary Physiology Laboratory, Veterans Affairs Medical Center, Washington

John A. Michos, M.D.
Pulmonary Fellow, George Washington University School of Medicine and Health Sciences, Washington

Richard A. Nicklas, M.D.
Clinical Professor of Medicine, Division of Pulmonary Diseases and Allergy, George Washington University School of Medicine and Health Sciences; Attending Physician, George Washington University Medical Center, Washington

James V. Palazzolo, M.D.
Senior Fellow in Pulmonary and Critical Care Medicine, George Washington University School of Medicine and Health Sciences, Washington

Donn Quinn, M.D.
Pulmonary Fellow, George Washington University School of Medicine and Health Sciences, Washington

David P. Remy, M.D.
Fellow in Pulmonary and Critical Care Medicine, George Washington University School of Medicine and Health Sciences, Washington

Prashant K. Rohatgi, M.D.
Associate Professor, Department of Medicine, George Washington University School of Medicine and Health Sciences; Staff Physician and Associate Chief, Pulmonary Disease Section, Veterans Affairs Medical Center, Washington

Harris Andrew Sachs, M.D.
Pulmonary Fellow, George Washington University School of Medicine and Health Sciences, Washington

Samuel V. Spagnolo, M.D.
Professor, Department of Medicine, George Washington University School of Medicine and Health Sciences; Director, Division of Pulmonary Diseases and Allergy, and Attending Physician, George Washington University Medical Center; Chief, Pulmonary Disease Section and Attending Physician, Veterans Affairs Medical Center, Washington

John F. Wiley, M.D.
Fellow in Pulmonary and Critical Care Medicine, George Washington University School of Medicine and Health Sciences, Washington

Philip Witorsch, M.D.
Clinical Professor of Medicine, Division of Pulmonary Diseases and Allergy, George Washington University School of Medicine and Health Sciences, and Adjunct Professor, Department of Pharmacology, Georgetown University School of Medicine; Attending Physician, George Washington University Medical Center, and Medical Director, Center for Environmental Health and Human Toxicology, Washington

Edward S. Yanowitz, M.D.
Assistant Professor of Medicine, Division of Pulmonary Diseases and Allergy, George Washington University School of Medicine and Health Sciences; Attending Physician, George Washington University Hospital, Washington

Preface

We have labored to produce a concise and useful book for all practicing physicians, housestaff, medical students, nurses, and respiratory therapists who are faced with questions regarding current drug therapy for their patients with pulmonary problems. The contents represent a synthesis of our own knowledge and experience with an in-depth appreciation of current medical literature. Due to the continuing rapid changes that are taking place in therapy, we have continued to update various chapters until the last possible moment before publication.

With the recent dramatic increase in tuberculosis cases, we felt strongly that the book include an extensive and separate chapter on the treatment of that infection. A chapter on lung cancer provides the reader with a straightforward approach to understanding the principles of cancer chemotherapy for this increasingly common clinical problem. Although the treatment of deep venous thrombosis and pulmonary thromboembolism remains controversial, separate sections on the use and monitoring of heparin, warfarin, urokinase, and streptokinase provide a simplified approach to therapy. As lung transplantation increases, more non-university hospitals will be performing this procedure and use of cyclosporin, antilymphocytic globulin, and azothioprine, agents necessary for suppressing the immune response, will increase. Thus, there is increasing need for information such as provided in the chapter on lung transplantation. Kaposi's sarcoma and asthma during pregnancy were special situations where separate chapters were necessary to assist the reader in understanding our current approach to treatment.

Although we appreciate that drug management is frequently difficult and complex, we have attempted to simplify this task as much as possible. Each chapter includes drugs that are effective and a simple rationale for their usage. Nevertheless, we recognize that adverse effects and drug interactions are common in seriously ill patients and for these reasons the reader is advised to consult other reference material, including the *Physicians' Desk Reference* and standard pharmacology and medical textbooks. Suggestions for additional reading are in the reference sections at the end of each chapter.

We gratefully acknowledge our colleagues and contributors for their dedication and willingness to participate in this undertaking and Patricia Allen and Carol DeBonis for their secretarial, administrative, and moral support. Special thanks also goes to our editorial consultants, Laurie Anello and Kellie Cardone of Little, Brown and Company, for keeping the manuscript moving and for their excellent editorial suggestions.

S.V.S.
R.A.N.
P.W.

Handbook of Pulmonary Drug Therapy

Notice

1

Asthma

Richard A. Nicklas
Edward S. Yanowitz

Definition

The features of asthma (Table 1-1) that tend to separate this condition from other diseases involving the lower airways are (1) reversibility, usually defined as a 15% or greater improvement in forced expiratory volume in 1 second (FEV_1) spontaneously or after administration of a bronchodilator some patients with chronic bronchitis or emphysema may have a reversible component) and (2) the presence of bronchial hyperresponsiveness, as demonstrated by response to methacholine or some other pharmacologic or nonpharmacologic bronchoprovocation; a positive methacholine challenge can occur in a small number of patients who do not have asthma.

Asthma is a chronic condition, although the chronicity may vary tremendously from patient to patient, and is a form of bronchitis, characterized by eosinophil infiltration and desquamation of the bronchial epithelium.

Symptomatically, asthma is characterized by recurrent episodes of wheezing, cough, chest tightness, and/or dyspnea, reflecting a significant increase in resistance to airflow due to airway obstruction.

Pulmonary function tests — FEV_1, forced vital capacity (FVC), and maximal midexpiratory flow (MMEF) — may be less than 50% of predicted during a symptomatic period and will usually improve to more than 80% of predicted when the patient is asymptomatic.

Table 1-1. Characteristics of asthma

Reversibility
Bronchial hyperresponsiveness
Bronchial inflammation
Symptoms of wheezing, cough, dyspnea, and tightness in the chest
Pulmonary function
Broad spectrum of severity
Capricious
Heterogeneous with multiple triggers
- Allergens
- Irritants
- Viral infections
- Reactive chemicals
- Exercise
- Foods, additives
- Emotional factors
- Sinusitis
- Possibly gastroesophageal reflux

A presumptive diagnosis of asthma can be made if the patient presents with the symptoms noted previously, induced or exacerbated on at least two occasions by exposure to recognized allergens (e.g., recurrent symptoms during the same season or after exposure to a cat), especially if associated with positive skin tests for the suspected allergen.

Clinically, asthma is characterized by a broad spectrum of severity; some patients are asymptomatic, and others experience life-threatening exacerbations. Changes in severity may occur spontaneously or as a result of therapy.

Pathophysiology and Mechanisms

Although the pathophysiology of asthma is diversified and complex, inflammation plays a central role. The interaction of inflammatory cells, mediators released from these and other cells, and tissues present in the airways result in bronchoconstriction, reduced mucociliary clearance, increased mucus secretion, mucosal edema, cellular infiltration, vasodilation, and increased vascular permeability.

Goals of Therapy

Asthma is a heterogeneous disease process that can be initiated by a wide array of factors — irritants (indoor and outdoor pollutants, cigarette smoke, odors), specific allergens (dust mites, animal proteins, mold spores, pollens), reactive chemicals, exercise, viral infections, foods and additives, emotional factors, sinusitis, and probably gastroesophageal reflux. One goal of therapy is to minimize exposure as much as possible to specific triggers or to modify the response to these triggers by allergen immunotherapy with well-standardized extracts. Treatment must be individualized in regard to choice of medication, taking into account the patient's age, concomitant medical conditions, degree of airflow obstruction, the cause of airflow obstruction, and other medications being taken concomitantly. The variable clinical pattern and natural history of asthma determine the need for individualization of treatment. This requires an initial definition of realistically attainable goals of therapy (treatment objectives) for each patient. The relative safety of the therapeutic alternatives influences the therapeutic decisions that are made in striving for these goals. Table 1-2 lists the specific goals of treatment for asthmatic patients. The probability of greater morbidity from the disease in some patients may justify a greater therapeutic risk, provided sufficient benefit can be obtained.

Asthma is a capricious disease. The perception of asthma is changing from a condition that is easily controlled and highly predictable to one that is multifaceted, individualistic, and subject to sudden unexpected changes. In part, this perception has been fostered by recognition of a gradual increase in asthma mortality in the United States over the past 12 years, at a time when mortality from other chronic diseases has generally been on the decline. There has also been a substantial increase in hospitalization for asthma, not only

Table 1-2. Goals of treatment for asthmatic patients

Individualization of treatment
Prevention of morbidity and mortality
  Reduction of emergent care
  Reduction of hospitalization
  Prevention of nocturnal symptoms
Improvement in quality of life
  Tolerance of physical activity
  Decreased loss of time from school or work
  Improved self-image
Reversal of airflow obstruction, improvement in pulmonary function
Prevention of airway inflammation
Optimal asthma control with utilization of the least amount of medication
Adequate monitoring
Sequential selection of treatment
Education of patient/parents

in the United States but elsewhere, during a period when there has been tremendous emphasis on the outpatient management of patients with chronic disease. The responsibility of those involved in the treatment of asthma is not only the prevention of morbidity and mortality but also improvement in quality of life for each patient.

Successful pharmacologic management requires two major strategies: (1) reversal of acute and chronic airflow obstruction and (2) long-term attenuation and prophylaxis of the intrabronchial sequelae of inflammatory cells and their mediators. Treatment of airway obstruction usually requires the administration of antagonists of smooth muscle contraction and occasionally administration of medications that counteract neurogenic imbalance (cholinergic overload), bronchial edema, and hypersecretion of mucus. In addition to their antiinflammatory effect, long-term administration of antiinflammatory drugs lessens airway obstruction by decreasing the exudative reaction in the bronchi and providing a local environment that is more conducive to regeneration of bronchial epithelium.

A determination of when and how long to use specific medications should be based on a number of factors, including the severity of the patient's asthma. Occasional and isolated episodes of asthma rarely require more than as-needed inhalation of a $beta_2$ agonist.

Cognizant of the need for individuality of treatment, outcome goals might include (1) reduction of emergency care, (2) reduction in hospitalization, (3) prevention of nocturnal symptoms that interfere with sleep and reflect the severity of asthma, (4) tolerance of physical activity appropriate for the patient's age, (5) improvement in pulmonary function to an extent that it is either normal or can be normalized with recommended doses of an inhaled beta agonist bronchodilator, (6) minimization of time lost from work or school and other daily activities, (7) improved self-image based on a full understanding of the disease and confidence in outlined approaches to treatment, (8) optimal control of asthma with utilization of the least medication possible, administered in a manner that permits the most normal life-style, and/or (9) general improvement in the quality of life of the patient.

Adequate patient monitoring is essential for assessing the continued efficacy, safety, and need for long-term medication. There should be appropriate review for compliance, correct technique for medication administration, drug interactions, and potential anomalies in drug absorption or elimination.

When initial measures are suboptimal, the sequential selection of further medication should proceed in an orderly manner that is understandable to the patient and based on mutually agreed upon objectives. In addition, patient monitoring of peak flow can be important in analyzing the day-to-day and within-day variability of pulmonary function seen in asthmatic patients. They supplement more complete pulmonary function tests, which should be performed periodically.

Adrenergic Agonists (Sympathomimetics)

Epinephrine

Parenteral epinephrine is still occasionally useful but has largely been replaced in the acute management of obstructive lung disease by inhaled relatively beta_2 selective agonists.

PHARMACOLOGY AND CLINICAL INDICATIONS

Epinephrine is a sympathomimetic drug, acting on both alpha and beta receptors on effector cells. Epinephrine is used to relieve respiratory distress due to bronchospasm.

DOSE AND ADMINISTRATION

In pediatric patients, 0.01 ml/kg/dose to a maximum of 0.50 ml sc, repeated every 15 minutes to a maximum of 3 doses can be given. In adults, a dose of 0.1–0.3 mg (0.1–0.3 cc of a 1:1000 dilution) has been utilized.

ADVERSE REACTIONS

Transient and minor side effects of anxiety, headache, and palpitations often occur at therapeutic dosages, especially in patients with hyperthyroidism. Reports have also been received of increased blood pressure, cardiac arrhythmias, and gastrointestinal symptoms after administration of epinephrine.

Ephedrine

Ephedrine, a non-beta_2 selective agonist, is rarely used now but has been employed combined with a fixed dose of theophylline and a sedative in a tablet form. It has demonstrable but relatively weak bronchodilator properties. The usual dose of 25 mg readily crosses the blood-brain barrier and is often associated with significant side effects. As a result, the benefit : risk profile is poor compared with $beta_2$ specific agonists.

Isoproterenol

Inhaled isoproterenol (Isuprel), a non-$beta_2$ selective agonist, has a rapid onset (usually within 5 minutes) and a duration of effect of 2 hours or less. There is little indication for inhaled isoproterenol at the present time because of the longer duration of action and more favorable side effect profile of newer $beta_2$ selective agonists.

PHARMACOLOGY

Isoproterenol reverses bronchospasm by its action on beta receptors in bronchial smooth muscle. It is metabolized mainly in the liver by catecholomethyltransferase.

INDICATIONS

Inhaled isoproterenol can be utilized for the relief of bronchospasm associated with acute and chronic asthma.

DOSE AND ADMINISTRATION

To reverse symptoms, 1–2 inhalations, 1 full minute apart, can be used. Repeated use requires further evaluation of the patient's overall asthma control.

ADVERSE EFFECTS

Occasional transient throat irritation has been reported, as well as nervousness, headaches, dizziness, weakness, nausea, vomiting, tachycardia, palpitations, angina, skin flushing, tremor, diaphoresis, and paradoxical bronchospasm.

Isoetharine

PHARMACOLOGY

Isoetharine is a sympathomimetic with affinity for beta and $beta_2$ adrenegic receptor sites of bronchial and arteriolar smooth muscle.

INDICATIONS

For use as a bronchodilation in asthma and reversible bronchospasm that may occur with bronchitis and emphysema.

ADMINISTRATION

Administration of Isoetharine is 0.5 ml diluted with 2.5 ml of saline for nebulization, to be repeated usually no more frequently than every 4 hours in 24 hours.

ADVERSE EFFECTS

Adverse effects seen with isoetharine are consistent with those seen with other sympathomimetic amines.

Beta$_2$ Selective Agonists

Beta-adrenergic agonists — metaproterenol, terbutaline, albuterol, pirbuterol, and bitolterol — are extensively used to produce bronchodilation and prevent bronchoconstriction in patients with reversible obstructive airway disease (Fig. 1-1). In addition to being used in the treatment of asthma, they are also used in the treatment of patients with chronic bronchitis, emphysema, and cystic fibrosis if these patients demonstrate an element of reversible airway obstruction. Beta$_2$ agonists reduce airway obstruction by relaxing airway smooth muscle, increasing mucociliary clearance, decreasing vascular permeability, and possibly modulating mediator release from mast cells and basophils.

CLINICAL PHARMACOLOGY

Single doses of inhaled beta$_2$ agonists produce clinically significant bronchodilation within 5 minutes in most patients, a peak effect 30–60 minutes after drug administration, and a duration of effect of 3–4 hours in many patients and up to 6 hours in some patients. (For doses and administration, see Table 1-3.)

Metaproterenol

Inhalation aerosol: 2–3 inhalations every 3–4 hours; no more than 12 inhalations daily.

Inhalation solution: 5% solution administered by nebulizer or an intermittent positive pressure breathing apparatus, 3–4 times daily for the treatment of reversible airway disease. In addition, there are 0.4% and 0.6% unit dose vials, 1 vial per nebulization treatment, administered 3–4 times a day.

Syrup: Children 6–9 years of age or under 60 pounds, 1 teaspoon 3–4 times daily. Children over 9 years of age or weighing more than 60 pounds, 2 teaspoons 3–4 times daily.

Tablets: Adults and children over 9 years of age or weighing more than 60 pounds, 20 mg 3–4 times a day. Children 6–9 years or under 60 pounds, 10 mg 3–4 times a day.

Table 1-3. Recommended dose for $beta_2$ agonists

Drug	Route of administration	Dose
Metaproterenol	Metered-dose inhaler	2–3 inh q3–4h, up to 12 inh/24h
	Nebulization solution	0.3 ml in 2.5 ml saline tid-qid for patients 12 years and older; 0.1 ml in 3 ml saline
	Syrup	1 tsp tid-qid for patients 6–9 years of age or under 60 lb; 2 tsp tid-qid in patients 9–12 years or over 60 lb
	Tablets	20 mg tid-qid in patients over 9 years or over 60 lb; 10 mg tid-qid in patients 6–9 years or under 60 lb
Terbutaline	Metered-dose inhaler	2 inh q4–6h up to 12 inh/24h
	Tablets	5 mg q6h; 2.5 mg q6h in patients 12–15 years
	Injection	0.25 mg SQ for acute asthma, repeated in 15–30 min if necessary
Albuterol	Metered-dose inhaler	1–2 inh q4–6h up to 12 inh/24h 2 inh 15 min prior to exercise for EIB
	Nebulized solution	2.5 mg tid-qid
	Rotocaps	200 μg q4–6h 200 μg 15 min prior to exercise for EIB
	Syrup	1–2 tsp tid-qid in patients under 14 years; 1 tsp tid-qid for patients 6–14 years; 0.1 mg/kg tid for patients 2–6 years
	Tablets	2–4 mg tid-qid in patients 12 years and older; 2 mg tid-qid in patients 6–11 years
Pirbuterol	Metered-dose inhaler	1–2 inh q4–6h up to 12 inh/24h in patients 12 years and older
Bitolterol	Metered-dose inhaler	2 inh q8h up to 12 inh/24 hours in patients 12 years and older
	Nebulized solution	Up to 1 ml (2 mg) tid

inh = inhalations

Terbutaline

Inhalation aerosol: 2 inhalations separated by a 60-second interval, repeated every 4–6 hours, not to exceed 12 inhalations in 24 hours.

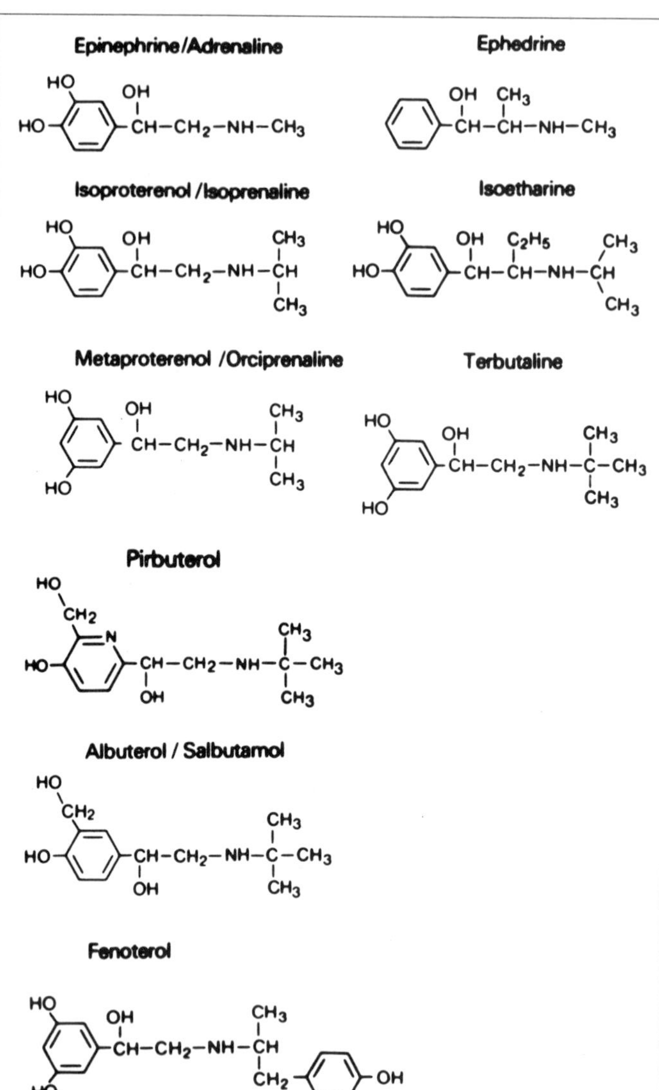

Fig. 1-1. Chemical structures of adrenergic agonist medications. (Reproduced by permission from: E. Weiss and M. Stein(eds.), *Bronchial Asthma: Mechanisms and Therapeutics* (3d ed). Boston: Little, Brown, 1993.)

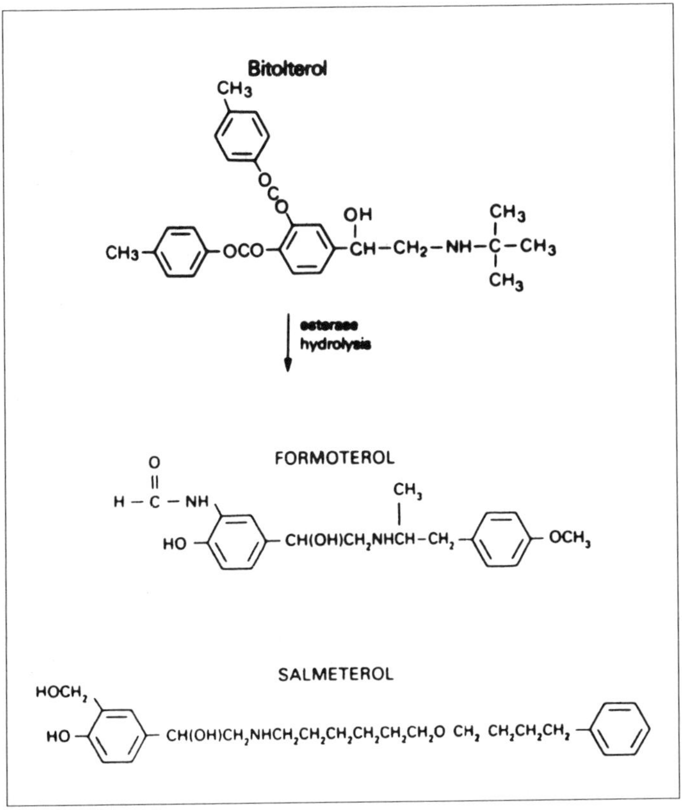

Fig. 1-1. (continued)

Tablets: The usual adult dose is 5 mg at 6-hour intervals, 3 times daily during waking hours. If side effects are disturbing or patients are 12 to 15 years of age, 2.5 mg 3 times daily may be an appropriate dose.

Injection: Subcutaneously 0.25 mg into the lateral deltoid area; if there is no significant clinical improvement with 15–30 minutes, a second 0.25 mg dose can be considered; do not exceed a total of 0.5 mg within any 4-hour period. If significant improvement is not achieved, other therapeutic approaches must be considered.

Albuterol (Ventolin, Proventil)

Inhalation aerosol: 1–2 inhalations repeated every 4–6 hours in adults and children 4 years of age and older not to exceed 12 inhalations in a 24-hour period; for prevention of exercise-induced bronchospasm (EIB): 2 inhalations 15 minutes before exercise in patients 12 years and older.

Inhalation solution: 2.5 mg administered 3–4 times daily by nebulization in patients 12 years and older; either dilute 0.5 ml of the 0.5% inhalation solution with 2.5 ml of sterile normal saline solution or give the contents of 1 sterile unit dose capsule (3 ml of 0.083% inhalation solution.)

Ventolin Rotocaps (200 μg capsule): The contents of 1 capsule inhaled every 4–6 hours using a rotahaler inhalation device. For EIB prevention in patients over 12 years of age, inhalation of the contents of 1 capsule 15 minutes before exercise.

Syrup: 2–4 mg (1–2 teaspoons) 3–4 times a day in adults and children over age 14 as a starting dose. For children 6–14 years of age, 2 mg (1 teaspoon) 3–4 times a day as a starting dose. For children 2–6 years, dosing should be initiated at 0.1 mg per kilogram of body weight, 3 times a day, not to exceed 2 mg (1 teaspoon) 3 times a day.

Tablets: 2–4 mg, 3–4 times a day in patients 12 years of age and older as a starting dose. For children 6–11 years of age, 2 mg 3–4 times a day, not to exceed 24 mg/day.

Pirbuterol (Inhalation Aerosol)

For patients 12 years of age and older; 1–2 inhalations (0.4 mg) every 4–6 hours, not to exceed 12 inhalations in a 24-hour period.

Bitolterol

Inhalation aerosol: For patients age 12 years and older, 2 inhalations every 8 hours, not to exceed 12 inhalations in a 24-hour period.

Inhalation solution 0.2%: Up to 1 ml (2 mg) 3 times a day by intermittent-flow nebulization or continuous-flow nebulization.

ADVERSE EFFECTS

Pharmacologic

The most common adverse effects seen after the administration of beta agonists — tremor, CNS effects, and tachycardia — are directly related to their pharmacologic activity (Table 1-4). The frequency of side effects depends on the route of administration. Parenteral administration of beta agonists produces the most adverse effects, and oral preparations generally produce more adverse effects than inhaled beta agonists.

Cardiovascular

Beta agonists, even inhaled relatively $beta_2$ selective agonists, have the potential to produce clinically significant increases in blood pressure and pulse rate, hemodynamic changes, and, in some patients, dysrhythmias and electrocardiographic evidence of myocardial necrosis. Although individual patients may sustain significant adverse cardiac effects from the administration of beta agonists, serious adverse cardiac effects due to the administration of $beta_2$ selective

Table 1-4. Partial list of adverse effects associated with beta agonist use

Tremor
CNS effects
Tachycardia
Palpitations
Cardiac arrhythmias (rare)
Hypokalemia
Tolerance
Myocardial necrosis (rare)
Paradoxical bronchospasm (inhaled formulations)
Hypoxemia

agonists in conventional doses are rare with oral administration and even more rare when administered by inhalation.

Tremor

Tremor produced by the administration of $beta_2$ selective agonists results from stimulation of $beta_2$ receptors on skeletal muscle. It is not uncommonly seen after the administration of $beta_2$ agonists but may decrease with continued treatment.

CNS Effects

With the exception of ephedrine, beta agonists cross the blood-brain barrier poorly. Nevertheless, headache and irritability may occur after their administration.

Paradoxical Bronchospasm

A paradoxical increase in airway obstruction can be seen in some patients with asthma after inhalation of epinephrine or beta agonists. Although the cause of most cases of drug-induced paradoxical bronchospasm is unclear, sulfites and other preservatives, emulsifying agents, and propellants have been implicated in some cases. Paradoxical bronchospasm may occur after the first use of a new canister or bottle in patients who have previously used the same product without difficulty.

Hypoxemia

Beta agonists can decrease arterial pO_2 due to ventilation-perfusion mismatches that occur despite improvement in airway obstruction.

TOLERANCE

After repetitive administration of oral or inhaled beta agonists, the peak effect may decrease, and the duration of clinically effective bronchodilation may be reduced from 4–6 hours to 2–3 hours after treatment for several months.

INDICATIONS FOR USE

Acute Asthma

Adrenergic agents are considered first-line therapy for the treatment of acute asthma in adults. Inhalation therapy with a nebulized $beta_2$ selective agonist produces bronchodilation equivalent to parenteral therapy with epinephrine and terbutaline but with fewer side effects; therefore, it should be considered the treatment of choice for most adult patients with acute asthma. Clinical studies have shown that inhaled $beta_2$ agonists are more effective than IV aminophylline in the treatment of acute asthma. Although the concomitant use of an adrenergic agonist and aminophylline may be effective in some patients, there continues to be debate about the routine use of these drugs concomitantly in the treatment of acute asthma.

Careful monitoring is often necessary in patients being treated for acute asthma, including spirometry or peak flow measurements before and after treatment if possible, ECG monitoring in patients at risk of adverse cardiovascular events, and measurement of serum potassium before and after treatment.

Oral beta agonists are not indicated in the treatment of acute asthma because (1) the onset of action is too slow, (2) there is no evidence for an increased bronchodilator effect over inhaled beta agonists, and (3) the risk of systemic effects is greater than with the use of inhaled beta agonists.

Chronic Asthma

Use of inhaled $beta_2$ agonists by metered-dose inhaler (MDI) on an as-needed basis is appropriate when only occasional pharmacologic intervention is necessary to control episodic bronchoconstriction. In general, if regular use of inhaled $beta_2$ agonists is required, particularly at doses greater than recommended, the patient should be considered to have more than mild asthma and requires careful evaluation and follow-up.

DRUG INTERACTIONS

$Beta_2$ agonists can be used alone or concomitantly with theophylline, cromolyn, corticosteroids, or anticholinergic agents, since many patients with moderate asthma require a combination of medications for effective control of symptoms and maintenance of pulmonary function. It is essential to recognize that the use of $beta_2$ agonists does not lessen the need for routine use of antiinflammatory drugs, preferably inhaled corticosteroids. Patients with nocturnal asthma are most likely to benefit from regular use of antiinflammatory medications, although an evening dose of an oral $beta_2$ agonist or theophylline can be considered.

If a patient requires more than 8 inhalations per day of an inhaled beta agonist to control symptoms and/or maintain pulmonary function or fails to achieve a rapid and sustained response to an inhaled $beta_2$ agonist during an exacerbation of asthma, treatment with oral corticosteroids or even hospitalization may be required.

ORAL BETA AGONISTS

Oral beta agonists are widely used in the treatment of chronic asthma in children. They may provide a distinct advantage in children because less frequent administration may lead to improved compliance.

SEVERE INTRACTABLE ASTHMA

Beta agonists may also be administered by injection, but whether given parenterally or by inhalation, they should be given with oxygen because of their ability to produce transient increase in ventilation-perfusion mismatches and worsening hypoxemia. Aqueous epinephrine and terbutaline sulfate when given subcutaneously are equally effective and unlikely to be associated with adverse cardiovascular effects in patients less than age 45 years. Nevertheless, continuous ECG monitoring should be used during treatment of severe intractable asthma whenever possible.

Inhaled beta agonists can be delivered by continuous nebulization or intermittently 2–3 times in the first hour of treatment. If no adverse effects are noted, the dose of nebulized beta agonist administered after the initial hour of treatment will depend on the patient's course and response to individualized treatment. Generally, repeated nebulizations are used every 20–60 minutes, with the interval between administration gradually lengthened until they are being given every 4–6 hours. However, in some patients with particularly severe exacerbations, repeated nebulizations every 20 minutes may not be adequate and be indicative of impending respiratory failure. Recently, continuous nebulization of terbutaline and albuterol has been used in this setting.

Intravenous beta-adrenergic agonists have also been used in this setting, although they should not be used unless absolutely necessary to prevent intubation and mechanical ventilation because of the risk of myocardial injury.

EXERCISE-INDUCED BRONCHOSPASM (EIB)

The medications of choice for the prevention of exercise-induced asthma are $beta_2$ selective agonists and/or cromolyn, but $beta_2$ agonists are usually the more effective of the two options. Because of ease of use, decreased potential for adverse effects, and demonstrated effectiveness, oral inhalation of beta agonists by an MDI is preferred over other routes of administration. The usual dose is 2 inhalations (although in some patients 1 inhalation may be sufficient) administered 15–20 minutes prior to exercise. Syrups have a slower onset of action, and the response may be variable. Nevertheless, they may be useful in children too young to use inhalers. Longer-acting dosage forms may be indicated before prolonged exercise or when it is inconvenient to take medication just before exercise.

LONG-ACTING BETA$_2$ SELECTIVE AGONISTS

Salmeterol

Salmeterol is a long-acting beta$_2$ selective adrenergic agonist bronchodilator, delivered by oral inhalation, which, like albuterol, is a saligenin derivative of the catecholamine nucleus common to all beta agonists (see Fig. 1-1). Its long duration of action has been demonstrated in clinical studies, where the duration of action is 12 hours in many patients. It is characterized by a long lipophilic nonpolar N-substituent side chain, which allows for high-affinity binding to the hydrophobic region of the cell membrane adjacent to the beta$_2$ receptor (termed an exoreceptor), while the phenylethanolamine portion of the molecule attaches to the beta receptor. Furthermore, studies have demonstrated its ability to produce long-acting protection against exercise-induced asthma. Because of its long duration of action, not only is there potential for improved compliance associated with twice-daily dosing, but salmeterol may be particularly valuable in the management of nocturnal asthma. Salmeterol has not been approved for use in the United States. It is marketed in the United Kingdom and other countries. The recommended dose is 50 μg (2 inhalations) every 12 hours by MDI.

Formoterol

Formoterol is a catecholamine derivative with beta$_2$ selectivity (see Fig. 1-1), a rapid onset of action, and a long duration of effectiveness (10–12 hours in most patients). Formoterol, like salmeterol, has been shown in clinical studies to produce a higher baseline pulmonary function, less use of additional medications, and better control of asthma symptoms than albuterol. The potential benefits from administration are the same as noted for salmeterol: twice-daily dosing may lead to improved compliance and may improve the ability to manage nocturnal asthma. Formoterol, like salmeterol, has not been approved for use in the United States. It is available for use in other countries.

Inhaled beta agonists have a wide therapeutic range and a favorable side effect profile. These agonists are indicated for the treatment of chronic asthma and the prevention of exercise-induced bronchospasm and are the treatment of choice for acute asthma. Beta agonists are generally safe, although they have the potential to produce life-threatening cardiovascular and respiratory side effects in some patients. Inhaled beta agonists used on an as-needed basis should be considered in the daily management of patients with chronic asthma because of the favorable benefit : risk ratio and the rapid onset of action. It is essential to recognize, however, that the use of this class of drugs does not lessen the need for antiinflammatory medications to control airway inflammation.

POINTS TO REMEMBER

1. Treatment of the asthmatic patient must be individualized.
2. Use of a $beta_2$ selective agonist is preferable to a nonselective beta agonist because of the longer duration of action and lower incidence of cardiovascular side effects.
3. Except when a longer duration of effect is desired or the patient does not tolerate inhaled $beta_2$ agonists, administration of $beta_2$ agonists by inhalation is preferable to oral administration in the treatment of chronic asthma because of their rapid onset of action, infrequency of adverse reactions, and comparable efficacy to other routes of administration.
4. If possible, while maximizing control of asthmatic symptoms, inhaled $beta_2$ agonists should be administered on an as-needed basis rather than a regular basis in the treatment of chronic asthma.
5. Inhaled $beta_2$ agonists are generally the safest and most effective treatment for acute asthma.
6. The use of $beta_2$ agonists in the treatment of acute or chronic asthma is not a substitute for the administration of antiinflammatory drugs, especially corticosteroids.
7. Since a large percentage of patients fail to use inhaler devices correctly, patients must be carefully instructed, often more than once, in the administration of inhaled beta agonists.
8. Inhaled $beta_2$ agonists are generally considered the treatment of choice for prevention of exercise-induced bronchospasm and should be administered 15–30 minutes prior to exercise.
9. Tolerance to $beta_2$ agonists, which is usually reversible after administration of corticosteroids, develops in some patients after continued use and may be associated with unrecognized decrease in efficacy and delay in seeking medical attention.
10. Bronchial hyperreactivity may increase in patients receiving inhaled $beta_2$ agonists on a regular basis and should be considered in patients whose asthma is becoming worse on a regimen that includes the regular use of these drugs.
11. Serious adverse effects resulting from the administration of $beta_2$ agonists, when administered in recommended doses, are rare when given orally and extremely uncommon when administered by inhalation. Nevertheless, both $beta_2$ agonists and nonselective beta agonists, when administered by the inhaled route, can produce a sudden paradoxical increase in bronchospasm in some asthmatic patients that can be life threatening.

Corticosteroid(s)

Corticosteroids are the most effective antiinflammatory drugs used in the treatment of asthma. Corticosteroids are 21-carbon molecules derived from hydrocortisone. Minor modifications in their structure change their potency, duration of action, and mineralocorticoid action significantly (Table 1-5). Steroids bearing a 1-ketone group (cortisone, prednisone) must first be converted to an 11-hydroxy molecule for glucocorticoid activity (cortisol and prednisolone).

Table 1-5. Corticosteroid properties

Steroid	Antiinflammatory relative potency	Plasma half-life (hr)	Biologic half-life (hr)	Equivalent dose (mg)	Sodium-retaining potency
Short acting					
Hydrocortisone	1	2	12	20.0	2+
Cortisone	0.8	0.5	*	25.0	2+
Intermediate acting					
Prednisone	3.5	1	*	5.0	1+
Prednisolone	4	2–3.5	12–36	5.0	1+
Triamcinolone	5	2–3.5	12–24	4.0	0
Methylprednisolone	5	2–3.5	12–36	4.0	0
Prolonged acting					
Betamethasone / Dexamethasone	25–30	5	24–48	0.6–0.75	0

Prednisone and cortisone must be first converted to prednisolone and hydrocortisone before being active; the half-lives are then compared to the initial compound.
Source: Reproduced with permission from E. Weiss and M. Stein (eds.), *Bronchial Asthma: Mechanisms and Therapeutics*, (3d ed). (Boston: Little, Brown, 1993).

CLINICAL PHARMACOLOGY

Corticosteroids are lipophilic compounds that are well absorbed and clinically effective when given orally, intravenously, or topically. More than 90% of circulating cortisol and its synthetic analogues bind to plasma proteins. Corticosteroids are metabolized primarily in the liver prior to excretion; as a result, liver disease and drugs or other chemicals that modify liver function can affect the half-life of corticosteroids. Corticosteroids are excreted in the urine as glucuronides, sulfates, or unconjugated compounds.

CLINICAL USE

Corticosteroids are essential for the control of bronchial inflammation in asthmatic patients. Improvement in pulmonary function can be seen within 3 hours after starting oral corticosteroids in patients with asthma. The peak effect generally occurs 6–12 hours after initiating treatment.

SYSTEMIC CORTICOSTEROIDS

Any patient with asthma severe enough to require hospitalization should receive systemic corticosteroids. If the patient requires oral corticosteroids, alternate-day treatment is preferable to daily treatment if the patient's asthma is adequately controlled since it lessens the chance of systemic side effects. Short-term systemic corticosteroid therapy can be initiated with 40–80 mg of prednisone daily in adults or 1–2 mg/kg/day in children and usually tapered over 5–7 days if there is no exacerbation of asthma. Treatment with systemic corticosteroids should be maintained until pulmonary function has returned to predicted normal or is acceptably close to the patient's personal best.

INHALED CORTICOSTEROIDS

Inhaled corticosteroids, which are relatively rapidly metabolized, have made it possible in many patients to maintain adequate asthma control with less risk of side effects (Note: inhaled CS does not reduce systemic side effects from systemic CS) than systemic corticosteroids. In patients with severe asthma who are already receiving oral corticosteroids, the introduction of inhaled corticosteroids may allow significant reduction of oral corticosteroids. Some patients, however, may still require oral corticosteroids in combination with inhaled corticosteroids. Oropharyngeal candidiasis, cough, and dysphonia have been reported after use of inhaled corticosteroids. Slow inspiratory rate during administration, gargling after use, and spacer units may reduce this risk. Inhaled corticosteroids may provide more effective symptomatic relief and a quicker return to acceptable pulmonary function by decreasing airway inflammation and hyperresponsiveness.

Inhaled corticosteroids available for administration by MDI in the United States, Canada, and Europe are beclomethasone (Vanceril, Beclovent, Becotide, Becloforte), betamethasone (Bextasol), budesonide (Pulmicort), flunisolide (Aerobid, Bronalide), and triamcinolone acetonide (Azmacort). The recommended doses for some of the products that are available in the United States are as follows:

Azmacort
- Patients over age 12 years: 2 inhalations tid-qid, not to exceed 16 inhalations/day
- Patients 6–12 years of age: 1–2 inhalations tid-qid, not to exceed 12 inhalations/day

Beclovent and Vanceril
- Patients over age 12 years: 2 inhalations tid-qid, not to exceed 20 inhalations/day
- Patients 6–12 years of age: 1–2 inhalations tid-qid, not to exceed 10 inhalations/day

Aerobid
- Patients over age 15 years: 2 inhalations bid, not to exceed 4 inhalations bid
- Patients 6–15 years of age: 2 inhalations bid, not to exceed this dose.

ADVERSE EFFECTS

Systemic corticosteroids primarily, but also inhaled corticosteroids at high doses in some patients, can produce CNS effects, including mood changes (ranging from euphoria to psychosis, irritability, depression), increased appetite, and suppression of the hypothalamic-pituitary-adrenal (HPA) axis. Chronic use of corticosteroids can produce buffalo hump, moon facies, posterior subcapsular cataracts, osteoporosis, hypertension, easy bruisability, striae, muscle wasting of the extremities with proximal muscle weakness, decreased wound healing, increased susceptibility to infection, hyperglycemia, acne, hirsutism, skin atrophy, myopathy, peptic ulcer disease, growth failure in children, pancreatitis, hypogonadism, hypercalcuria, and avascular necrosis of the head of the femur. Too rapid withdrawal of corticosteroids can produce exacerbation of asthma or signs of adrenal insufficiency in patients receiving systemic corticosteroids for longer than short periods. In addition, termination of corticosteroids after long-term use can cause a withdrawal syndrome consisting of fever, general malaise, arthralgias, abdominal pain, nausea, emesis, and affective changes. The effect of inhaled corticosteroids on growth in children must be evaluated very carefully (Table 1-6).

Theophylline

Theophylline is an effective bronchodilator for the treatment of acute and chronic asthma. It is a methyl xanthine similar in structure to the commonly consumed xanthines, caffeine and theobromine. Dosage and labeling of theophylline salts is related to anhydrous theophylline, which in the case of aminophylline is 86%.

CLINICAL PHARMACOLOGY

When theophylline enters the circulation, approximately 40% is bound to plasma protein, with the remainder being distributed

Table 1-6. Adverse effects associated with corticosteroid use

Musculoskeletal
- Myopathy
- Osteoporosis — vertebral compression fractures
- Aseptic necrosis of bone

Gastrointestinal
- Peptic ulceration (often gastric)
- Gastric hemorrhage
- Intestinal perforation
- Pancreatitis

Central nervous system
- Psychiatric disorders
- Pseudotumor cerebri

Ophthalmologic
- Glaucoma
- Posterior subcapsular cataracts

Cardiovascular and renal
- Hypertension
- Sodium and water retention—edema
- Hypokalemic alkalosis

Metabolic
- Precipitation of clinical manifestations of genetic diabetes mellitus, including ketoacidosis
- Hyperosmolar nonketotic coma
- Hyperlipidemia
- Induction of centripetal obesity

Endocrine
- Growth failure
- Secondary amenorrhea
- Suppression of hypothalamic-pituitary-adrenal system

Inhibition of fibroplasia
- Impaired wound healing
- Subcutaneous tissue atrophy

Suppression of the immune response
- Superimposition of a variety of bacterial, fungal, viral, and parasitic infections in steroid-treated patients

Source: Reproduced by permission from E. Weiss and M. Stein (eds.), *Bronchial Asthma: Mechanisms and Therapeutics* (3d ed). (Boston: Little, Brown, 1993).

throughout the body. Serum concentration reaches equilibrium with drug tissue concentrations within 1 hour after an IV injection. Theophylline crosses the placenta and passes into breast milk, but only minor adverse effects have been found in infants indirectly exposed to theophylline.

Between 85% and 90% of theophylline is metabolized in the liver. It is transformed by the cytochrome P450 enzyme system into relatively inactive metabolites, which are rapidly excreted in the urine. The elimination rate is reduced by liver disease, congestive heart failure, febrile illnesses, and drugs that reduce the rate of clearance, such as cimetidine, erythromycin, quinoline antibiotics, troleandomycin (TAO), allopurinol, propranolol, influenza A vaccine, oral contraceptives, and a low protein–high carbohydrate diet (Table 1-7). On the other hand, some drugs increase the rate of theophylline clearance and thereby decrease the serum concentration for a given theophylline dose. These include carbamazepine (Tegretol), aminoglutethimide, IV isoproterenol, phenobarbital, phenytoin (Dilantin), rifampin, and sulphinpyrazone (see Table 1-6). Increased clearance also results from cigarette smoking and low carbohydrate–high protein diets, including ingestion of charcoal-broiled meats.

INTERPATIENT DIFFERENCES

Interpatient differences in theophylline metabolism may require periodic measurement of serum levels, especially if higher therapeutic levels are needed or if conditions exist that are known to alter theophylline metabolism. In individuals greater than 120% of ideal body weight for age and height, the initial theophylline dose should be based on the ideal rather than the actual weight to avoid toxicity, since theophylline does not distribute into adipose tissue. Serum theophylline levels may need to be monitored when a patient begins therapy, if the expected bronchodilator effect of an apparently therapeutic regimen is not achieved, if the patient, develops adverse effects on recommended doses.

DOSAGE AND ADMINISTRATION FOR ACUTE BRONCHODILATION

An inhaled $beta_2$ agonist such as albuterol or terbutaline provides greater bronchodilation with fewer side effects than theophylline when administered for the treatment of acute asthmatic symptoms. When the addition of theophylline is required, IV aminophylline provides rapid relief of symptoms in most patients.

On average, each milligram per kilogram (ideal body weight) of theophylline loading dose administered as an IV 30-minute infusion results in an average 2 μg/ml ± 30% incremental increase in serum concentration. However, the initial level depends on the distribution volume, which varies unpredictably (a loading dose of 6 mg of aminophylline per kilogram of total body weight results in about 12 μg of theophylline/ml blood level). When a loading dose is required in

Table 1-7. Medications affecting serum theophylline levels

Decreasing	Increasing
Phenobarbital	Cimetidine
Phenytoin	Troleandomycin
Isoproterenol	Erythromycin
Rifampin	Quinolone
Carbamazepine	Allopurinol
	Propranolol
	Ciprofloxin
	Oral contraceptives

a patient who has received theophylline in the past 24 hours, estimation of the serum concentration based on the history is unreliable, and an immediate measurement of the serum concentration is indicated. The loading dose (LD) can then be determined as follows:

LD = (desired concentration − measured concentration) × (0.5 liter/kg)
where 0.5 liter/kg is the mean volume of distribution.

The serum concentration obtained 30 minutes after an IV loading dose when distribution is complete, can be used to assess the need for and size of subsequent loading dose if clinically indicated, and for guidance of continuing therapy. A recommended initial dose is 0.4 mg/kg/hour in nonsmokers and 0.7 mg/kg/hour in smokers. Once a serum concentration of 8–15 μg/ml has been achieved, a constant IV infusion is then started at an appropriate rate. Because of the large interpatient variability in theophylline clearance, serum concentrations will rise or fall when the patient's clearance is significantly different from the mean population value used to calculate the initial infusion rate. Therefore, a second serum concentration is obtained 4–6 hours in children and 8 hours in adults after starting the constant infusion to determine whether the concentration is increasing or decreasing from the post–LD level. If the level is decreasing as a result of a greater-than-average clearance, an additional loading dose can be administered and the infusion rate increased. In contrast, if the second sample demonstrates a higher level, accumulation of the drug can be assumed and the infusion rate should be decreased. Additional samples can be obtained 12–24 hours later and then at 24-hour intervals to determine whether further adjustments are required.

DOSAGE AND ADMINISTRATION FOR CHRONIC THERAPY

It has been suggested that the appropriate dose for the treatment of chronic asthma should be established using an immediate-release preparation with slow titration to determine the best dose for each patient. Then the total 24-hour dose can be given at half the daily dose every 12 hours. In patients who are young, smokers, or rapidly metabolize theophylline, one-third of the daily dose can be given at 8-hour intervals. The recommended starting dose for short-acting preparations are 4 mg/kg q6h in children 6 to 9 years of age; 3 mg/kg q6h in children 9 to 12 years of age and 3 mg/kg q8h in otherwise healthy, nonsmoking adults. Dose adjustments should be guided by clinical response and serum theophylline levels.

Alternatively, a long-acting preparation can be given initially to adults and children over 25 kg at a dose of 200 mg q12h. If the desired clinical response is not achieved and there are no adverse reactions, the dose can be increased by 25% at 3-day intervals, with clinical response being assessed after every dose adjustment.

If the serum theophylline level can be measured approximately 8 hours after a dose when no doses have been added or missed for at least 3 days, the following actions should be taken:

1. If the level is 25–30 μg/ml, skip the next dose and decrease subsequent doses by 25% and recheck the serum level in 3 days.
2. If the level is 20–25 μg/ml, decrease the dose by 10%, and recheck the level in 3 days.
3. If the level is more than 30 μg/ml, skip the next 2 doses, decrease the subsequent dose by 50%, and recheck the serum level in 3 days.
4. If the level is 5–7.5 μg/ml, increase the dose by 25%.
5. If the level is 7.5-10 μg/ml, increase the dose by 25%.

Once-a-day dosing may be possible in certain adult, nonsmoking patients.

Serum theophylline levels should be rechecked at 6–12-month intervals at least in patients on chronic therapy.

SIDE EFFECTS

Theophylline has a wide range of potential side effects, reflecting a relatively narrow therapeutic index. Caffeinelike effects, such as CNS stimulation and GI manifestations, are not uncommon during the initiation of therapy, and become more prominent with higher serum concentrations. Adults with cardiac decompensation or liver dysfunction have impaired theophylline clearance and are more likely to develop toxic serum concentrations. In this setting, theophylline-induced convulsions may occur and are not always preceded by evidence of CNS stimulation. In addition, theophylline can cause (1) arrhythmias, especially in adults, (2) relaxation of the detrusor muscle leading to dysuria in older men with prostatic hypertrophy, (3) dehydration in children, (4) excess gastric acid secretion in patients with peptic ulcer disease, (5) hyperglycemia, and (6) hypokalemia. Urticaria, exfoliative dermatitis, and asthma have been associated with exposure to the ethylene diamine preservative in aminophylline. Most studies have shown that the addition of therapeutic doses of theophylline to treatment with inhaled beta agonists provides little additional benefit while increasing the likelihood of side effects.

Overdose

In the event of theophylline overdose, the drug should be discontinued and if less than 30 minutes has elapsed, the patient should be promptly treated with syrup of ipecac, followed by activated charcoal. If more than 30 minutes has elasped since ingestion of theophylline, ipecac should *not* be given, and activated charcoal alone should be administered. The serum levels should be measured frequently and if the level is over 30 μg/ml, the patient should be followed in an intensive care unit. If the serum theophylline level falls slower than expected or if it rises, repeated doses of activated charcoal can be administered and repeated every 2–4 hours until the serum level falls below 20 μg/ml. If the serum theophylline concentration is over 40 μg/ml, charcoal hemoperfusion may be used to remove theophylline rapidly, even in the absence of obvious signs of toxicity. In addition, IV phenobarbital prophylactically may prevent seizures in patients with serum theophylline levels over 40 μg/ml. If seizures develop, they should be rapidly treated with IV diazepam, paraldehyde, thiopental, or a general anesthetic if needed, while adequate oxygenation and respiratory support are maintained.

POINTS TO REMEMBER

1. For the treatment of acute severe asthma, theophylline is less effective than inhaled $beta_2$ selective agonists.
2. Maintenance therapy with theophylline is effective in reducing the frequency and severity of symptoms of chronic asthma. Effectiveness may be similar to cromolyn or $beta_2$ agonists, and long-acting preparations allow for effective control of nocturnal symptoms.
3. The rate of theophylline metabolism varies greatly among patients and is influenced by numerous medical conditions and pharmaceutic interventions.
4. The rate of theophylline metabolism is reduced, thereby leading to increased serum levels and increased potential for toxicity, in the presence of such conditions as cardiac decompression, respiratory failure, hepatic cirrhosis, sustained high fever, viral infections, hypothyroidism and after administration of cimetidine, oral contraceptives, TAO, erythromycin, ciprofloxacin, and disulfiram. In contrast, such factors as cigarette or marijuana smoking, hyperthyrodism, rifampin, phenytoin, cambamazepine, and phenobarbital increase the rate of metabolism.
5. Oral slow-release formulations generally provide stable serum concentrations and favor patient compliance. However, the rate and extent of absorption vary among formulations, among individuals, and possibly in the same individual from time to time. Food ingestion also may affect the rate of absorption in different ways, depending on the specific formulation.
6. Dosage for chronic therapy is based on the principle of slowly titrating the dose over several days to circumvent transient caffeine like side effects. Final dosage is usually based on the peak serum concentration measurement obtained at steady rate.
7. Elevated blood levels may produce neurologic, gastrointestinal, or cardiovascular side effects.
8. Orally administered activated charcoal or charcoal hemoperfusion dialysis should be considered at toxic theophylline concentrations. With theophylline overdosage, intravenous phenobarbital should also be considered to prevent seizures; diazepam, but not phenytoin, should be used to terminate seizures.

Cromolyn Sodium

Cromolyn sodium is available for delivery from an MDI, as a powdered capsule delivered by a spinhaler, and as a solution for nebulization. The MDI is generally more convenient to use and is less likely to produce irritation of the respiratory tract. The spinhaler, however, does not contain propellants and emulsifying agents found in the MDI and therefore is an acceptable alternative to the MDI in the occasional patient who develops reactions to these excipients. Moreover, the spinhaler may be helpful in patients who have difficulty coordinating use of the MDI. The comparable effectiveness of the MDI, spinhaler, and nebulized solution has been demonstrated.

CLINICAL PHARMACOLOGY

Cromolyn is minimally absorbed from epithelial surfaces, is rapidly eliminated from the serum, and has almost identical distribution and elimination phases. The mean percentage of inhaled cromolyn that is absorbed by patients with asthma is between 1% and 15%. Within 5–30 minutes after inhalation, peak plasma levels may be detected. Although the duration of action is considered to be 4–6 hours, clinical studies have demonstrated a substantial carryover effect for several weeks after drug administration. There is no known interaction between cromolyn sodium and other medications.

CLINICAL USE

As demonstrated in many clinical studies, cromolyn is effective for the treatment of mild and moderate asthma in some patients, with a degree of control comparable to that of theophylline. Based on an assessment of the benefit : risk ratio, many clinicians believe that cromolyn should be considered a first-line medication for the treatment of chronic asthma, although its effectiveness is less predictable than inhaled corticosteroids when used in the treatment of asthma and a 4–6-week period of administration may be necessary to demonstrate efficacy in individual patients. Cromolyn may be effective in patients with nonallergic as well as allergic asthma and can effectively prevent cough-variant asthma. It can also be effective in preventing exercise-induced asthma if administered 15 minutes prior to exercise alone or in combination with an inhaled beta agonist. Often cromolyn is most effective when taken for 1 week before anticipated allergen exposure (e.g., pollen season) or 30 minutes before a brief allergen exposure (e.g., visiting someone who has a cat).

DOSAGE AND ADMINISTRATION

The usual starting dose for cromolyn sodium, if administered by spinhaler, MDI, or as a solution for nebulization, is the contents of 1 capsule, 2 inhalations, or the contents of 1 ampule, respectively, tid or qid at regular intervals. Failure of the patient to take the drug as prescribed is probably an important reason for lack of efficacy. Clinical observation suggests that cromolyn may need to be administered for at least 8 weeks in an individual patient before concluding that it is ineffective.

For prevention of exercise-induced bronchospasm, the dose is 2 inhalations of the MDI given 10–15 minutes, but not more than 60 minutes prior to exercise.

ADVERSE EFFECTS

Serious side effects have not been noted following extensive clinical experience except in rare individuals and could be related in some cases to reactions to excipients in the drug product. Most of the side effects that have been described have been mild; they include irritation of the throat, hoarseness, dryness of the mouth, and other signs of local irritation.

POINTS TO REMEMBER

1. Although individual variation in response must always be considered, in general, comparable efficacy can be achieved when cromolyn is administered by spinhaler, MDI, or nebulized solution.
2. The efficacy of cromolyn in the management of some patients with mild or moderate asthma, alone or in conjunction with bronchodilators and or inhaled corticosteroids, has been demonstrated.
3. Cromolyn can be effective in preventing exercise-induced asthma in many patients and is most likely to be effective when given 15–30 minutes prior to exercise.
4. Cromolyn has been shown to be extremely safe and has a favorable benefit : risk ratio.

Anticholinergic Agents

With a growing understanding of the importance of the autonomic nervous system in normal and pathologic lung function and with the development of synthetic anticholinergic agents with significantly fewer side effects, interest in the use of this class of drugs for the treatment of asthma is increasing.

All anticholinergic medications are either tertiary or quaternary ammonium compounds. Atropine, a tertiary compound, and ipratropium bromide, the synthetic *N*-propyl derivative of atropine, a quaternary ammonium compound, differ significantly in their pharmacologic properties.

Ipratropium is not absorbed from the GI tract in appreciable amounts and is not capable of crossing the blood-brain barrier; atropine is well absorbed from the GI tract and readily crosses the blood-brain barrier. In the inhaled form, ipratropium bromide produces negligible serum levels because more than 90% is swallowed and minimally absorbed from the GI tract. Unlike atropine, ipratropium has no effect on mucus production, mucus transport, or ciliary activities.

CLINICAL USE

Both atropine and ipratropium have been shown to produce significant bronchodilation. In addition, all anticholinergic drugs prevent bronchoconstriction produced by cholinergic agents, such as methacholine, in a dose-related fashion. On the other hand, there is only partial protection against bronchospasm produced by irritants, such as sulfur dioxide, carbon dust, citric acid, and tobacco smoke, as well as bronchoconstriction after inhaled histamine. Ipratropium is also partially protective at high doses against bronchospasm induced by prostaglandin F_2 alpha and prostaglandin D_2 but does not consistently inhibit respiratory response to serotonin, bradykinin, or ultrasonically nebulized distilled water. Anticholinergic medication at any dose does not protect against allergen-induced bronchospasm.

Atropine and ipratropium bromide are generally ineffective in the treatment of patients with acute asthma.

Ipratropium is not effective in the management of most children and adults with chronic asthma. Nevertheless, ipratropium bromide appears to be more efficacious than beta agonists in a small subset of patients with mild or moderate asthma (FEV_1 over 50%). (Patients with chronic obstructive pulmonary disease with a reversible component appear to benefit the most from the regular use of anticholinergic drugs.)

Combined therapy with ipratropium bromide and other asthma medications (beta agonists, theophylline, cromolyn sodium, and cromolyn plus corticosteroids) has shown that anticholinergic agents are most effective when they are combined with beta agonists; in this case, the efficacy of the combination is equal to or greater than the efficacy of the medications administered separately.

Ipratropium bromide has been shown to be effective in some patients with allergic and nonallergic asthma. Anticholinergic therapy may be particularly useful in patients with bronchospasm, which occurs secondary to beta blockade, "psychogenic asthma," and cough-variant asthma.

DOSAGE AND ADMINISTRATION

The initial effect of atropine can be seen within 15 minutes after inhalation and the maximal response within 100–200 minutes. In adults, the duration of action is 3–5 hours. The usual dose is 0.4–0.8 μg every 3–4 hours. Ipratropium bromide is marketed in the United States in a MDI (Atrovent) that delivers 18 μg per actuation. The usual dose is 1–2 inhalations qid. Patients should not receive more than 12 inhalations in a 24-hour period. After 2 inhalations of ipratropium (38 μg), most patients who respond will do so within 15 minutes; by 30 minutes, 75–85% of maximal bronchodilation has been attained, with the peak effect usually occurring within 1–2 hours. There is a variable duration of effect of 4–6 hours. The area under the time-response curve (a measure of overall drug effectiveness) is generally less, the onset slower, and the duration longer after administration of ipratropium than after administration of beta agonists.

SIDE EFFECTS

Bradycardia and dry mouth are the major side effects of atropine and can be seen with a dose as low as 0.5 mg. At higher doses (2–5 mg), tachycardia, mydriasis, urinary retention, dry flushed skin, difficulty with speech, dysphagia, excitement, drying of respiratory secretions, blurred vision, and fever can be noted. Delirium and coma may occur with atropine poisoning. Atropine should not be used in patients with narrow-angle glaucoma, bladder-neck obstruction, or prostatic hypertrophy. Ipratropium has very low bioavailability when inhaled and therefore does not produce the side effects noted after atropine administration. Occasionally, inhaled ipratropium may produce life-threatening paradoxical bronchospasm, probably due to components of the drug product other than the drug itself, particularly benzalkonium chloride in the solution for nebulization. The MDI also contains propellants and soya lecithin. Patients should be warned that inadvertent spraying into the eyes may produce temporary blurring of vision and may be associated with acute glaucoma.

POINTS TO REMEMBER

1. Inhaled anticholinergic medications are not indicated as the primary therapeutic modality for acute or chronic asthma.
2. Inhaled anticholinergic medications, especially ipratropium, appear to be effective in some patients with chronic mild or moderate reversible airflow obstruction.
3. Inhaled anticholinergic medications, especially ipratropium, could be considered for patients in whom alternative medications (1) have not been sufficiently effective, (2) are inappropriate because of other medical conditions, or (3) have produced unacceptable side effects.
4. The chronic administration of anticholinergic medications, especially ipratropium, appears to be most effective in patients with chronic obstructive pulmonary disease who have partially reversible airflow obstruction.

Antihistamines

For over 40 years it has been known that allergen exposure triggers histamine release and subsequent bronchoconstriction. Inhalation challenge with histamine can be used to establish the degree of airway hyperresponsiveness in patients with asthma.

CLINICAL INDICATIONS AND USAGE

There has been renewed interest in the use of antihistamines for the management of asthma with the recent development of antihistamines that are not only generally nonsedating but also can produce bronchodilation. Recent studies with terfenadine and astemizole indicate that approximately 50% of acute airflow obstruction after allergen exposure is due to histamine. Furthermore, repetitive-dose studies suggest that terfenadine and astemizole are effective in preventing pollen-induced asthma. It has also been shown that pretreatment with terfenadine will partially protect against allergen inhalation challenge, to a degree similar to that seen after pretreatment with cromolyn sodium.

It has been postulated that H_1 antagonists may lessen asthmatic symptoms through two postulated mechanisms: (1) direct inhibition of histamine-induced bronchoconstriction and (2) inhibition of histamine-induced increase in nasal resistance, preserving nasal filtration of allergen in patients who also have allergic rhinitis. Whatever the mechanism, patients with asthma can improve dramatically when antihistamines are utilized to control nasal symptomatology.

LABELING ISSUES

Some early clinical studies utilizing H_1 antihistamines raised concern about the potential for this class of drugs to produce bronchospasm in certain individuals. In addition, antihistamines could have a drying effect on bronchial mucus through their anticholinergic properties, although this effect has never been confirmed. As a result, the labeling for this class of drugs indicates that antihistamines should not be used in patients with asthma. Some studies, however, have demonstrated that asthmatic patients benefit from the use of antihistamines. Therefore, there is no general contraindication to the use of antihistamines in patients with asthma. In fact, antihistamines may be useful additions to the treatment program for many patients with asthma.

DOSAGE AND ADMINISTRATION

Terfenadine: 1 tablet (60 mg) twice daily for patients 12 years of age and older.

Astemizole: 1 tablet (10 mg) once daily for patients 12 years of age and older. Astemizole should be taken on an empty stomach at least 2 hours after a meal or 1 hour before food intake.

ADVERSE EFFECTS

Data are accumulating on the ability of terfenadine and astemizole to produce prolongation of the QT_c interval on ECG monitoring, which could lead to ventricular arrhythmias such as torsades de pointes. This possibility is particularly likely if the patient has been receiving ketoconazole or macrolide antibiotics concomitantly or has significant liver or cardiovascular disease.

POINTS TO REMEMBER

1. Antihistamines can be safely used in most patients with asthma.
2. Some antihistamines can produce bronchodilation or prevent bronchoconstriction, thus alleviating asthmatic symptoms by a direct effect on the bronchial passageways.
3. There is a strong clinical impression that improvement in upper respiratory symptoms by use of antihistamines, in patients who have allergic rhinitis as well as asthma, may facilitate the treatment of lower respiratory symptoms.
4. Antihistamines, if used in the treatment of asthma, should be considered adjunctive therapy, since histamine is not the only mediator responsible for the clinical manifestations of asthma.

Expectorants and Mucolytics

CLINICAL USE

Iodides have been used extensively in the past for the treatment of asthma, but their therapeutic value is unproven. The National Asthma Education Program states that there is no available evidence to support their use as a mucolytic agent in severe exacerbations of asthma; moreover, they can worsen cough or airflow obstruction and therefore should be avoided.

ADVERSE EFFECTS

Iodides have significant side effects, including a metallic taste, nausea, vomiting, pyrosis, acneiform rash, parotiditis, nasal congestion, and rarely erythema nodosum, urticaria, bullous eruptions, fever, and hypersensitivity angiitis. Development of goiter in children on chronic therapy and hypothyroidism have also been seen.

Investigational Agents and Combinations

To a large degree, investigational medications or combinations of already-approved drugs are an attempt to provide practicing physicians with additional options for the management of patients on long-term corticosteroid therapy, some of whom may be inadequately controlled despite high-dose systemic corticosteroids. The choice of such therapy should be based on the experience of the physician as well as the specific problems of the patient and might include troleandomycin, methotrexate, gold, IV gamma globulin, or even mediator antagonists or investigational medication combinations. Only physicians knowledgeable in the use of these drugs should consider their administration to patients.

Troleandomycin

CLINICAL INDICATIONS

Studies have demonstrated that troleandomycin (TAO) can decrease sputum production and reduce the need for other medications, unrelated to an antibiotic effect, in some patients with asthma. Clinical improvement has been shown when TAO was added to the treatment regimen of patients with severe asthma who were not responding to high-dose daily corticosteroids. If the patient is receiving prednisone, he or she should be switched to methylprednisolone prior to initiating therapy with TAO, since pharmacokinetic studies show that methylprednisolone and theophylline elimination but not prednisolone elimination is significantly impaired in the presence of TAO. Consistent with these findings, the clinical response is greater when TAO is added to a treatment program in which patients are receiving methylprednisolone rather than one in which patients are receiving prednisolone or prednisone.

DOSAGE AND ADMINISTRATION

Doses of TAO lower than 1 g/day may reduce the severity of asthma in adults, but even low doses require careful monitoring of liver function (at least every other week initially) since TAO can produce significant hepatotoxicity and exacerbation of corticosteroid-related adverse effects. Theophylline levels must also be monitored, since

TAO may increase theophylline levels by 25–50% within the first 12 hours of treatment.

Methotrexate

CLINICAL INDICATIONS

It has been demonstrated in a double-blind, placebo-controlled study that methotrexate may facilitate reduction in the dose of corticosteroid and the risk of adverse corticosteroid effect. On the other hand, a recent double-blind, placebo-controlled study failed to show a significant reduction in corticosteroids in patients treated with methotrexate. Methotrexate's efficacy and safety remain controversial and need to be further demonstrated in controlled blinded studies.

ADVERSE EFFECTS AND CONTRAINDICATIONS

Interstitial Pneumonitis

Methotrexate can produce interstitial pneumonitis. Therefore, patients with asthma should be carefully evaluated for the presence of other forms of respiratory disease before starting treatment with this agent. Methotrexate is contraindicated in patients who have significant renal or hepatic function abnormalities, are pregnant, have liver disease or a strong history of alcohol consumption, have severe liver dyscrasias, immunodeficiency, or active infectious disease, and/or are likely to be noncompliant.

Liver Toxicity

Because of the potential for liver toxicity, consultation with a hepatologist and consideration of a liver biopsy is recommended after reaching a cumulative dose of 2 g. Evaluation of liver function, including prothrombin time and serum albumin, should be done every 3–6 months.

PRECAUTIONS

Laboratory tests, including blood chemistries and CBC with differential and platelet count, should be done at least every 4 weeks and more frequently during periods when doses are increased weekly.

With a low-dose protocol, adverse effects are minimal, but patients nevertheless must be monitored carefully. Gastrointestinal symptoms, stomatitis, and hematologic effects, especially leukopenia, are the most frequent adverse effects seen after methotrexate administration. Since these are usually dose related, they are often alleviated by temporarily reducing the dose or discontinuing the drug. Patients should be advised against alcohol consumption and pregnancy while receiving methotrexate. In addition, the risk of methotrexate toxicity may be increased by medications such as salicylates, sulfonamides, and penicillin, which decrease renal elimination.

Gold

CLINICAL USE

Studies suggest that gold administration may improve symptoms in asthmatic patients, allow for reduction in mean daily dose of corticosteroids, and diminish bronchial hyperresponsiveness to methacholine.

DOSAGE AND ADMINISTRATION

The effects of gold administration in some patients can be seen after a total daily dose of 1500 mg of parenteral gold sodium thiomalate administered for 6–12 months. More recently, auranofin, an oral gold compound, has been studied in an open trial at a dose of 3 mg twice daily for 20 weeks in 20 steroid-dependent asthmatic patients who demonstrated a decrease of approximately 35% in mean maintenance corticosteroid dose and a correlating decrease in bronchial hyperresponsiveness to methacholine, despite no change in spirometry.

ADVERSE EFFECTS

Adverse effects have been limited to mild diarrhea, dermatitis, and proteinuria, which resolved with temporary discontinuation or dose reduction.

PRECAUTIONS

Because of the difficulty in interpreting efficacy in an open study, controlled clinical studies are necessary to demonstrate whether oral gold is efficacious in patients with asthma. Furthermore, there are no data on the efficacy and safety of gold therapy in children.

Intravenous Gamma Globulin

CLINICAL USE

Parenteral immunoglobulins may be beneficial in the treatment of asthma since (1) low doses increase serum antibody levels and can protect individuals with impaired immunity, (2) high doses IV may act as an immunomodulator, providing passive protection and potentially assisting the immune system in reducing the production of specific immunoglobulin E (IgE), (3) in a small number of patients, pulmonary function has improved and bronchial reactivity has decreased after administration, and (4) the IV use of immunoglobulin in patients with recurrent sinus disease, asthma, and deficiency in one or more immunoglobulin G (IgG) subclasses provides benefit. Because there is a strong association among chronic sinus disease, recalcitrant asthma, and immunodeficiencies, speculation that treatment of the underlying antibody deficiency could improve asthma requires further evaluation.

Thus IV gamma globulin may improve asthma by (1) reducing chronic bacterial sinusitis, (2) reducing persistent infection in the lower respiratory tract in patients with immunodeficiency, or by (3) immunomodulation in severe, steroid-dependent patients.

Mediator Antagonists

There has been extensive study of mediator antagonists, specifically leukotriene, kinin, and platelet-activating factor antagonists, but none of these compounds has been approved for use in the United States. They include a wide array of complex chemical structures that have provided variable degrees of efficacy.

Combination Inhaled Medications

The combination of ipratropium, a synthetic (quaternary ammonium derivative of atropine) anticholinergic bronchodilator, and albuterol, a $beta_2$ selective agonist, has been evaluated in the treatment of asthma. Both drugs are approved for use by inhalation by MDI or as a solution for nebulization and are frequently used concomitantly in the treatment of asthma. Studies have also been done with a combination product that contains ipratropium and fenoterol, a combination that, like ipratropium-albuterol, is marketed in other countries.

Most studies have demonstrated that the response to a combination product of ipratropium and albuterol was greater than the response to either administered alone.

References

1. Benstein D. I., et al. An open study of Auranofin in the treatment of steroid-dependent asthma. *J. Allergy Clin. Immunol.* 81:6, 1988.
2. Blumenthal, M.N., et al. A multicenter evaluation of the clinical benefits of a cromolyn sodium inhaled by metered-dose inhaler in the treatment of asthma. *J. Allergy Clin. Immunol.* 81:681, 1988.
3. Brenner, M., and Szefler, S. T. Troleandomycin in the treatment of severe asthma. *Immunol. Allergy Clin. N. Amer.* 11:92, 1990.
4. Chervinsky, P. Concomitant bronchodilator therapy and ipratropium bromide. *Am J. Med.* 81:67, 1986.
5. Eigen, H. et al. Evaluation of the addition of cromolyn sodium to bronchial maintenance therapy in the long-term management of asthma. *J. Allergy Clin. Immunol.* 80:612, 1987.
6. Fanta, C. H., et al. Treatment of acute asthma: Is combination therapy with sympathomimetics and methylxanthines indicated? *Am. J. Med.* 85:5–10, 1986.
7. Guidelines for the diagnosis and management of asthma; National

Heart, Lung & Blood Institute National Asthma Education Program; expert panel report. *J. Allergy Clin. Immunol.* 88:477, 1991.

8. Holgate, S. T., et al. Astemigole and other H, antihistamine drug treatments of asthma. *J. Allergy Clin. Immunol.* 76:375, 1985.
9. Kemp, J. P. New drugs in the treatment of asthma. *Immunol. Allergy Clin.* 11:1, 1991.
10. Kemp, J. P. Editorial: Antihistamines — is there anything safe to prescribe? *Ann. Allergy* 69:276, 1992.
11. Kurland, G., et al. Fatal myocardial toxicity during continuous infusion of intravenous isoprotenerol therapy of asthma. *J. Allergy Clin. Immunol.* 63:407, 1979.
12. Mager, B. D., and Gelfand, E. W. An open label study of high dose intravenous immunoglobulin in severe childhood asthma. *J. Allergy Clin. Immunol.* 87:976, 1991.
13. Moler, F. W., et al. Improvements in clinical asthma score and $PaCO_2$ in children with severe asthma treated with continuous nebulized terbutaline. *J. Allergy Clin. Immunol.* 81:1101, 1988.
14. Mullarky, M. F., et al. Methotrexate in the treatment of corticosteroid-dependent asthma. *N. Engl. J. Med.* 318:603, 1988.
15. Nelson, H. S. Adrenergic therapy of bronchial asthma. *J. Allergy Clin. Immunol.* 77:771–785, 1986.
16. Nicklas, R. A. Paradoxical bronchospasm associated with the use of inhaled beta agonists. *J. Allergy Clin. Immunol.* 95:959–964, 1990.
17. Reed, C. E. Beta agonists: Adrenergic bronchodilators: pharmacology and toxicology. *J. Allergy Clin. Immunol.* 76:335, 1985.
18. Schlueter, D. P. Ipratropium bromide in asthma. *Am. J. Med.* 81:55, 1986.
19. Settipane, G. A., et al. Adverse reactions to cromolyn. *JAMA* 241:811, 1979.
20. Siegel, D. et al. Aminophylline increases the toxicity but not the efficacy of an inhaled beta-adrenergic agonist in the treatment of acute exacerbations of asthma. *Am. Rev. Respir. Dis.* 132:283, 1985.
21. Windom H. H., et al. The pulmonary and extrapulmonar effects of inhaled B-agonists in patients with asthma. *Clin. Pharmacol. Ther.* 48:296, 1990.
22. Wolthers, O. D., and Pederson, S. Growth of asthmatic children during treatment with budesonide: A double-blind trial. *Br. Med. J.* 303:163, 1991.
23. Wong, C. S., et al. Bronchodilatation, cardiovascular, and hypokalemic effects of fenoterol, salbutamol, and terbutaline in asthma. *Lancet* 336:1396, 1990.
24. Wrenn, K., et al. Aminophyline therapy for acute bronchospastic disease in the emergency room. *Ann. Intern. Med.* 115:2, 1990.

Bronchitis, Bronchiolitis, and Chronic Obstructive Lung Disease with Respiratory Failure

Harris Andrew Sachs
Samuel V. Spagnolo

Overview and Definitions

The respiratory tract is divided into upper and lower systems, with the vocal cords separating the two areas. Infections of the upper respiratory tract include the common cold, sinusitis, pharyngitis, and tonsillitis. Infections of the lower respiratory tract can involve the airways, lung parenchyma, or pleural space. **Acute infectious bronchitis** is defined as infection involving the large airways with symptoms reflective of this localization: cough, sputum production, and often wheezing. The term **chronic bronchitis** has been defined by the American Thoracic Society as persistence of cough and excessive mucus secretion for most days out of 3 months in at least 2 successive years. **Bronchiolitis** is a term used to describe inflammation involving primarily smaller, more peripheral airways. This condition has traditionally involved children and is usually caused by a viral infection, but an adult version, possibly initiated by an infectious agent, has been recognized and may lead to bronchiolitis obliterans with or without associated organizing pneumonia.

Numerous noninfectious agents may result in acute and chronic bronchitis and bronchiolitis. Treatment of these conditions will depend on the clinical setting, the Gram's stain of expectorated sputum, the appearance of sputum, the findings on physical examination, and the offending agent.

Respiratory failure occurs when gas exchange is impaired. Mild degrees of respiratory failure with hypoxemia or hypercarbia may be present for many years without apparent serious physiologic consequences because of the body's normal compensatory mechanisms. The severity of respiratory failure and the need for urgent therapeutic intervention depend on the rate and degree of deterioration in gas exchange as reflected in the arterial blood gases (ABG). Life-threatening, acute respiratory failure occurs when gas exchange is deteriorating rapidly, with accelerated alterations in acid-base chemistry. Abrupt alterations in gas exchange (occurring over minutes to several days) that lower the PaO_2 below 55 mm Hg or lower the pH below 7.30 (by raising the $PaCO_2$ above 50 mm Hg) require rapid and aggressive therapy.

Life-threatening respiratory failure occurs most frequently in patients with underlying severe, chronic airflow obstruction (CAO), primarily caused by emphysema and chronic bronchitis, who previously functioned in a compensated state of chronic respiratory insufficiency.

Physiologic Considerations and Compensatory Responses

A variety of medical and/or surgical insults can precipitate acute respiratory failure in patients with chronic pulmonary insufficiency. Often a viral or bacterial infection leads to increased airflow obstruction. With such infections, bronchial mucus is secreted into the airways at a faster rate than it can be cleared; in addition, there is frequently an increase in spasm of bronchial smooth muscle. Additional factors precipitating acute respiratory failure are listed in Table 2-1. As a consequence of any of these events, ventilation-perfusion ratios (V/Q) are further altered throughout the lung, causing increased arterial hypoxemia and hypercarbia. The degree of hypercarbia and hypoxemia is determined by the severity of the increased airway resistance and the ability of the lung's compensatory mechanisms to match ventilation (airflow) with perfusion (blood flow). The patient's initial compensatory response to the worsening of pulmonary gas exchange is an increase in respiratory rate; this elevated respiratory rate is an attempt to raise minute ventilation. In addition, the actual muscular work of breathing increases because the pump (lung) works against higher resistance. These compensatory ventilatory responses can be blunted for several reasons. First, the respiratory muscle work required to overcome the high airway resistance and maintain adequate ventilation is too great for many patients to sustain. Second, some patients with CAO have abnormal central and peripheral respiratory chemoreceptor responses, and consequently, a falling PaO_2 and rising $PaCO_2$ may stimulate less central ventilatory activity (output).

In addition to these airflow and central respiratory drive problems, chronic and acute alveolar hypoxia causes constriction of pulmonary arterioles. As a result, pulmonary vascular resistance rises and right-heart failure (cor pulmonale) can occur suddenly. Although patients with a chronically reduced PaO_2 appear to tolerate acutely lowered levels of PaO_2 better than normal people, these levels cannot be tolerated for long and eventually lead to tissue and cell death. When the PaO_2 persists below 30 mm Hg, irreversible brain and myocardial damage occurs. Most patients with CAO develop chronic daily cough and produce varying amounts of sputum. Many of these patients will slowly progress to a condition of chronic dyspnea, frequently associated with a feeling of chest tightness and wheezing. When further acute decompensation of respiratory function occurs

Table 2-1. Factors commonly precipitating acute decompensation in patients with chronic airflow obstruction

Viral or bacterial bronchitis	Pulmonary emboli
Viral or bacterial pneumonia	Pleural effusion
Spontaneous pneumothorax	General anesthesia
Left heart failure	Sedative drugs
Abdominal or thoracic surgery	Poor compliance with prescribed medications

in these patients, they will become aware of increasing shortness of breath and wheezing, along with marked difficulty in raising sputum. Patients will note that their sputum has changed color, usually from a clear white to yellow or green.

Treatment

Several basic physiologic principles are involved in the therapy of patients with acute, life-threatening respiratory failure and CAO. There should be an immediate attempt to improve tissue oxygenation by improving the PaO_2 utilizing controlled low-flow oxygen therapy. Simultaneously with oxygen administration, measures should be taken to improve V/Q by clearing the airways of secretions, relieving bronchospasm and inflammation, and treating the frequently associated acute bronchitis or pneumonia. Oxygen administration usually results in reducing pulmonary vascular resistance and improving cardiac output.

Reducing Pulmonary Vascular Resistance

The correction of alveolar hypoxia with administration of supplemental oxygen is often effective in decreasing acute elevation in pulmonary artery pressure. The use of a vasodilator agent such as nifedipine may decrease pulmonary artery pressure but should be used only with continuous monitoring of the pulmonary pressure.

Improvement in Cardiac Output

Biventricular failure is occasionally a prominent feature in severely decompensated respiratory failure. Measurement of pulmonary capillary pressure is often required to identify left heart failure. In the absence of left heart failure, right heart failure is often due to acute and chronic pulmonary hypertension. In order to improve cardiac output, a variety of different treatment modalities have been used, including cautious diuresis; oxygen therapy, which may reduce pulmonary artery pressure and improve ventricular function; and digitalis, which may be dangerous secondary to its potential for serious cardiac arrhythmias in the hypoxic patient.

Reducing Bronchospasm and Inflammation

Bronchodilators are given to reduce lower airway resistance. Even the patient without appreciable wheezing may benefit from bronchodilator therapy. Patients with severe, acute bronchospasm may have little or absent wheezing secondary to significantly reduced airflow. Small changes in airway resistance can significantly improve airflow, ventilation, and gas exchange.

Bronchodilator Agents

Theophylline

PHARMACOKINETICS

Theophylline is a member of the class of methylxanthines, with actions that include the relaxation of smooth muscle, notably bronchial muscle, CNS stimulation, excitation of cardiac muscle, and action on the kidney to produce diuresis. The side effect/benefit comparison of theophylline has been the focus of recent controversy. Aminophylline is the IV solution of theophylline that contains approximately 80% theophylline.

CLINICAL USE

Theophylline is a weak bronchodilator compared with the inhaled anticholinergic or adrenergic drugs. An additional role of theophylline has been evaluated, including relief from respiratory muscle fatigue, stimulation of mucociliary transport, and improvement of respiratory drive in chronic obstructive pulmonary disease (COPD) patients. The data over the years have been very controversial as to the level of benefit provided. Theophylline has a marked variability in pharmacokinetics, which makes accurate estimate of serum concentration difficult. With the wide side-effect profile and narrow therapeutic range, the role of this drug as a therapeutic agent may require reexamination. If aminophylline is used in the setting of acute respiratory failure, the IV route is recommended in order to achieve stable blood levels.

DOSAGE AND ADMINISTRATION

The recommended IV **loading dose** of aminophylline is 6 mg/kg unless the patient is currently on theophylline, then the loading dose should be reduced to 3 mg/kg. (**Note:** We do not recommend loading dosage if a patient is on theophylline therapy.)

The recommended IV **maintenance dosage** of aminophylline is 0.6 mg/kg/hour or 0.3 mg/kg/hour if the patient is taking theophylline. **Caution:** These dosages are guidelines only. Final dosing should be adjusted based on theophylline level.

Aminophylline is supplied as IV solution of 250 mg/10 cc single vial.

ADVERSE EFFECTS

Gastrointestinal upset, headache, seizures, palpitations, and arrhythmias have been noted with theophylline, especially with blood levels greater than 20/mg/dl.

SUMMARY

Theophylline levels can be significantly altered by drug interactions. Increased theophylline levels have been noted with allopurinol, cimetidine, erythromycin, lithium, oral contraceptives, ciprofloxacin, and propranolol. Decreased theophylline levels have been noted with phenytoin and rifampin. Pregnancy Category C (risk cannot be ruled out) pertains.

Adrenergic Agents

PHARMACOKINETICS

Adrenergic agents play a major role in the treatment of acute respiratory failure. The primary action of beta-adrenergic agents is to stimulate adenylate cyclase, which results in increased cyclic adenosine monophosphate (cAMP) which mediates cellular response. $Beta_2$ receptors are the predominant receptors on the bronchial smooth muscle; therefore, these $beta_2$ selective agents provide the optimal effect with limited systemic effects from $beta_1$ receptors. Despite the availability of oral adrenergic agents, the primary mode of administration for respiratory failure is through inhalation, by metered-dose inhaler (MDI) or by aerosol nebulization.

Albuterol

CLINICAL USE

Albuterol (Proventil, Ventolin) is effective in the treatment of bronchospasm. Clinical trials have noted that the use of albuterol, as well as many of the other adrenergic agents, are most effective in patients with bronchial asthma versus patients with chronic obstructive lung disease. The goal in therapy with these agents is reduced airway obstruction and improved airflow.

DOSAGE AND ADMINISTRATION

Albuterol is given by MDI using 1–2 puffs q4–6h. This dosage may be increased as tolerated, watching for side effects or toxicity. Many clinicians have recommended the initial use of 4 puffs q4–6h in an attempt to optimize drug delivery. When albuterol is given by nebulizer, the recommended dosage is 2.5 mg q6–8h. The albuterol oral tablet may be given to adults and children over age 12 years using 2 mg or 4 mg q6–8h. For children aged 6–12 years, it is recommended that only 2 mg q6–8h be given. Albuterol is available as an MDI delivering 0.09 mg/puff (90μg/puff). Nebulizer solution is available as a 5% solution. Oral tablets are available in 2-mg or 4-mg tablets. Sustained-release tablets (Proventil Repetabs) are also available. The use of reservoir devices (InspirEase, Aerochamber) has provided improvement in optimal delivery of medication via MDI to appropriate sites of action, the alveoli.

ADVERSE EFFECTS

Cardiovascular disease, arrhythmias, and hypertension are noted with adrenergic agents, especially those taken orally.

SUMMARY

Many recent studies have described the equivalent response to MDI (with spacer devices) as to nebulizers in the treatment of reversible airflow obstruction. The use of MDIs instead of nebulizers has shown significant cost reduction. Oral albuterol plays very little role in the acute setting but plays an increasing role in chronic therapy.

The Proventil Repetabs have been shown to provide benefit for nocturnal asthma. The dosing is recommended either twice a day or at bedtime.

Metaproterenol

CLINICAL USE

Metaproterenol (Alupent, Metaprel) is another adrenergic agent used in the treatment of airway bronchospasm. In comparison with isoproterenol, metaproterenol has been noted to have a prolonged duration of action and apparently decreased incidence and severity of adverse cardiac side effects. Metaproterenol is less $beta_2$ selective than albuterol.

DOSAGE AND ADMINISTRATION

Metaproterenol is given by MDI using 2–3 puffs q3–4h. This dosage may be increased as tolerated, noting side effects and toxicity. When metaproterenol is given by nebulizer, the recommended dosage is 0.3 cc of 5% solution with 2.5 cc saline. The oral metaproterenol dosage for adults and children older than age 9 years (or weighing more than 60 pounds) is 20 mg q6–8h. For children aged 6–9 years or weighing less than 60 pounds, the recommended dosage is 10 mg q6–8h. Metaproterenol is supplied as MDI with 0.65 mg/puff, 5% nebulizer solution, or oral tablets of 10 or 20 mg.

ADVERSE EFFECTS

Cardiovascular disease, arrhythmias, and hypertension are side effects that have been noted, especially when taken orally.

SUMMARY

Many clinicians have noted fewer cardiovascular side effects with albuterol use as compared to metaproterenol.

Isoetharine

CLINICAL USE

Isoetharine (Bronkometer, Bronkosol) is used for symptomatic relief of reversible bronchospasm. This agent was the first widely used medication with $beta_2$ selectivity; however, its degree of selectivity for the $beta_2$ receptor does not approach that of the newer agents (albuterol or metaproterenol). In the light of the availability of more $beta_2$ selective agents, we do not recommend this agent as first-line therapy.

DOSAGE AND ADMINISTRATION

Isoetharine is given by MDI using 1–2 puffs q4h. In severe cases, the frequency of dosing may be increased, paying close attention to potential side effects. The MDI dosage is 0.34 mg/puff. A 1% nebulizer solution is available with recommended dosage of 0.025–0.5 cc solution in 2–3 cc saline q4h.

ADVERSE EFFECTS

Isoetharine contains a sulfite and is therefore contraindicated in patients with sulfite allergy. Cardiovascular disease, arrhythmias, hypertension, and hyperthyroidism have been noted with isoetharine.

Anticholinergic Agents

PHARMACOKINETICS

Anticholinergics prevent the increase in intracellular concentration of cyclic guanosine monophosphate (cGMP) that is caused by the muscarinic receptors on bronchial smooth muscle. Therefore, these agents appear to inhibit vagally mediated reflexes by blocking the effects of acetylcholine. Many recent studies have shown that ipratropium provides a more significant improvement in flows in patients with emphysema or bronchitis versus asthma. These agents are administered through inhalation with minimal systemic side effects.

Atropine

CLINICAL USE

Atropine produces a variety of systemic effects, including bronchodilation. Unlike the newly developed quaternary ammonium structure anticholinergic agents with decreased mucosal absorption, atropine is well absorbed through the bronchial mucosa. This increased absorption across mucosal membranes has led to systemic anticholinergic side effects, which has limited the effective use of this agent for bronchodilation.

DOSAGE AND ADMINISTRATION

Atropine is administered via nebulizer with a dosage of 0.4–0.8 mg q3–4h; yet frequency of administration and quantity of medication is often limited by systemic side effects. We recommend that the use of atropine be limited. We prefer to utilize ipratropium or glycopyrrolate as first-line therapy in nonasthmatic patients.

ADVERSE EFFECTS

Atropine administration through nebulizer has been associated with significant systemic anticholinergic side effects, including tachycardia, dry mucous membranes, dilated pupils, hypertension, and urinary retention.

Glycopyrrolate

CLINICAL USE

Glycopyrrolate (Robinul), a quaternary ammonium–structured anticholinergic agent, has historically been used as a parenteral preanesthetic, antimuscarinic agent during reversal of neuromuscular blockade. In addition, glycopyrrolate has been demonstrated to result in significant bronchodilator action. Most clinical studies have evaluated the role of glycopyrrolate in asthmatic patients, yet many clinicians have noted significant broncodilator effects in patients with chronic obstructive lung disease. In comparative studies of glycopyrrolate, atropine, and metaproterenol, it has been noted that in asthmatics, glycopyrrolate has fewer side effects and longer duration of action. Yet of the anticholinergic agents, glycopyrrolate has a slower onset of action.

DOSAGE AND ADMINISTRATION

Glycopyrrolate is administered via nebulizer with dosage of 0.4–0.8 mg q3–4h as needed. This medication is supplied as 0.2 mg/ml vials.

ADVERSE EFFECTS

Side effects of glycopyrrolate, although rare, include tachycardia, hypertension, dry mucosal membranes, and dilated pupils.

SUMMARY

Although not specifically indicated or approved by the Food and Drug Administration (FDA) for bronchodilator therapy, many studies have shown improvement in bronchial airflow with minimal adverse side effects.

Ipratropium

CLINICAL USE

Ipratropium bromide (Atrovent) is a synthetic quaternary ammonium congener of atropine. The use of ipratropium has shown improvement in the bronchial airway flow in patients with chronic obstructive airway disease and to a lesser extent in patients with asthma. Many clinicians have used either beta agonists or anticholinergics in evaluating the optimal agent for their patients. Occasionally, patients show benefit from a combination of beta agonists and anticholinergic agents.

DOSAGE AND ADMINISTRATION

The starting dosage of ipratropium is 2 puffs q6h. It is adjusted as needed up to 12 puffs per 24 hours. Studies are evaluating the benefit of higher dosages. This agent is currently supplied as MDI with 0.018 mg/puff. Under FDA consideration is a solution for nebulization.

ADVERSE EFFECTS

Nervousness, headache, GI upset, dry mouth, and cough are the most commonly noted side effects. Caution must be exercised when it is used in patients with narrow-angle glaucoma, prostatic hypertrophy, and bladder-neck obstruction.

Antimicrobial Agents

Antibiotics appear helpful in patients seriously ill with chronic obstructive lung disease. Most of these patients have heavy sputum production and bacterial colonization in the lower respiratory tract. Further disruption of airway defense mechanisms may permit these bacteria and other microbes (*Mycoplasma pneumonia, Chlamydia,* anaerobic bacteria, and other gram-negative bacteria) to invade tissues, possibly resulting in acute bronchopneumonia.

The choice of appropriate antibiotic(s) must be chosen to treat suspected organism(s). In general, the antimicrobial agent(s) used in the acutely decompensated patient with respiratory failure will depend on whether acute bronchitis, overt clinical pneumonia, or both, is present. The treatment of acute pneumonia is fully described in Chapters 3–5.

For the patient with only acute or worsening chronic bronchitis, the antimicrobial agent(s) chosen for treatment should be effective against the bacteria identified by Gram's stain of a lower-respiratory-tract specimen (sputum). Bacteria found most often by Gram's stain in this setting include *Streptococcus pneumoniae, Haemophilus influenzae,* and *Moraxella catarrhalis* (formerly *Branhamella catarrhalis*). If there are increased number of polymorphonuclear leukocytes (PMNs) in the sputum, this suggests a bacterial etiology, and antimicrobial administration can be predicted on the predominant organism seen on the smear. When a suspected organism cannot be identified, empiric therapy is often directed against the probable microorganism for the specific clinical setting.

Here we examine the common antimicrobials used in the treatment of acute bronchitis.

Ampicillin

See page 67.

Azithromycin

Azithromycin (Zithromax) is the first azalide antibiotic released in the United States for the treatment of acute exacerbation of chronic bronchitis, community-acquired outpatient pneumonia, pharyngitis, skin infections, and nongonococcal urethritis.

ANTIMICROBIAL ACTIVITY

Azithromycin has in vitro spectrum of activity against gram-positive aerobic bacteria, including *S. pneumoniae* and *S. pyogenes;* gram-negative aerobic bacteria, including *H. influenza, M. catarrhalis,* and *Legionella pneumophilia;* intracellular organisms such as *Mycoplasma pneumoniae;* and anaerobic bacteria such as *Bacteroides bivis.*

PHARMACOKINETICS

After oral dosing, azithromycin is rapidly absorbed and distributed widely throughout the body. The rapid absorption of azithromycin from serum into tissues and its high and sustained serum tissue levels distinguish it pharmacologically from oral antimicrobial agents whose tissue concentrations are usually lower than or similar to their serum concentration. Following the initial dose of azithromycin, the serum concentration peaks in 2–3 hours; tissue levels will peak later (approximately 48 hours). Although azithromycin is a weak base upon entering the cell, it becomes concentrated in the acidic compartments, i.e., lysosomes. Uptake of azithromycin within phagocytes leads to increased drug levels at the site of infection.

CLINICAL USE

In clinical trials, comparison of azithromycin with cefaclor showed that the 5-day/5-dose course of treatment with azithromycin is as effective as cefaclor 3 times a day for 10 days in the treatment of acute bacterial exacerbations of chronic bronchitis or treatment of community-acquired pneumonia.

DOSAGE AND ADMINISTRATION

For adults and children older than age 16 years, the recommended dosage of azithromycin is 2 250-mg tablets on day 1 followed by 1 250-mg tablet daily for days 2–5. Azithromycin should be taken either 1 hour before meals or 2 hours after meals.

ADVERSE EFFECTS

Precaution in administering this agent includes use in patients with known hypersensitivity to azithromycin, erythromycin, or any macrolide. It is to be used with caution in renal or hepatic impairment. It is Category B in pregnancy: No evidence of risk in humans.

SUMMARY

Many of the generic antibiotics, which include the penicillins, erythromycin, tetracycline, and the combination of trimethaprim and sulfamethoxazole, should usually be considered first-line therapy if a bacterial etiology is suspected. In the event of poor response to the initial antimicrobial trial, treatment with azithromycin may provide a broader spectrum of coverage. Patients who have been treated with a variety of antimicrobials may develop resistant organisms that may respond to a new exposure to azithromycin. In a patient whose compliance may be a problem, azithromycin provides convenient dosing with broad-spectrum coverage, though with increased cost.

Cefaclor

ANTIMICROBIAL ACTIVITY

Cefaclor (Ceclor) is a second-generation cephalosporin with activity against a variety of common pathogens. In vitro studies demonstrate bactericidal against *S. pneumonia*, *S. pyogenes* (group A beta-hemolytic streptococci), *M. catarrhalis*, *H. influenza*, *Escherichia coli*, *Proteus mirabilis*, *Klebsiella pneumoniae*, *Citrobacter diversus*, *Neisseria gonorrhoea*, *Peptococci*, and *Peptostreptococci*.

PHARMACOCKINETICS

Cefaclor is well absorbed after oral administration to the **fasting** patient. Total absorption is the same whether the drug is taken on an empty stomach or after eating. In patients who have taken this medication with food, the peak concentration achieved is 50–75% less than that observed in the fasting individual. The serum half-life in normal subjects is 0.6–0.9 hours. In patients with complete renal failure, the half-life of cefaclor is 2.3–2.8 hours. The bactericidal activity of cefaclor results from inhibition of cell wall synthesis.

CLINICAL USE

Cefaclor is indicated in the treatment of otitis media, lower respiratory tract infections, pharyngitis, tonsillitis, urinary tract infections, and skin infections, provided the offending organism is sensitive to cefaclor.

DOSAGE AND ADMINISTRATION

The standard dosage of cefaclor is 250 mg q8h. For more severe infections, the dosage may be increased to 500 mg q8h.

ADVERSE EFFECTS

The most common side effects to cefaclor are gastrointestinal upset, skin rash, and mild leukopenia. Serum sickness–like reactions have also been noted in 1–2% of patients taking cefaclor. This reaction involves joint aches, erythema multiforme, and purpura and will last 3–4 days after discontinuation of the drug.

SUMMARY

Many factors often influence the selection of a specific antimicrobial agent use in the treatment of bronchitis. Of primary concern is the efficacy of the selected agent against a suspected organism. Once the field of agents is narrowed, cost, frequency of dosing, side effects, and convenience of dosing must be considered. Many of the generic antimicrobials provide adequate coverage of suspected organisms yet are associated with increased side effects and decreased convenience.

Cefixime

Cefixime (Suprax) is a recent oral semisynthetic third-generation cephalosporin available in the United States for treatment of acute bronchitis and acute exacerbations of chronic bronchitis.

ANTIMICROBIAL ACTIVITY

Cefixime appears to inhibit bacterial cell wall synthesis and is beta-lactamase stable. It is active in vitro and in clinical situations caused by *S. pneumoniae* and *H. influenzae*. The drug is also active in vitro against *M. catarrhalis, E. coli,* and *P. mirabilis*.

Note: Pseudomonas species, strains of group D streptococci (including enterococci), *Listeria monocytogenes,* most strains of staphylococci (including methicillin-resistant strains), and most strains of *Enterobacter* are resistant to cefixime. Also, most strains of *Bacteroides fragilis* and *Clostridia* are resistant to cefixime.

SUSCEPTIBILITY TESTING

A specific disk is available for testing susceptibility to cefixime; the class disk for cephalosporins (the cephalothin disk) will not yield reliable susceptibility information for this drug.

PHARMACOKINETICS

Cefixime is 40–50% absorbed, and a single 200-mg tablet of cefixime produces an average peak serum concentration of approximately 2 mg/ml. The oral suspension will produce an average peak concentration approximately 25–50% higher than the tablets. This increased absorption must be considered if the oral suspension is to be substituted for the tablet. In animal studies, approximately 50% of the absorbed dose is excreted unchanged in the urine in 24 hours. Cefixime is also excreted in the bowel in excess of 10% of the administered dose. In individuals with moderate impairment of renal function (20–40 ml/minute creatinine clearance), the average serum half-life of cefixime is prolonged from 6 to 7 hours. The drug is not cleared significantly from the blood by hemodialysis or peritoneal dialysis.

CLINICAL USE

In clinical trials, cefixime is effective in treating acute bronchitis and acute exacerbations of chronic bronchitis caused by *S. pneumoniae* and *H. influenzae* (beta-lactamase positive and negative strains). Appropriate cultures and susceptibility studies should be performed to determine the causative organism and its susceptibility to cefixime; however, initial therapy may be given while awaiting the results of susceptibility studies.

DOSAGE AND ADMINISTRATION

The recommended adult dosage of cefixime is 400 mg daily, or 8 mg/kg/day of the suspension for children. The 400-mg adult dosage may be given as a single dose or as a 200-mg tablet q12h. The oral suspension may be given as a single dose or in two divided doses, as 4 mg/kg q12h. Patients with creatinine clearance between 21 and 60 ml/minute may be given 75% of the standard dosage at the standard dosing intervals (300 ml daily).

ADVERSE EFFECTS

Cefixime is generally well tolerated. Adverse effects include clinically mild gastrointestinal side effects — diarrhea, abdominal pain, nausea, dyspepsia, and flatulence — in 20% of all patients. Some patients have developed documented pseudomembranous colitis, and some patients have required hospitalization.

DRUG-LABORATORY TEST INTERACTIONS

A false reaction for ketones and glucose in the urine may result using Clinitest, Benedict's solution, or Fehling's solution. Clinitix or test tape should be used for testing the urine for glucose in these patients. A false-positive Coombs test has also been reported during treatment with cephalosporin antibiotics.

Cefprozil

Cefprozil (Cefzil), a new oral second-generation cephalosporin, was recently released in the United States for treatment of bronchitis, pharyngitis otitis media, and skin infections.

ANTIMICROBIAL ACTIVITY

Cefprozil is similar in antibacterial activity to cefaclor (Ceclor) and cefuroxime axetil (Ceftin). It is active in vitro against most gram-positive cocci, including beta-hemolytic streptococci, *S. pneumoniae,* and methicillin-susceptible *S. aureus* but not against methicillin-resistant *S. aureus.* The drug is also active in vitro against *H. influenzae,* including beta-lactamase-producing strains, *M. catarrhalis,* and some strains of *K. pneumoniae, E. coli, Salmonella,* and *Shigella. Enterobacter, Serratia, Proteus, Pseudomonas,* and *Bacteroides fragilis* are resistant to cefprozil.

SUSCEPTIBILITY TESTING

A specific disc is available for testing susceptibility to cefprozil; the class disc for cephalosporins (cephalothin) will not yield reliable susceptibility information for the new drug.

PHARMACOKINETICS

Cefprozil is 95% absorbed from the GI tract; absorption is unaffected by the presence of food. The drug is excreted mainly by the kidney. It has a half-life of at least 1.3 hours. Peak serum concentrations and half-life are both prolonged in patients with impaired renal function, and the dosage should be halved in patients with a creatinine clearance of less than 30 ml/minute. Cefprozil is removed by hemodialysis; a postdialysis booster dose should be given.

CLINICAL USE

In randomized controlled trials, cefprozil has been effective in treating bronchitis, pharyngitis, otitis media, and impetigo in both adults and children. It has been about as effective in these infections as erythromycin, cefaclor, cefuroxime axetil, or amoxicillin-clavulanic acid. Studies comparing cefprozil with trimethoprim-sulfamethoxazole are unavailable.

DOSAGE AND ADMINISTRATION

The recommended adult dosage of cefprozil is 250 or 500 mg twice daily and 15 mg/kg bid for children. For group A streptococcal pharyngitis, 500 mg once daily has been effective.

ADVERSE EFFECTS

Cefprozil is generally well tolerated. Adverse effects include rash, diarrhea, nausea, and vomiting. In controlled trials, the new drug has caused less diarrhea than amoxicillin–clavulanic acid and less GI discomfort than erythromycin.

Cefuroxime Axetil

ANTIMICROBIAL ACTIVITY

Cefuroxime axetil (Ceftin) is a second-generation cephalosporin that has a bactericidal activity against a wide range of common pathogens, including many of the beta-lactamase strains. In vitro testing shows that cefuroxime is active against gram-positive organism, including *S. aureus* (except methicillin-resistant *Staphylococcus*), *S. pneumoniae,* and *S. pyogenes* (group A beta-hemolytic streptococci). Certain strains of enterococci are resistant to cefuroxime. In addition to the in vitro studies for gram-positive organisms, cefuroxime shows activity against gram-negative organisms (*M. catarrhalis, E. coli, H. influenza,* and *K. pneumoniae*). Most anaerobic organisms are resistant to cefuroxime.

PHARMACOKINETICS

After oral administration, cefuroxime axetil is readily absorbed through the GI tract and hydrolyzed by enzymes in the intestinal mucosa and blood to release this agent into the bloodstream. Studies to evaluate the effect on absorption with regard to ingestion of this medication on an empty stomach versus with food present showed that differences in absorption exist in these two settings, but clinical and bacteriological differences were not noted to be significant. The bactericidal action of cefuroxime results from the inhibition of cell wall synthesis by binding to essential target proteins.

CLINICAL USE

Cefuroxime axetil is indicated for the treatment of pharyngitis tonsillitis, otitis media, lower respiratory tract infections, urinary tract infections, and skin infections (provided organisms show sensitivity to cefuroxime). A study comparing the efficacy of cefuroxime, dosed q12h, compared to cefaclor, dosed q8h, in lower respiratory tract infections showed at least equivalent therapeutic efficacy of both medications.

DOSAGE AND ADMINISTRATION

The standard dosage for otitis media, pharyngitis, and respiratory infections is 250 mg orally q12h. For more severe infections that do not require IV therapy, an oral dosage of 500 mg q12h may be used.

ADVERSE EFFECTS

The most significant observed side effect of cefuroxime is diarrhea (3.5%), followed by nausea, vomiting, hypersensitivity rash, and urticaria. In patients with history of penicillin reaction, 2.9% had a reaction.

Erythromycin

See page 85.

Lomefloxacin

ANTIMICROBIAL ACTIVITY

Lomefloxacin (Maxaquin) is a difluorinated quinolone with virtually complete oral absorption and a half-life of 7–8 hours of antimicrobial activity. Spectrum of coverage includes excellent antimicrobial activity against enterobacteriaceae, haemophilus, and moraxella species and inhibits *Pseudomonas aeruginosa* and *S. aureus*. The drug is less active against *S. pneumoniae* and hemolytic streptococcus. Lomefloxacin has no antianaerobic activity.

PHARMACOKINETICS

The dosage of lomefloxacin must be adjusted for renal impairment with a creatine clearance less than 30–40 ml/minute. In severe renal failure — creatine clearance less than 40 ml/minute — the serum half-life is 21 hours compared to 8 hours with normal renal function. Liver disease does not require dosing adjustment.

CLINICAL USE

Lomefloxacin is effective in the treatment of acute exacerbation of chronic bronchitis due to gram-negative bacteria. Based on in vitro studies, lomefloxacin cannot be considered appropriate treatment of pneumococcal infections.

DOSAGE AND ADMINISTRATION

The recommended adult dosage of lomefloxacin is 400 mg once daily.

ADVERSE EFFECTS

The most frequently noted adverse effects are nausea, headache, photosensitivity, and dizziness, with nausea being the most frequent at 3.7%.

SUMMARY

Lomefloxacin offers improved patient compliance due to its once-daily dosing. Theophylline, unlike many of the other quinolones, does not require dosing adjustment with lomefloxacin.

Ofloxacin

Ofloxacin (Floxin) is a new fluoroquinolone antimicrobial agent for treatment of a variety of infections, including the lower respiratory tract, genitourinary tract, GI tract, and skin, secondary to susceptible organisms.

ANTIMICROBIAL ACTIVITY

In vitro activity of ofloxacin is highly active against *H. influenzae, M. catarrhalis, Meningococci,* and *Gonococcus*. Ofloxacin is also highly active against most of the bacterial causes of enteritis. Although ofloxacin shows in vitro activity against staphylococcus and many streptococcus organisms, activity is much less than cephalosporins or penicillins. In vitro activity against anaerobes is poor. Ofloxacin has activity against *Legionella pneumophilia, M. pneumonia, C. trachomatis,* and *Mycobacterium tuberculosis*. A cephalosporin or penicillin is recommended for the treatment of known or suspected streptococcal or pneumococcal infection.

PHARMACOKINETICS

Oral ofloxacin is 98% bioavailable. Serum concentrations reach a peak 1–2 hours after the oral dose. The half-life of this agent in the body is 5–8 hours. Dosage adjustments are recommended when creatine clearance falls below 50 ml/hour. Unlike ciprofloxacin, ofloxacin does not cause significant increase in serum concentration of theophylline.

CLINICAL USE

In the treatment of chronic bronchitis, ofloxacin is effective in the infections secondary to *H. influenzae, Legionella* species, and *M. catarrhalis*. In cases in which a pneumococcal or streptococcal infection is suspected, cephalosporins or penicillins are more appropriate antimicrobial agents. Ofloxacin has been noted to be as effective as ciprofloxacin and trimethoprim-sulfamethoxazole in the treatment of acute exacerbation of bronchitis in patients with chronic obstructive pulmonary disease.

DOSAGE AND ADMINISTRATION

The recommended dosage for patients with infections of the lower respiratory tract is 400 mg daily for 10 days.

ADVERSE EFFECTS

Side effects of ofloxacin include nausea, insomnia, headache, dizziness, diarrhea, hypersensitivity, rash, pruritis, and nervousness. This medication is not recommended for patients less than age 18 years or pregnant or nursing women.

Tetracycline

See pages 110–111.

Trimethoprim-Sulfamethoxazole

See pages 103–104.

Antitussive Agents

Cough is a significant physiologic mechanism for clearing the tracheobronchial tree, and suppression of cough can lead to increased mucus plugging and delayed clinical improvement. Cough suppression should be instituted only when the cough is dry, profoundly irritating to the patient, or prevents sleep. The cough reflex is a complex mechanism involving central and peripheral nervous systems, as well as the smooth muscle of the bronchi. It has been suggested that irritation of the bronchial mucosa causes bronchoconstriction, which stimulates the cough receptors in the bronchial tree. Afferent conduction from these receptors is via the vagus nerve. Antitussive agents may have a pharmacologic effect on various sites.

Benzonatate Perles

PHARMACOKINETICS

Benzonatate perles (Tessalon Perles) are believed to exert their antitussive action on the stretch receptors in the lungs and the pleura by dampening their activity and decreasing the cough reflex at its source. Action begins within 15–20 minutes and lasts for 3–8 hours.

CLINICAL USE

Benzonatate perles are used for the symptomatic relief of cough. This agent is ideal when the use of narcotic agents is contraindicated. The duration of action, up to 8 hours, provides a benefit in decreasing nocturnal cough and allowing improvement in sleep.

DOSAGE AND ADMINISTRATION

The standard dosage of benzonatate perles is 100 mg PO tid prn, up to 600 mg daily.

ADVERSE EFFECTS

Adverse effects have included sedation, headache, dizziness, GI upset, and pruritus. This agent is not recommended for children less than age 10 years or pregnant or lactating women.

Codeine

PHARMACOKINETICS

Codeine exerts its main effect on the CNS. The actual mechanism of action with regard to antitussive action is unclear.

CLINICAL USE

Codeine is an effective cough suppressant, and it also causes sedation. It is an ideal choice as a cough suppressant for patients who are unable to sleep due to a persistent cough. Codeine is a narcotic with addictive potential. Therefore, it is intended for a short course of therapy, not chronic use.

DOSAGE AND ADMINISTRATION

The recommended dosage of codeine is 10–20 mg q4–6h. The daily maximum dosage is 120 mg. Although this low dosage is ineffective for analgesia, it has a demonstrated antitussive action.

ADVERSE EFFECTS

The use of codeine in patients with pulmonary, renal, or hepatic dysfunction may lead to respiratory depression or depressed mental status. Constipation and sedation are the most common side effects.

Dextromethorphan with Guaifenesin (Robitussin DM)

PHARMACOKINETICS

Dextromethorphan-guaifenesin (Robitussin DM) is a combination product. Dextromethorphan is a codeine analogue of levorphanol but has no analgesic or addictive properties. This drug acts centrally. Sites that bind dextromethorphan with high affinity have been identified in various regions of the brain. At therapeutic dosage, this drug does not inhibit ciliary activity in the tracheobronchial tree. Guaifenesin is an expectorant that loosens secretions by decreasing their viscosity. Guaifenesin is readily absorbed from the GI tract and excreted through the kidney.

CLINICAL USE

Dextromethorphan-guaifenesin is an agent, like many of the other antitussives described in this chapter, that is used as a nonaddictive, nonsedating cough suppressant. This medication, unlike the tessalon perles, is taken in a liquid form. This agent must be used with caution since suppression of cough may lead to worsening of bronchitis symptoms by inhibiting the clearance of bronchial secretions. The presence of guaifenesin, an expectorant, allows for effective clearance when a patient does attempt to cough.

DOSAGE AND ADMINISTRATION

The recommended dosage of Robitussin for adults and children older than age 12 years is 2 teaspoons q4h prn. For children aged 6–12 years, the recommended dosage is 1 teaspoon q4h prn. For children aged 2–6 years, ½ teaspoon q4h prn is the current recommended dosage. The use of dextromethorphan is not approved for children less than age 2 years.

ADVERSE EFFECTS

Noted side effects of dextromethorphan include GI upset, drowsiness, and headache. The use of dextromethorphan is contraindicated within 14 days of monoamine oxidase inhibitors secondary to increased sympathomimetic effects.

Codeine with Guaifenesin and Alcohol (Robitussin AC)

PHARMACOKINETICS

See codeine for pharmacokinetics.

CLINICAL USE

The clinical use is otherwise the same as for codeine.

DOSAGE AND ADMINISTRATION

The recommended dosage of Robitussin AC for adults and children older than age 12 years is 2 teaspoons q4h prn. For children aged 6–12 years, the recommended dosage is 1 teaspoon q4h prn. Extreme caution must be taken in patients under age 6 years. This agent is not approved for patients under age 2 years. Each 5 ml (1 teaspoonful) contains 10 mg codine phosphate.

ADVERSE EFFECTS

The use of Robitussin AC in patients with pulmonary, renal, or hepatic dysfunction may lead to respiratory depression or depressed mental status. The elderly metabolize narcotics more slowly, leading to accumulation of the drug for an extended period of time. Codeine is not recommended for patients with urinary obstruction or increased intracranial pressure. Pregnant and lactating women should use it with caution. This drug is contraindicated within 14 days of monoamine oxidase inhibitors secondary to increased sympathomimetic effects. Sedation and constipation are the most commonly reported side effects, and dizziness, nausea, and vomiting have been reported.

Antiinflammatory Agents: Glucocorticoids

The role of glucocorticoids is to stabilize lysosomal membranes, reduce capillary permeability, and decrease chemotaxis and phagocytosis. Glucocorticoids are well absorbed after oral administration and clinically effective systemically when given by this route. The activity of glucocorticoids depends on entry into the cell cytoplasm, binding to specific intracytosol receptors to then enter the nucleus. Prednisone, the most commonly used glucocorticoid, is converted to its active metabolite prednisolone in the liver.

Prednisone

CLINICAL USE

Prednisone (Deltasone, Prednisone) is commonly given in the initial treatment of acute bronchiolitis in an attempt to decrease bronchospasm and lessen inflammation. The use of prednisone in the treatment of acute bronchitis is limited to patients with COPD who have shown benefit from long-term corticosteroid therapy. Yet in bronchiolitis, prednisone is the drug of choice. A prominent feature of bronchiolitis is the presence of a bronchiolar inflammatory process. It is likely that the ultimate improvement in lung function with steroid therapy will depend on the relative degree of inflammation versus fibrosis that is present at the onset of treatment.

DOSAGE AND ADMINISTRATION

Most patients with bronchiolitis respond to a 3-month course of prednisone (1 mg/kg/day) with gradual tapering of steroids to a lower daily dosage, and then alternate-day regimens after the initial 3 months for a total period of 1–2 years of therapy.

In patients with an acute exacerbation of COPD with respiratory failure, the use of prednisone for a short course has provided benefit in improving symptoms. Initial daily treatment with prednisone 40–60 mg has been shown to provide improvement in airflow and sputum clearance. The dose of prednisone is tapered, often over a 2–3-week period, carefully noting any worsening of symptoms as the dosage of glucocorticoids is decreased.

ADVERSE EFFECTS

The most frequently noted major side effects of prednisone are peptic ulcer disease, hypertension, and psychiatric disturbance; they have been noted to occur in almost 30% of patients. The minor side effects include moon facies, acne, and weight gain. The vast majority of side effects will resolve with reduction in dosage or withdrawal of therapy. All patients with latent or positive tuberculin reactivity should receive chemoprophylaxis during prolonged steroid therapy. Fluid retention may require diuretic therapy to alleviate symptoms. Glucose homeostasis may be altered in diabetics, requiring adjustment in diet, oral agents, or insulin.

Expectorants and Mucolytics

In the treatment of patients with acute bronchitis and bronchiolitis, it is important to clear the airways of excessive secretions. In a select group of patients who are unable to clear secretions due to increased viscosity of airway mucus, mucolytics and/or expectorants may be useful.

Acetylcysteine

PHARMACOKINETICS

Acetylcysteine (Mucomyst) is used traditionally in the treatment of acetaminophen overdose. In patients with severe mucoid impaction of the airways, acetylcysteine has been noted to lyse mucopeptide disulfide bonds. This action decreases the viscosity of mucoid sputum, which improves clearance of the airways.

CLINICAL USE

Acetylcysteine is indicated as adjunctive therapy for use in patients with thick, retained mucoid or mucopurulent secretions. These conditions include acute and chronic bronchopulmonary disorders, infectious atelectasis secondary to mucus obstruction, and pulmonary complications of cystic fibrosis. It has not been established that acetylcysteine provides any advantage over properly performed saline instillation or adequate hydration.

DOSAGE AND ADMINISTRATION

The suggested starting dosage of acetylcysteine is 4 ml of 10% solution by nebulizer q2–6h. **Caution:** In the light of significant bronchospasm with this agent, administration of concomitant bronchodilator is recommended.

ADVERSE EFFECTS

Noted side effects of acetylcysteine include severe bronchospasm and excessive liquefication of dried, retained secretions, stomatitis, nausea, and hypersensitivity.

Guaifenesin

PHARMACOKINETICS

Guaifenesin (Humabid) loosens the secretion by reducing its viscosity. It is readily absorbed from the GI tract and excreted through the kidney. Plasma half-life is 1 hour. The major metabolite is beta-(2-methoxyphenoxy) lactic acid.

CLINICAL USE

The use of guaifenesin has been shown to be effective in reducing viscosity of bronchial secretions and allowing more effective expectoration. This agent is often found in combination with cough suppressants. Since cough suppression is often an undesired side effect, this has resulted in the availability of guaifenesin as a single agent.

DOSAGE AND ADMINISTRATION

Guaifenesin is available in two forms: tablets and sprinkles. The dosage recommendation for the tablets varies with age. In adults and children older than age 12 years, the dosage is 1–2 tablets q12h prn. For children aged 6–12 years, the dosage is 1 tablet q12h prn. The recommended dosage for children aged 2–6 years is ½ tablet q12h prn.

The dosage for sprinkles varies with age also. In adults and children older than age 12 years, the dosage is 2–4 tablets q12h prn. In children aged 6–12 years, the dosage is 2 tablets q12h prn. The recommended dosage in children aged 2–6 years is 1 tablet q12h prn.

ADVERSE EFFECTS

No serious side effects have been reported in the use of guaifenesin. This medication is listed as a Category C in pregnant patients: a drug in which risk cannot be ruled out. It has an unclear effect on the lactating mother and is contraindicated within 14 days of monoamine oxidase inhibitors due to increased sympathomimetic effects.

Iodinated Glycerol

PHARMACOKINETICS

Iodinated glycerol (Organidin) is a mixture of several iodinated compounds formed by a reaction of iodine and glycine. Iodides are readily absorbed from the GI tract and concentrated primarily in the secretions of the respiratory tract. The mechanism of action of this agent is unclear.

CLINICAL USE

Iodinated glycerol may be helpful as a mucolytic expectorant.

DOSAGE AND ADMINISTRATION

The recommended dosage of iodinated glycerol in adults is 2 tablets (30 mg) q6h prn with liquid; or 1 teaspoon of elixir q6h prn; or 20 drops of solution q6h prn. The recommended dosage in children is ½ the adult dosage based on weight.

ADVERSE EFFECTS

Gastrointestinal irritation, thyroid enlargement, and acute parotitis are noted side effects with iodinated glycerol. This medication is contraindicated in pregnancy and during lactation. We urge extra caution in its usage until more information is available.

20. McCarty, J. M., and Renteria, A. Treatment of pharyngitis and tonsillitis with cefprozil: Review of three multicenter trials. *Clin. Infect. Dis.* 14:S224–S230, 1992.

21. Nolen, T. M. Clinical trials of cefprozil for treatment of skin and skin-structure infections. *Clin. Infect. Dis.* 14:S255–S263, 1992.

22. *Physician's Desk Reference for Nonprescription Drugs.* Montvale, N.J.: Medical Economics Data, 1992.

23. Pomerleau, O. F. Nicotine on the central nervous system: Biobehavioral effects of cigarette smoking. *Am. J. Med.* 93(Suppl. 1A):2–7, 1992.

24. Robson, R. A. The effects of quinolones on xanthine pharmacokinetics. *Am. J. Med.* 92 (Suppl. 4A):108–113, 1992.

25. Schleupner, C. J., et al. Blinded comparison of cefuroxime to cefaclor for lower respiratory tract infections. *Arch. Intern. Med.* 148:343–348, 1988.

26. Shrestha, M., et al. Decreased duration of emergency department treatment of chronic obstructive pulmonary disease with the addition of ipratropium bromide to beta-agonist therapy. *Ann. Emerg. Med.* 20:1206–1209, 1991.

27. Shyu, W. C., et al. Pharmacokinetics of cefprozil in healthy subjects and patients with hepatic impairment. *J. Clin. Pharmacol.* 31:372–376, 1991.

28. Spagnolo, S. V., and Medinger, A. E. *A Handbook of Pulmonary Emergencies.* New York: Plenum, 1986.

29. Sturani, C., et al. Oral nifedipine in chronic cor pulmonale secondary to severe chronic obstructive pulmonary disease — short and long term hemodynamic effects. *Chest* 84:135–142, 1983.

30. Tenholder, M. F., et al. A model for conversion from small volume nebulizer to meter dose inhaler aerosol therapy. *Chest* 101:634–637, 1992.

31. Transdermal Nicotine Study Group. Transdermal nicotine for smoking cessation. *JAMA* 266:3133–3138, 1991.

32. Wise, R., and Lockley, M. J. The pharmacokinetics of ofloxacin and a review of its tissue penetration. *Antimicrob. Chemother.* 22(Suppl. C):59–64, 1988.

3

Pneumonia

Infections of the Lung: Overview and General Considerations

Philip Witorsch

Infection of the lung parenchyma pneumonia, can be caused by various microorganisms, including bacteria of different types (gram-positive, gram-negative, aerobic, anaerobic), mycobacteria, mycoplasma, chlamydia, and numerous viruses, as well as protozoans and other parasites. The likelihood of one or another etiologic agent as the cause of pneumonia will be influenced to some extent by the location of the patient in the community versus in the hospital and the patient's underlying state of health, particularly the presence or absence of certain risk factors. Risk factors that may be associated with pneumonia caused by certain organisms include advanced age, cardiac disease, alcoholism, diabetes mellitus, mechanical ventilation, chronic obstructive pulmonary disease (COPD), certain immune defects, and particular therapies. These associations may be helpful when taken together with other information, such as clinical features, radiographic findings, other initial laboratory studies, and preliminary microbiologic determinations — such as smears — in directing initial antimicrobial therapy pending definitive identification of the infecting organism(s).

Thus, community-acquired pneumonia in otherwise generally healthy individuals is commonly caused by viral agents, pneumococcus, Mycoplasma, or Legionella. Alcoholics and insulin-dependent diabetics appear to be particularly prone to infection with *Klebsiella pneumoniae;* alcoholics are also especially likely to develop anaerobic infections, including lung abscess.

Bacterial pneumonia following immediately on the heels of viral influenza is commonly due to infection with pneumococcus, *Haemophilus influenzae,* or *Staphylococcus aureus*. The most common cause of pneumonia in patients with AIDS is Pneumocystis carinii; such patients are also at greatly increased risk of infection with *Mycobacterium tuberculosis* or *M. avium-intracellulare,* as well as cytomegalovirus and certain fungi, especially cryptococcus. Patients with underlying COPD appear to have an increased risk of pneumonia due to pneumococcus, *H. influenzae* and *Moraxella catarrhalis*. Immunocompromised patients with abnormal T-lymphocyte function have an increased risk of pneumonia due to cryptococcus, pneumocystis, toxoplasma, cytomegalovirus, mycobacteria, and legionella, among other organisms. On the other hand, patients who have abnormal B-lymphocyte function or who have had a splenectomy appear to be at greater risk of infection by encapsulated bacteria, such as *Streptococcus pneumoniae* and *H. influenzae,* among others. Prolonged use of corticosteroids predisposes patients to a variety of infections, including pneumonia due to fungi, parasites — such as pneumocystis — and a variety of bacteria, including gram-negative bacilli.

Hospital-acquired pneumonias are commonly caused by gram-negative bacilli, particularly in patients who have been on antimicrobials, receiving mechanical ventilation, or have tracheostomies, especially when such patients are in intensive care units.

Appropriate antimicrobial therapy depends on the specific infecting pathogen(s). Definitive identification of the infecting organisms, however, may require several days and, thus, therapy must be empiric and directed against the most likely pathogen(s) pending specific identification, especially in patients in whom any delay in therapy would be hazardous. In such a setting, the best estimate is based on all of the available data including clinical findings, x-ray findings, results of smears and other quick microbiologic determinations, other laboratory studies, knowledge regarding the patient's preexisting, underlying medical conditions and medications, and recognition of the setting in which the infection occurs. The decision is very much individualized and will depend on a variety of the foregoing factors, as well as considerations of relative efficacy and toxicity of various drugs.

Pneumonias may be complicated by other conditions that affect the response to antimicrobial therapy, may require the use of ancillary measures and may alter the prognosis. These complications include: pleural effusion, including parapneumonic effusion and empyema; bronchial obstruction with atelectasis; respiratory failure, including adult respiratory distress syndrome (ARDS); and necrosis with abscess formation.

Parapneumonic effusion and empyema are discussed in detail in Chapter 5. Both conditions may cause persistence of fever in spite of appropriate antimicrobial therapy, both require thoracentesis for diagnosis, and empyema requires drainage for definitive treatment.

Necrosis with abscess formation is also discussed in detail under anaerobic lung infections. Commonly associated organisms include anaerobic bacteria, staphylococci, and gram-negative enteric bacilli. Treatment usually requires definitive and prolonged antimicrobial therapy and often may necessitate bronchoscopy, both for diagnosis of bronchial obstruction and treatment.

Significant atelectasis (i.e., lobar or greater) may occur with or without bronchial obstruction. Bronchial obstruction may be the result of a foreign body, a tumor, or inspissated secretions. Bronchoscopy is often necessary for diagnosis and therapy, although occasionally vigorous chest physical therapy alone will result in improvement when the atelectasis is solely the result of secretions.

When respiratory failure complicates pneumonia, it necessitates the administration of supplementary oxygen and, in many cases, requires endotracheal intubation and assisted mechanical ventilation. When respiratory failure is the result of ARDS complicating pneumonia, additional therapy usually includes the implementation of positive end-expiratory pressure, as well as very careful fluid management.

Two other complications that may develop are not a direct result of the infection per se but rather a result of the treatment: drug reactions and fluid overload. The former, including fever, skin rash, liver toxicity, hematologic toxicity, and renal toxicity related to the antimicrobial agents being administered should always be kept in mind when such problems develop. Large volumes of fluid is sometimes necessary for the administration of IV antimicrobials. Additionally, some antimicrobials that are administered as a sodium salt entail the administration of large amounts of sodium. These factors should be kept in mind in patients with marginal cardiac reserve who may be at particular risk for such complications.

Gram-Positive Pneumonias

John A. Michos
Samuel V. Spagnolo

Streptococcus Pneumoniae

Streptococcus pneumoniae is a nonmotile, nonsporulating, encapsulated gram-positive organism which may cause pneumonia as well as bacteremia with seeding of the pleural space and CSF in the susceptible host. *S. pneumoniae* are aerobic, facultatively anaerobic, and produce alpha hemolysis on blood agar. Only the capsulated or smooth form is virulent. More than 83 different types have been speciated based on unique capsular polysaccharides. The Danish system of typing serotypes is based on antigenic similarities of the capsular polysaccharides (e.g., Danish group 9 includes 9N and 9V, which are antigenically similar), while the American system of typing is based on sequence of discovery (lower-numbered serotypes were usually the most virulent and earliest to be discovered). Most common serotypes implicated in disease are types 3, 4, 14, and 19; while the most common types to cause epidemic pneumonia or bacteremia in the setting of pneumonia are types, 1, 2, 3, 5, and 8. *S. pneumoniae* is the leading cause of pneumonia in non-hospitalized patients with between one half and three quarters of patients hospitalized for this disease.

TRANSMISSION

S. pneumoniae is isolated from the upper respiratory tract of as many as 60% of normal persons. Carriage of the microorganism varies with the season (maximal October-April in the Northern hemisphere) and with close cohabitation. Pneumonia results from either inhalation of organisms in crowded or poorly ventilated regions or from aspiration of secretions from the oropharynx. There are approximately 150,000–570,000 cases per year in the United States, with an incidence of 68–260 cases per 100,000. The attack rate is highest in the population 30–50 year-age group, but serious infection is most prevalent in the extremes of life. The incidence of pneumococcal pneumonia is increased in patients with impaired humural immunity and in patients with altered mechanisms of clearance such as chronic obstructive pulmonary disease (COPD) and bronchitis. The incidence of pneumococcal bacteremia in patients with AIDS is 200-fold greater than that of the young adult population at large. Thus, patients with AIDS, COPD, bronchitis, malignancy, splenic dysfunction, cirrhosis, multiple myeloma, hypogammaglobulinemia, nephrotic syndrome, ethanol abuse, congestive heart failure, diabetes, and liver or kidney disease are at increased risk for infection.

PRESENTATION

Pneumococcal pneumonia is classically described as a sudden single shaking chill followed by fever to 39°–41°C, pleuritic chest pain, and productive cough. This classic description may typify the presentation in the young, healthy adult; at the extremes of age, these symptoms are attenuated. In patients with COPD, an increase in cough or change in color and sputum production may herald the onset of disease. A more abrupt presentation is seen in patients following splenectomy in whom rapid bacteremia and death may occur secondary to an impaired humoral immunity. Absence of fever, hypothermia, white blood cell count less than 4,000, hypotension, and PO_2 less than 50 mm Hg portend a poor prognosis. The physical examination may be significant for fever, while examination of the lung may reveal E to A changes, dullness to percussion, bronchial breath sounds, as well as splinting with decreased respiratory excursions of the chest wall. New murmurs may indicate endocarditis. Mental confusion raises the suspicion of meningitis. Radiographic findings are typically significiant for a segmental lobar or multilobar presentation, with 20% of patients presenting with a pleural effusion. Laboratory findings generally reveal a leukocytosis, and sputum Gram's stain is significant for numerous WBC's with ovoid gram-positive cocci in diploids or short chains.

TREATMENT

Penicillin

Penicillins are the agents of choice in the treatment of pneumococcal pneumonia. Discovered by Fleming in 1928 and tried therapeutically in 1943, penicillin consists of a thiazolidine ring connected to a beta-lactam ring to which a side chain is attached. The nucleus is the source of antibacterial activity; the side chain determines many of the pharmacologic and antibacterial characteristics of each particular type of penicillin.

MECHANISM OF ACTION AND PHARMACOKINETICS

Bacterial cell walls are composed of peptidoglycans, which are heteropolymers that confer mechanical stability. In gram-positives, the cell wall is 50–100 molecules thick but is only one or two molecules thick in gram-negative bacteria. Penicillins act not only by inhibiting transpeptidases involved in the synthesis of cell walls but also by binding to other proteins needed to maintain cell integrity. The proteins affected by penicillins are termed penicillin-binding proteins (PBP).

Oral administration of penicillin (PCN) G results in one third of the drug absorbed by the GI tract with maximal serum concentration attained 30–60 minutes after ingestion. A pH less than 2.0 destroys the antimicrobial and ingestion of food interferes with its absorption. Thus, tablets should be ingested 30 minutes before a meal or 2 hours after. Oral PCN V has similar properties to PCN G except for better stability in acidic media.

Parenteral administration of PCN G through the IM route achieves peak concentrations 15–30 minutes after injection. Volume of distribution is approximately 0.35 liters/kg, while 60% of PCN G is reversibly bound to albumin.

Excretion is mainly from the kidneys; while anuria increases the half-life from 30 minutes to 10 hours.

MECHANISMS OF RESISTANCE

Resistance to penicillin occurs through either one of three mechanisms: (1) production of beta lactamases, (2) mutation of sites in PBP's, and (3) inability to penetrate to its site of action. Pneumococcal pneumonias highly resistant to PCN's (MIC 2.0 mg/ml) have been reported at an incidence of less than 1%. These resistant strains have been reported in a number of European countries and have also been proved to be resistant to chloramphenicol, erythromycin, and clindamycin, but sensitive to vancomycin.

ADVERSE REACTIONS

The overall incidence of adverse reactions to penicillins is estimated at 0.7–10%. The most common cause of drug reaction is a hypersensitivity reaction, which has ranged in order of decreasing frequency from a maculopapular rash to fever, dermatitis, and anaphylaxis. Long-term use of the semi-synthetic penicillins (2 weeks or greater) has also been known to cause neutropenia, believed to be either secondary to a hypersensitivity reaction or a toxic dose–related suppression of white blood cell precursors.

Penicillin G & V

CLINICAL INDICATIONS

Penicillin G (Penicillin G Potassium) and Penicillin V (Betapen-VK, Ledercillin VK, Pen-Vee K, Penicillin V Potassium, Veetids) are highly active against gram-positive cocci such as pneumococcus. They are readily hydrolyzed by penicillinase and are ineffective against most strains of *Staphylococcccus aureus*. Pneumococci of all serologic types are, in general, highly susceptible to PCN G and V.

PREPARATIONS AND DOSAGES

Oral Preparations

Penicillin G Potassium tablets are available in 125 mg, 250 mg, and 500 mg strengths.

Penicillin V Potassium tablets are available in 250 mg and 500 mg strengths. Each 250 mg tablet is equivalent to 400,000 units of PCN

V or G. Each 500 mg tablet is equivalent to 800,000 units of PCN V or G.

Penicillin G and V Potassium solutions are available from reconstituted powder forms. Penicillin G Potassium syrup and Penicillin V Potassium solutions are available at dosages of 125 mg/5 cc and 250 mg/5 cc. Both Penicillin G and V Potassium solutions must be kept refrigerated.

Therapy for children under 12 years of age who are able to swallow tablets is 15–56 mg/kg/day. For mild to moderately severe pneumococcal infections 250–500 mg PO qid is the recommended adult dosage.

Aqueous Solution

PCN G IV may be infused at a rate of 6–20 million units/day in 4–6 divided doses (1 million units of PCN G K^+ is equivalent to 1.7 milliequivalents K^+).

PCN G procaine and Penicillin G benzathine suspension

Bicillin, Wycillin, are available for IM injection and supply 300,000 units per cc of PCN G (150,000 units PCN G benzathine and 150,000 units PCN G procaine). This is supplied in multiple dose vials of 10 cc. In pneumococcal infections (except pneumococcal meningitis) approximately 600,000 to 1.2 million units IM every day should be given until the temperature is normal for at least 48 hours, then switching to PO and completing a 7–10 day course. However, in severe infections, IV penicillin is recommended.

Semisynthetic Penicillins

The semisynthetic penicillins were developed from *Penicillum chrysogenum* cultures depleted of their side chain precursors. Thus, side chains could be added which alter the antimicrobial activity and pharmacologic properties of the drug as well as alter the compound to inactivating enzymes such as beta lactams.

Ampicillin

CLINICAL INDICATIONS

Ampicillin (Ampicillin capsule; Omnipen suspension, Polycillin) is a semisynthetic penicillin which extended the coverage of the penicillins to include gram-negatives such as *H. influenzae, Escherichia coli, Proteus,* as well as including pneumococcus in its spectrum of coverage. Ampicillin, however, is rapidly destroyed by beta lactamases and is, thus, not recommended for beta lactam-producing strains of *Haemophilus influenzae.* It offers no advantage over penicillin in the treatment of *S. pneumoniae* pneumonia.

Ampicillin is well absorbed after oral administration. A dose of 500 mg peaks at 3 μg/ml after 2 hours. It is stable in acidic media but is affected by meals. Clearance of the drug is through renal as well as enterohepatic mechanisms. Adjustment of dosage is needed in renal dysfunction.

DOSAGE AND ADMINISTRATION

Ampicillin is available in 250 mg and 500 mg strength tablets. Ampicillin oral suspension is available in 125 mg and 250 mg suspension per 5 cc. For respiratory infections, the usual dosage is 250 mg PO qid, while for more severe infections 6–12 grams IV per day is recommended.

Beta Lactam–Binding Antibiotics

Augmentin and Timentin are agents with a beta lactam structure that contains substrates that can bind to beta lactamases and inactivate them, thus enabling the beta lactam antimicrobial to bind to cell wall proteins. An example of a beta lactam binder is clavulanic acid. It is well absorbed by mouth, can be given parenterally, and when combined with amoxicillin or ticarcillin is known as Augmentin or Timentin, respectively.

Amoxicillin-Clavulanic Acid

CLINICAL INDICATIONS

Amoxicillin-clavulanic acid (Augmentin) is effective for pneumococcus as well as for beta lactam–producing strains of *staphylococcus, H. influenzae,* and *gonococci.* Augmentin's pharmacologic properties are similar to ampicillin except that it is less affected by food and is more rapidly absorbed from the GI tract. Augmentin is recommended over Penicillin G or V if beta lactam–producing *H. influenzae* is a supected agent of pneumonia. Amoxicillin-clavulanic acids wholesale cost at the lowest usual recommended dosage for 10 days of treatment is approximately $50.00 while the wholesale cost for generic Penicillin V is about $2.00 for a 10-day course. Thus, if pneumococcus is isolated, PCN V or G is recommended, given the wide discrepancy in cost.

DOSAGE AND ADMINISTRATION

The usual dosage of amoxicillin-clavulanic acid is 0.75–1.5 g/day in 3 divided doses (oral). Augmentin is available in 250 mg and 500 mg tablets. Each 250 mg contains 250 mg of amoxicillin and 125 mg of clavulanic acid. Augmentin oral suspension is also available in 125 mg and 250 mg per 5 cc solution. Augmentin 500 mg PO tid is recommended for serious infections of the respiratory tract.

Ticarcillin-Clavulanic Acid

Ticarcillin-clavulanic acid (Timentin) is effective for aerobic gram-negative bacilli and staphylococcus. Timentin is generally used IV for pseudomonal infections at a dosage of 200–300 mg/kg in 4–6 divided portions. However, in the treatment of severe pneumococcal infections, IV penicillin is the preferred agent.

Prevention of Pneumococcal Pneumonia: Pneumococcal Vaccine

The pneumococcal vaccine (Pneumovax 23; Pnu-Immune 23) has been a controversial area of study in its use for reducing the incidence of pneumococcal disease. From the first three serotype preparations administered by Lister up to the early field trials in South African gold, diamond, and copper miners, the incidence of pneumococcal pneumonia was found to decrease with its use. However, in patients who are immunocompromised or hosts who have chronic disease, the ability to mount an adequate antibody response to the vaccine is less than adequate.

The current pneumococcal vaccine contains 23 serotypes of which 25 μg of each polysaccharide antigen is injected. The 23 valent dosage compromises 88% of all the virulent strains causing pneumococcal disease in the United States. The vaccine was initially licensed in 1977 as a 14 valent vaccine, but now includes Danish types 1, 2, 3, 4, 5, 6B, 7F, 8, 9N, 9V, 10A, 11A, 12F, 14, 15B, 17F, 18C, 19F, 19A, 20, 22F, 23F, and 33F.

RECOMMENDATIONS FOR USE

1. Immunocompetent adults at increased risk of pneumococcal infection because of chronic illness such as coronary artery disease, COPD, diabetes mellitus, alcohol abuse, cirrhosis, or age greater than 65 years.
2. Immunocompromised adults such as patients with malignancy, multiple myeloma, HIV disease, chronic renal failure, splenic dysfunction, or nephrotic syndrome.
3. Persons living in crowded or poorly ventilated rooms at high risk for pneumococcal disease.

ADMINISTRATION

The pneumococcal vaccine is given IM and is generally well tolerated. Humoral antibody response is generally 2–3 weeks; thus, the vaccine should be given 2 weeks before splenectomy and in anyone about to receive immunosuppression, as in chemotherapy. Safety in pregnant women has not been evaluated, altough women at high risk of pneumococcal disease should ideally be vaccinated before pregnancy. Revaccination should be considered in patients who received the vaccine more than 6 years ago and who are in high-risk situations. Revaccination with the 23 valent vaccine should be strongly considered for persons who received the 14 valent vaccine and who are at highest risk for fatal pneumococcal infection (e.g., asplenic patients). The pneumococcal vaccine can be given at the same time as the influenza vaccine using different injection sites without increasing side effects. The pneumococcal vaccine should be delayed in patients having febrile illness or other active infection. As mentioned earlier, the pneumococcal vaccine is a long-term vaccination with revaccination occurring only under special circumstances.

ADVERSE REACTIONS

Erythema and pain occur in 50% of patients at site of injection. Severe systemic reactions such as anaphylaxis are less than 1%.

Staphylococcus Aureus Pneumonia

S. aureus is responsible for most cases of staphylococcal disease in humans. Staphylococci are nonspore-forming, nonmotile, gram-positive cocci. They are characteristically grouped in clusters, and some may possess distinct capsules. On blood agar, *S. aureus* produces beta hemolysis. *Staphylococcal pneumoniae* tends to occur in one of three settings: (1) among hospitalized patients, (2) in IV drug abusers who inject unsterile material into their veins; and (3) following epidemic influenza. About 33% of healthy adults are colonized by *S. aureus* and transmission to lower airways in presumed to be secondary to microaspiration of colonized secretions.

PRESENTATION

Staphylococcal pneumoniae is heralded by high fevers, shaking chills, and purulent secretions. Hematogenous staphylococcal pneumonia may manifest by rapidly cavitating small nodules, while *nosocomial staphylococcus pneumoniae* may present as an ill-defined infiltrate with fever, chills, and leukocytosis. Diagnosis is established by culturing sputum, blood, and pleural fluid, while Gram's stain of sputum showing many WBC's with gram-positive cocci in clusters is suggestive of the disease.

TREATMENT

Most isolates of *S. aureus* are resistant to penicillins. Thus, initial treatment should be with a penicillinase-resistant drug such as nafcillin or an antibiotic such as vancomycin if penicillin allergy is suspected. However, if antibiotic susceptibility tests demonstrate that the organism is sensitive to penicillin, use of this agent is preferable since it is the most convenient and inexpensive to administer.

Nafcillin

PHARMACOKINETICS AND USAGE

Nafcillin (Nafcil, Nafcillin, Unipen) is indicated for penicillinase-producing *S. aureus*. It is inactivated by an acidic medium and is, thus, given in IV form. Ninety percent of the drug is bound to plasma protein. Doses for *S. aureus* pneumoniae range from 6–12 g IV q4h in divided doses. Adverse reactions are similar to the other penicillins and range from a rash to as severe as anaphylaxis. Decreased prothrombin times have also been reported in patients treated with warfarin and nafcillin, thus requiring close observation of coagulation times in patients requiring anticoagulation.

Vancomycin

CLINICAL INDICATIONS

Vancomycin (Vancomycin, Vancocin) is a tricyclic glycopeptide with a molecular weight of 1500. It is active against gram-positive bacteria including strains of methicillin-resistant *S. aureus* (MRSA). Synergism between vancomycin with an aminoglycoside has also been demonstrated in vivo against *S. aureus* and MRSA. Use is primarily for MRSA pneumonia, empyema, as well as in patients allergic to pencillins or cephalosporins.

MECHANISM OF ACTION

Vancomycin inhibits the synthesis of cell wall production by binding with high affinity to the D-alanyl-D-alanine portion of the cell wall precursor units.

RESISTANCE

Resistance to vancomycin as shown by enterococci is presumed to be secondary to expression of a unique cytoplasmic protein which reduces access of the antimicrobial to its source of action.

DISTRIBUTION

Vancomycin is poorly absorbed orally. A 1-g IV infusion produces plasma concentrations of 15–30 mg/ml within approximately 1 hour after infusion. The half-life is approximately 6 hours and 30% of the drug is bound to plasma protein. Ninety percent is excreted by glomerular filtration.

DOSAGES AND ADMINISTRATION

Vancomycin must be given IV over at least a 60 minute period. The dosage will vary from 500 mg IV q6h to 1 g IV q12h depending on the renal status of the patients. Anephric patients on dialysis should receive 1 g IV once per week.

ADVERSE REACTIONS

Adverse reactions have ranged from hypersensitivity reactions, such as rash and anaphylaxis to chills, fever, and a shocklike state termed red-man syndrome (rapid IV infusion–causing histamine release). Ototoxicity and nephrotoxicity can occur when concentrations are high (80–100 μg/ml); thus, caution should be used in conjunction with other agents such as the aminoglycosides with vancomycin peak and trough levels monitored closed.

References

PNEUMOCOCCAL VACCINE

1. Gable, C., et al. Pneumococcal vaccine, efficacy and associated cost savings. *JAMA* 264: 2910–2915, 1990.
2. Hager H., and Woolley, T. Review of recent pneumococcal infections with attention to vaccine and nonvaccine serotypes. *Rev. Infect. Dis.,* 12 (2): 267–272, 1990.
3. Jorgensen J. et al. Serotypes of respiratory isolates of streptococcus pneumoniae compared with the capsular types included in the current pneumococcal vaccine. *Journal of Infectious Diseases*. 163:644–646, 1991.
4. MMWR. Recommendations of the immunization practices advisory committee pneumococcal polysaccharide vaccine. *JAMA,* 261: 1265–1267, 1989.
5. Musher, D., et al. Pneumococcal vaccination: Work to date and future prospects. *Am. J. Med. Sci.* 300: 45–52, 1974.

STREPTOCOCCUS PNEUMONIAE

1. The Medical Letter, Vol. 34 (Issue 879), September 18, 1992 pp. 87–90.
2. Mufson, M. A. Pneumococcal infections. *JAMA,* 246: 1942–1948, 1981.
3. Musher, D. Infections caused by streptococcus pneumoniae: Clinical spectrum, pathogenesis, immunity, and treatment. *Clinic. Infect. Dis.,* 14: 801–809, 1992.
4. Pesola, G., and Charles, A. Pneumococcal bacteremia with pneumonia: Mortality in acquired immunodeficiency syndrome. *Chest,* 101: 150–154, 1992.
5. Walbroehl, G. S. Antibiotic-associated neutropenia. *Am. Fam. Physician,* 45: 2237–2241, 1992.

STAPHYLOCOCCUS PNEUMONIAE

1. Goodman, L. and Gillman, A. *The Pharmacological Basis of Therapeutics.* (8th ed.). New York: Pergamon Press, Inc., 1990.
2. Mandell, G. C., et al. *Principle and Practice of Infectious Diseases* (3d ed.). New York: Churchill Livingstone, 1990.
3. Peacock, J. E., et al. Methicillin-resistant staphylococcus aureus: Introduction and Spread within a Hospital. *Ann. Intern. Med.* 93:526–532, 1980.
4. Shovick, V. A. Re-created hypothrombinemic response to warfarin

secondary to the warfarin-nafcillin interaction. *DICP,* 25: 598–600, 1991.

5. Weinstein, A. Diagnosis and treatment of staphylococcal infections. *Hospital Medicine,* 11: 8–9, 1975.
6. Wise, R. Z. Modern management of severe staphylococcal disease. *Medicine,* 52(4): 295–304, 1973.

Gram-Negative Pneumonias

Jonathan G. W. Evans
Samuel V. Spagnolo

Many childhood bacterial infections are due to *Haemophilus influenzae,* and among adults, its increasing prevalence has made it a common cause of pneumonia in hospitalized patients. While *Klebsiella pneumoniae* (family Enterobacteriaceae) is the most common of all the gram-negative bacillary pneumonias, *Pseudomonas aeruginosa* is the most commonly acquired nosocomial pneumonia. Other common but less frequently encountered organisms are from the family Enterobacteriaceae, including *Escherichia, Proteus, Serratia, Enterobacter, Morganella, Providencia, Salmonella, Citrobacter, Erwina,* and *Hafnia.* These infections may be acquired in the community or nosocomially, and of these *Escherichia coli* is the bacterium most frequently encountered in the community.

Haemophilus influenzae Pneumonia

The clinical presentation of *Haemophilus* pneumonia is very much like that of other acute bacterial pneumonias, with bronchopneumonia (without bacteremia) typical. It may be preceded by upper respiratory tract infection followed by development of fever, dyspnea, and cough production of purulent sputum. Presentation may be subacute, with symptoms persisting for weeks prior to diagnosis.

The laboratory findings include leukocytosis in 75% of patients (generally 10,000–15,000 cells/mm^3), although leukopenia is occasionally seen in children and is associated with multilobar bronchopneumonia in 75% of cases to lobar consolidation in 38%. Parapneumonic effusions are common but are usually small and rarely progress to empyema or cavitation. The clinical course varies depending on other underlying disease.

Antimicrobial therapy has been changing with the emergence of beta-lactamase strains of *H. influenzae* (ampicillin resistance was documented in 50% of the isolates recovered from patients with chronic bronchitis in one study). As a result, cefuroxime, cefotaxime, or ceftazidime is recommended in serious cases of pneumonia, until sensitivities of the organism are known.

Cefuroxime

MECHANISM OF ACTION

Cefuroxime is a broad-spectrum second-generation semisynthetic cephalosporin. Cefuroxime axetil is administered orally; cefuroxime sodium is administered IV or IM. Its bactericidal action results from inhibition of cell wall synthesis. It is beta-lactamase stable and is active against numerous gram-negative organisms.

PHARMACOKINETICS

With PO, IM, or IV administration, the serum half-life is approximately 80 minutes. With concomitant oral probenecid administration, half-life is increased by 30%.

INDICATIONS

Cefuroxime sodium is one of the antimicrobials of choice for severe *H. influenzae* pneumonia. The minimum inhibitor concentration (MIC) 90 of cefuroxime for *H. influenzae* is 0.1–2 μg/ml. It is also indicated for treatment of pneumonias caused by *Streptococcus pneumoniae, Staphylococcus aureus* (penicillinase and nonpenicillinase producing), *Streptococcus pyogenes, Klebsiella* species, and *E. coli*. For less severe pneumonia or bronchitis, cefuroxime axetil (250 or 500 mg bid) is as effective as cefaclor (500 mg tid) or amoxicillin (500 mg bid).

Because cefuroxime is active against most strains of *H. influenzae* (ampicillin-resistant strains as well as most *Staphylococcus* and *Streptococcus* strains), it is thought by some that it can be used as initial empiric parenteral treatment in children and adults for pneumonia (rather than a combination therapy with penicillin and chloramphenicol). In vitro data indicate that the activity of cefuroxime and aminoglycosides may be synergistic in the treatment of Enterobacter, *E. coli, Klebsiella, Proteus mirabilis* and *Serratia marcescens*.

SIDE EFFECTS AND CONTRAINDICATIONS

Cefuroxime is contraindicated in patients with known hypersensitivity to cephalosoporin. Side effects include phlebitis (2%), rash (1%), positive Coombs (1%), decreased hematocrit (10%), eosinophilia (7%), and neutrophilia (1%). Liver effects include increased aspartate aminotransferase (4%), lactic dehydrogenase (1.5%) and alkaline phosphatase (2%).

DOSAGE AND ADMINISTRATION

The route and administration is PO, IM, or IV. Tablets of 250 mg and 500 mg are available. Adult oral dosage (cefuroxime axetil) is 250 mg q12h but may be increased to 500 mg q12h for more severe infections. The adult IM and IV dosage (cefuroxime sodium) is 750 mg–1.5 g q8h for 5–10 days depending on the severity of the infection. For severe infections, 1.5 g q6h may be needed. Reduced dosage is required when renal function is impaired. The cefuroxime axetil oral dosage for children is 125 mg bid for under age 2 years, and 250 mg bid up to age 12 years. Cefuroxime sodium dosing for infants and children over 3 months is 50–100 mg/kg/day (in equally divided doses 3–4 times/day), depending on the severity of the infection.

Cefotaxime

MECHANISM OF ACTION

Cefotaxime is a semisynthetic third-generation cephalosporin available only for parenteral administration. Its bacterial action results from inhibition of cell wall synthesis. It is beta-lactamase stable and has activity against a wide range of gram-negative organisms.

PHARMACOKINETICS

Cefotaxime has an elimination half-life of 1 hour. Sixty percent of a given dose can be found in urine during the first 6 hours following an infection; 20–36% of a given IV dose is renally excreted as unchanged and 15–25% as the desacetyl derivative, the major metabolite. This metabolite participates in this drug's bactericidal activity.

INDICATIONS

It is also an antimicrobial choice for severe *H. influenzae* pneumonia (as is cefuroxime and ceftazidime). The MIC 90 of cefotaxime reported for *H. influenzae* is 0.01–0.8 μg/ml. Additionally, it is indicated for pneumonias caused by *S. pneumoniae, S. pyogenes, S. aureus* (penicillinase and nonpenicillinase producing), *E. coli, Klebsiella* species, indole-positive *Proteus,* and *Pseudomonas* species. In combination with an aminoglycoside, cefotaxime has occasionally been found to be synergistic.

SIDE EFFECTS AND CONTRAINDICATIONS

Cefotaxime is contraindicated in patients who have proved hypersensitivity to cefotaxime or cephalosporins in general. Side effects include pain on IM injection (33%), phlebitis (3–10%), and hypersensitivity, including rash (2%), eosinophils (8%), hematologic (positive Coombs) (5%), and elevation of hepatic transaminases in 15%.

DOSAGE AND ADMINISTRATION

Cefotaxime may be administered IM or IV after reconstitution. Dosage route should be decided on severity of infection.

Children

Neonates age 0–1 week: 50 mg/kg q12h.
Neonates age 0–4 weeks: 50 mg/kg q8h.

1 month–12 years of age: daily dosage, 50–180 mg/kg, divided into 4–6 equal doses.

Adults

Recommended dosage is 1 g q8h up to 2 g q4h for severe infections. One gram q8h is sufficient for uncomplicated pneumonias of moderate severity such as *H. influenzae, K. pneumoniae,* and *E. coli* (nonpseudomonal pneumonias).

Ceftazidime

MECHANISM OF ACTION

Ceftazidime is a broad-spectrum, third-generation, semisynthetic, parenteral cephalosporin. Its bactericidal action results from inhibiting the enzymes that synthesize bacterial cell walls. It is active against many strains resistant to other cephalosporins (and to ampicillin) because it is beta-lactamase stable.

PHARMACOKINETICS

Eighty to ninety percent is excreted unchanged by the kidneys within 24 hours. The absorption and elimination rates are directly proportional to the size of the dosage. The half-life is significantly lengthened in patients with impaired renal function.

INDICATIONS

It is effective in the treatment of acute pneumonia caused by *Pseudomonas* sp., *Klebsiella* sp., *Enterobacter* sp., *Citrobacter* sp., *Serratia* sp., *H. influenzae* (including ampicillin-resistant strains), *S. pneumoniae,* and *S. aureus* (methicillin-susceptible strains). The MIC 90 of the drug for *H. influenzae* is 0.1–1 μg/ml. Concomitant use of ceftazidime and an aminoglycoside is synergistic against some strains of Enterobacteriaceae and *P. aeruginosa*. Nevertheless, studies have found ceftazidime alone to be as effective in the treatment of adult pneumonia caused by *Enterobacteriaceae* as combination therapy with an aminoglycoside and (another) cephalosporin or an aminoglycoside and an extended-spectrum penicillin.

It has also been found effective when used alone or in conjunction with an aminoglycoside for the treatment of bronchopulmonary *P. aeruginosa* infections in children, and adults with cystic fibrosis. However, treatment failures have been reported because of superinfection with resistant strains during therapy. Although ceftazidime is more active against *P. aeruginosa* than other cephalosporins, it has been found ineffective in reducing sputum colony counts of *Pseudomonas cepacia* in patients with cystic fibrosis.

SIDE EFFECTS AND CONTRAINDICATIONS

Ceftazidime is contraindicated in patients with known allergy to the drug. Side effects include phlebitis (1.5%), hypersensitivity rash (1.3%), eosinophilia (7%), and fever (0.4%). Hematologic side effects include positive Coombs (4%), neutropenia (1%), and thrombocytosis (2%). Other side effects include elevation of SGOT (6%) elevation of BUN (0.6%). Suprainfection with enterococci occurs in 3%.

DOSAGE AND ADMINISTRATION

Dosage by IM or IV administration is 1 g q8–12h. Route of administration is based on severity of infection and renal function of the patient. Dosage should be reduced when renal function is impaired.

Ciprofloxacin

MECHANISM OF ACTION

Ciprofloxacin is a broad-spectrum fluoroquinolone for oral and IV use. It demonstrates activity against many aerobic gram-negative bacteria. It is bactericidal due to inhibition of bacterial DNA gyrase (topoisomerase 11), an enzyme involved in DNA replication.

PHARMACOKINETICS

The half-life for IV ciprofloxacin is 5–6 hours, and 50–70% is excreted in the urine as unchanged drug. In patients with reduced renal function, slight dosage decrements may be required. Ciprofloxacin tablets are well absorbed from the GI tract, have a half-life of 4 hours, and are eliminated by the same route as IV ciprofloxacin.

INDICATIONS

Ciprofloxacin (IV and PO) is recommended for the treatment of upper and lower respiratory tract infections and is active against *S. pneumoniae,* beta-lactamase positive and negative *H. influenzae* (MIC 90 is 0.008–0.05 μg/ml), *Haemophilus parainfluenzae, Klebsiella pneumoniae, E. coli, Enterobacter cloacae, P. mirabilis,* and *P. aeruginosa.* It has been found to be active even when some organisms were resistant to penicillins. In controlled studies, oral ciprofloxacin was as effective as parenteral regimens using cephalosporins and aminoglycosides, azlocillin, and gentamicin (or tobramycin) for short-term, non-life-threatening treatment of acute exacerbations of *P. aeruginosa* infections in cystic fibrosis patients. However, resistant strains of *P. aeruginosa* have developed during treatment in cystic fibrosis patients, and relying solely on oral ciprofloxacin for treatment as a single agent in these patients is not recommended.

SIDE EFFECTS AND CONTRAINDICATIONS

This agent is contraindicated in individuals with known hypersensitivity to ciprofloxacin or any of the quinolone antibiotics and should not be used during pregnancy and breast-feeding. Side effects include CNS stimulation (insomnia, restlessness, dizziness). It interferes with theophylline metabolism (theophylline levels increase) and metabolism of caffeine (increases caffeine levels), causing increased CNS stimulation. Other side effects include crystalluria (rare) at higher dosages (750 mg twice a day), elevations of transamingses, nausea, vomiting, and diarrhea. Dosages should be decreased by 50% in patients with impaired renal function (creatinine clearance less than 50 ml/minute), and the dosing intervals should be increased to 18 hours in patients with creatinine clearance less than 30 ml/minute.

DOSAGE AND ADMINISTRATION

Ciprofloxacin is given by mouth 500 mg–750 mg bid (q12h) depending on the severity of infection. Tablets are available in 250-, 500-, and 750-mg sizes. Intravenous form comes as a premixed unit dose of 200 or 400 mg. Infusion time should be kept at 60 minutes. The optimal ciprofloxacin dose for *H. influenzae* is 400 mg IV q12h for 7–14 days. (See the previous section for dosage reductions in patients with renal disease.)

Other Gram-Negative Pneumonias

Gram-negative bacillary pneumonia refers to infections caused by organisms of the Enterobacteriaceae and Pseudomonadaceae families, as well as *other* nonfermentative, aerobic gram-negative bacilli. These organisms cause 9–20% of community-acquired pneumonias and 40–45% of hospital-acquired pneumonias. Most cases of gram-negative bacillary pneumonias result from aspiration of endogenous flora (in community-acquired and hospital-acquired infections). They are seen prominently in patients with altered mental status due to a variety of causes: alcohol, seizures, cerebrovascular accidents, or anesthesia.

The most common gram-negative bacillary pneumonia is that due to *K. pneumoniae,* causing 18–64% of community-acquired pneumonia and 30% of nosocomial gram-negative pneumonia. It is seen predominantly in men (> 90% of cases) over age 40 years and in association with alcoholism, diabetes mellitus, and chronic pulmonary diseases. Clinical presentation is similar to other acute bacterial pneumonias. Onset is sudden, with cough, productive thick, bloody sputum ("currant jelly"), dyspnea, pleuritic chest pain, and fever and chills. On physical examination, lung consolidation is typical. Laboratory findings include a wide range of leukocyte counts (25% with normal count), and radiographic upper lobes (frequently right). Clinical course often ends in death, and poor prognostic indicators are old age, bacteremia, and neutropenia. Patients who are seriously ill are best treated with a cephalosporin and an aminoglycoside, in combination.

P. aeruginosa is the most commonly acquired nosocomial pneumonia. It results from aspiration in debilitated patients and from bacteremia in oncologic/hematologic patients. Chronic obstructive pulmonary disease patients on chronic corticosteroids are also at increased risk. The clinical manifestations in nonbacteremic pneumonia include fever, chills and cough production of purulent sputum. Leukocytosis may or may not initially be present, and radiographically, bilateral, nodular, lower lobe infiltrates are typical. Abscess and empyema formation occur commonly. In bacteremic pneumonia, onset is sudden, with confusion, dyspnea, and fever. Cough is present but usually nonproductive. On physical examination, ecthyma gangrenosum may be present, representing pseudomonal vascular invasion. Chest examination is nonspecific, and leukopenia is frequently seen, presumably related to the immunosuppressed state of these patients (chemotherapy or corticosteroids). The chest roentgenogram may show minimal changes or bronchopneumonia with areas of cavitation. Prognosis is poorest in bacteremic patients (with mortality as high as 80% in some studies). Treatment is best achieved with *two* synergistic agents such as an aminoglycoside (gentamicin or tobramycin) and an antipseudomonal penicillin (ticarcillin–clavulanic acid) or broad-spectrum cephalosporin (ceftazidime).

Enterobactericeae and Pseudomonadaceae usually result from aspiration pneumonia due to other members of the oropharyngeal flora, although exceptions are *E. coli* and *S. pneumonia,* which result from hematogenous seeding. Mortality is high, ranging from 25–50%. Treatment will vary using ampicillin or an aminoglycoside for susceptible *E. coli, Proteus,* or *Morganella* to an aminoglycoside, and antipseudomonal penicillin for *Enterobacter* infections.

Piperacillin

MECHANISM OF ACTION

Piperacillin is a semisynthetic broad-spectrum penicillin antimicrobial used parenterally. It is bactericidal and demonstrates activity against a broad spectrum of gram-negative and gram-positive pathogens by inhibiting both septum and cell wall synthesis.

PHARMACOKINETICS

Piperacillin sodium is not absorbed by the GI tract and must be given IV or IM. Mean serum concentrations following IV infusion (given over 30 minutes of 6 g q6h) is 420 mg/ml, reached on the fourth day of administration in healthy adults with normal renal function. Its elimination half-life is 0.6–1.3 hours. It is excreted through bile and urine.

INDICATIONS

This agent is indicated in the treatment of lower respiratory tract infections due to *E. coli, Klebsiella* sp., *Enterobacter* sp., *Proteus vulgaris, Providencia retteer, P. aeruginosa, Serratia* sp., *H. influenzae, Bacteroides* sp., and anaerobic cocci. It is used in conjunction with an aminoglycoside to treat exacerbations of bronchopulmonary *P. aeruginosa* in cystic fibrosis patients.

CONTRAINDICATIONS

Piperacillin is contraindicated in patients with known hypersensitivity to the penicillins or cephalosporins due to the partial cross-allergenicity among penicillins and cephalosporins. Side effects include eosinophilia, rash (6%), fever, neutropenia (up to 6%), and diarrhea. Liver effects include increased SGOT and increased bilirubin; phlebitis, hypokalemia, and nephropathy are rarely seen.

DOSAGE AND ADMINISTRATION

The route and administration is slow IV injection or infusion or by deep IM injection.

For serious infections, the drug should be given IV. Adult dosage for uncomplicated community-acquired pneumonia is 100–125 mg/kg (6–8 g daily) given q6–12h, IM or IV. For more serious infections such as nosocomial pneumonia, adult dosage is 200–300 mg/kg (12–18 g daily, usual maximum dosage of 24 g daily), IV q4–6h. When used to treat *P. aeruginosa* in cystic fibrosis patients (in conjunction with an aminoglycoside), it can be given IV in a dosage of 300–600 mg/kg daily. The piperacillin dosage for children has not been approved by the U.S. Food and Drug Administration, but it has been used IM or IV in children age 1 month to 12 years in a dosage of 76–100 mg/kg daily, or 50 mg/kg q4h IV given over 30 minutes. Reduced dosage is required when renal function is impaired. For adults with serious pneumonias, the dosage is 4 g q8h with a creatinine clearance of 20–40 ml/minute and 4 g q12h with a creatinine clearance less than 20 ml/minute.

Ticarcillin and Clavulanic Acid

MECHANISM OF ACTION

Ticarcillin is a semisynthetic alphacarboxypenicillin. Clavulanic acid is a beta-lactamase inhibitor that, when combined with penicillins (or cephalosporins), has a synergistic effect, which broadens the spectrum of activity of the penicillin. Ticarcillin and clavulanerate (Timentin) is usually bactericidal in action.

PHARMACOKINETICS

Ticarcillin is not absorbed by the GI tract (though clavulanate is well absorbed orally), and consequently, the combination must be given IV. Following IV administration of ticarcillin and clavulanate in adults with normal renal function, the elimination half-life of ticarcillin is 1.1–1.2 hours and of clavulanate 1.1–1.5 hours. Ticarcillin and clavulanate are excreted through urine principally, although clavulanate is also excreted through bile.

INDICATIONS

Ticarcillin is indicated in the treatment of lower respiratory infections caused by beta-lactamase-producing stains of *S. aureus, H. influenzae, Klebsiella* spp., *Citrobacter, Enterobacter, E. coli, Pseudomonas,* and *Serratia.* It is particularly useful in treating nosocomial respiratory tract infections. The in vitro antibacterial activity of ticarcillin and aminoglycosides is synergistic against *P. aeruginosa.*

CONTRAINDICATIONS

Ticarcillin and clavulanate is contraindicated in patients with known hypersensitivity to the penicillins or cephalosporins due to the partial cross-allergenicity among these agents. Side effects include phlebitis, rash, eosinophilia, diarrhea, neutropenia, increased prothrombin time and SGOT, positive Coombs, and hypokalemia.

DOSAGE AND ADMINISTRATION

The route and administration is IV infusion. Dosage is expressed in grams of ticarcillin plus grams of clavulanic acid (to give grams of Timentin). Adult dosage for patients weighing 60 kg or more is 3.1 g of the 30 : 1 fixed ratio combination (3 g of ticarcillin and 100 mg of clavulanic acid) q4–6h. For children over age 12 years and adults and children weighing less than 60 kg, the dosage of the 30 : 1 fixed ratio combination is 200–300 mg of ticarcillin per kg daily in divided doses q4–6h. For children under age 12 years, thorough safety and efficacy have not been established, although dosages of 207 mg of ticarcillin per kg (mild-moderate infection) to 310 mg of ticarcillin per kg daily (severe infections) have been used in divided doses q4–6h.

For patients with renal impairment alone or hepatic and renal impairment (not hepatic impairment alone), the recommended adult dosage is 3.1 g of ticarcillin and clavulanate loading dose with a maintenance dosage based on creatinine clearance:

Creatinine clearance (ml/minute)	Dosage (Timentin)
30–60	2 g q4h
10–30	2 g q8h
< 10	2 g q12h

Gentamicin

MECHANISM OF ACTION

Gentamicin is a water-soluble aminoglycoside antimicrobial derived from *Micromonospora purpurea* (an actinomycete) for parenteral usage. Its bactericidal activity results from inhibition of normal protein synthesis in susceptible organisms.

PHARMACOKINETICS

When gentamicin is administered IV or IM, peak serum concentrations are reached within 30–60 minutes, with measurable levels lasting 6–8 hours. This agent may accumulate in patients with impaired renal function. In a normal patient, 70% of the gentamicin may be recovered in the urine within 24 hours.

INDICATIONS

Gentamicin used alone and in combination with other antimicrobial agents is effective in treating pneumonia caused by *P. aeruginosa, E. coli, Proteus* sp. (indole = negative and positive), *Enterobacter* sp., *Serratia* sp., and *Klebsiella* sp. Because of in vitro synergism, we recommend concomitant use of an extended spectrum penicillin with antipseudomonal activity (azlocillin, carbenicillin, mezlocillin, piperacillin, or ticarcillin) and an aminoglycoside (gentamicin or tobramycin) in treatment of serious pseudomonal lung infections.

SIDE EFFECTS AND CONTRAINDICATIONS

Gentamicin is contraindicated in patients with known hypersensitivity to it or other aminoglycosides. Side effects include nephrotoxicity (elevated BUN, proteinuria), ototoxicity (vestibular), fever, and rash. All aminoglycosides may cause increased neuromuscular blockage (apnea), and caution should be used in patients with myasthenia gravis, parkinsonism, botulism, patients on neuromuscular blocking drugs, or patients who have had massive transfusion of citrated blood. (6–8 units/24 hours).

DOSAGE AND ADMINISTRATION

It may be administered IV (preferred for serious infections) or IM, using the patient's pretreatment body mass for dosing. In patients with normal renal function, 3–5 mg/kg/day should be given in divided doses q8h. In patients with impaired renal function, the dosage intervals should be adjusted by monitoring serum concentrations.

Tobramycin

MECHANISM OF ACTION

Tobramycin is a water-soluble aminoglycoside parenteral antimicrobial derived from *Streptomyces tenebrarius*. Its bactericidal activity is a result of its inhibition of protein synthesis in susceptible organisms.

PHARMACOKINETICS

Tobramycin is quickly absorbed by IV or IM administration. By the IM route, peak serum concentrations are reached between 30 and 60 minutes. Similar concentrations are obtained via a 1-hour IV infusion. The usual serum half-life is 2 hours. Tobramycin is not well absorbed in the GI tract and remains almost completely intact when it is eliminated by granular filtration. In patients with normal renal function, 84% is recovered in the urine at 8 hours and 93% at 24 hours.

INDICATIONS

Tobramycin is effective in lower respiratory tract infections caused by *P. aeruginosa, Serratia* sp., *E. coli, Klebsiella* sp., *Enterobacter* sp., and *S. aureus* (penicillinase and nonpenicillinase infections).

SIDE EFFECTS AND CONTRAINDICATIONS

Tobramycin is contraindicated in patients with known allergies to it or other aminoglycosides. Side effects include nephrotoxicity (elevations of BUN, creatinine, proteinuria), ototoxicity (vestibular and auditory) fever, and rash. Additionally, all aminoglycosides may cause or increase neuromuscular blockade, and respiratory monitoring should be done when given to patients with myasthemia gravis, parkinsonism, or botulism and in patients receiving neuromuscular drugs or large amounts of citrated blood.

DOSAGE AND ADMINISTRATION

Tobramycin may be given IM or IV in the same dosage (IV for more serious infections). The patient's weight is used to determine proper dosage. In patients with normal renal function, 3–5 mg/kg day should be administered in divided doses q6–8h for 7–14 days. When renal function is impaired, a loading dosage of 1 mg/kg should be given followed by either reduced dosages q8h or the normal dosage at longer intervals. Serum concentrations should be monitored; if these values are unavailable, monitoring of the serum BUN and creatinine level is advised.

Cefuroxime

See page 74.

Ceftazidime

See page 76.

Cefotaxime

See page 75.

Ciprofloxacin

See page 77.

References

1. Arcieri, G. et al. Ciprofloxacin: An update on clinical experience. *Am. J. Med.* 82 (Suppl. 4A):381, 1987.

2. Cooper, T. J. A comparison of oral cefuroxime axetil and oral amoxicillin in lower respiratory tract infections. *J. Antimicrob. Chemother.* 16:373, 1985.

3. Kauffman, C. A., et al. Antimicrobial resistance of Haemophilus species in patients with chronic bronchitis. *Am. Rev. Resp. Dis. 120:1382–1385, 1979.*

4. *The Medical Letter. The Choice of Antimicrobial Drugs.* Vol. 32 (817): 41–48. May 4, 1990.

5. Murray, J. F., and Nadel, J. A. *Textbook of Respiratory Medicine.* Philadelphia: Saunders, 1988.

6. Pennington, J. E., et al. Pseudomonas pneumonia: A retrospective study of 36 cases. *Am. J. Med.* 55: 155–160, 1973.

7. Schleupner, C. J., et al. Blinded comparison of cefuroxime to cefaclor for lower respiratory tract infections. *Arch. Int. Med.* 148:343, 1988.

8. Trucksis, M., et al. Emerging resistance to fluoroquinolones in staphylococci: An alert. *Ann. Int. Med.* 114(5):424–426, 1991.

9. Valdivieso, M., et al. Gram negative bacillary pneumonia in the bacillary host. *Medicine.* 56:241–254, 1977.

Legionella Pneumonia

Peter C. Hill
Samuel V. Spagnolo

Legionnaires' disease derives its name from an outbreak of pneumonia at the 1976 American Legion Convention in Philadelphia. Thirty-four of the 221 individuals who developed pneumonia eventually died. The microorganism, *Legionella pneumophila,* was isolated 6 months after the epidemic. Since then, this pneumonia has been documented throughout the world, and over 30 species are now classified in the new family Legionellaceae.

L. pneumophila is a small, weakly staining gram-negative rod and is associated with fresh water supplies, such as air-conditioner condensers and cooling towers. It is estimated to account for between 1% and 5% of all pneumonias. Unlike other gram-negative pneumonias, symptoms may resemble viral or mycoplasmal infection early on in the course. The infection is often accompanied by relative bradycardia, fevers, elevated white blood cell count, proteinuria, and a "patchy" alveolar infiltrate that frequently progresses to lobar consolidation. A dry, irritating cough and pleural effusions are also common.

The diagnosis of Legionnaires' disease is usually based on a "positive" serology with a consistent clinical picture. A single-complement fixation titer of 128 or greater or a documented fourfold increase in the titer is considered diagnostic of an acute infection. Culturing *Legionella* is difficult since 3–4 days is required for growth, and special medias are needed. Sensitivity of sputum culture approaches 70% when dye-containing selective media are used in combination with the buffered yeast extract agar following acid pretreatment for contamination species. Direct fluorescent antibody stain of respiratory tract secretions or a tissue sample is a more rapid means of diagnosing *Legionella* infection, but there are false-negatives with this test.

Erythromycin

Erythromycin, produced from a strain of *Streptomyces erythraeus,* is classified as a macrolide antimicrobial since it contains a multimembered lactone ring with attached deoxy sugars. Macrolide antimicrobials inhibit protein synthesis by reversibly binding to 50s ribosomal subunits of sensitive organisms without affecting nucleic acid synthesis. Gram-positive bacteria accumulate nearly 100 times more erythromycin than gram-negative organisms.

PHARMACOKINETICS

Erythromycin readily forms salts with acids. The base, the stearate salt, and the esters are all poorly soluble in water, but they are suitable for oral administration. Gastric secretions inactivate erythromycin, so enteric coatings that dissolve in the duodenum are necessary. Diffusion into most body fluids occurs rapidly, with the exception of noninflamed meningeal membranes and the placental membrane.

Clearance of erythromycin is achieved primarily by the liver. In individuals with normal hepatic function, erythromycin is concentrated by the liver and excreted in the bile. Less than 5% of the activity of an oral dose can be recovered from the urine.

INDICATIONS

Erythromycin is the drug of choice for *Legionella* infection, and the clinical response is usually within 2 days. It is an excellent choice especially for outpatients with pneumonia since it provides adequate antimicrobial effect for common gram-positive pneumonias (streptococcal and staphylococcal [but not methicillin-resistant]), as well as "atypical" pneumonias (*Chlamydia pneumoniae* and *Mycoplasma pneumoniae*). It is also the drug of choice for streptococcal prophylaxis infections when the patient is allergic to penicillin.

SIDE EFFECTS AND CONTRAINDICATIONS

Most side effects of oral erythromycin — abdominal cramping and discomfort, nausea, vomiting, and diarrhea — are related to the GI tract. The symptoms are dosage related and decrease when the drug is taken with large amounts of water. Intravenous erythromycin is often followed by thrombophlebitis, although this side effect can be minimized by slowing the infusion rate.

Erythromycin will increase blood levels of theophylline when both drugs are given concurrently, so caution about theophylline toxicity is warranted.

DOSAGE AND ADMINISTRATION

For *Legionella* pneumonia, the usual dosage is 1.0 g q6h and should be given by the IV route when initiating therapy. Once the patient is afebrile and the white blood cell count is decreasing, the antimicrobial course may be completed with oral therapy. A 3-week course of therapy is recommended since relapses are common.

Rifampin

Rifampin is a macrocyclic antimicrobial, a semisynthetic derivative from rifamycin B that is derived from *Streptomyces mediterranei.* Rifampin works by inhibiting DNA-dependent RNA polymerase of sensitive organisms and is bactericidal for both intracellular and extracellular microorganisms.

PHARMACOKINETICS

Peak concentrations of rifampin occur 1–4 hours following oral ingestion. Drug distribution in bactericidal concentrations occurs in many organs and body fluids, including the cerebrospinal fluid. Rifampin turns body fluids (urine, tears, saliva, etc.) orange-red, and this effect can be used to help determine patient compliance. Elimination occurs rapidly through the bile and entrohepatic circulation deacetylation.

INDICATIONS

Rifampin is active against many gram-positive and gram-negative microorganisms, as well as numerous mycobacterium. Since the drug is highly active against *Neisseria meningitidis* and *Haemophilus influenzae,* it is used frequently for prophylaxis against these organisms. Rifampin has been shown to be strongly inhibitory to *Legionella* species in cell culture and animal models, and its effect is enhanced when used in combination with erythromycin.

SIDE EFFECTS AND CONTRAINDICATIONS

Rifampin has a low side effect profile. In a study with tuberculosis patients, less than 4% had significant adverse reaction. The most common were rash (0.8%), fever (0.5%), and nausea and vomiting (1.5%). The most serious reaction, although rare, is the occurrence of drug-induced hepatitis and jaundice, which has been fatal in several cases.

Since hepatic microsomal enzymes are induced by rifampin, increased clearance of many compounds, including sulfonylureas, colfibrate, metoprolol, propranolol, ketoconazole, digitoxin, quinidine, and prednisone, may occur. Methadone and coumadin also cleared more rapidly from the body when used with rifampin.

DOSAGE AND ADMINISTRATION

Rifampin is available in 150- and 300-mg capsules. The suggested dosage for *Legionella* pneumonia is 600–900 mg daily, given along with erythromycin. Rifampin should not be used alone because of the possibility of rapid development of resistance.

Ciprofloxacin

Ciprofloxacin belongs to a new class of antimicrobials, the fluoroquinolones, which are related to nalidixic acid. Its bactericidal activity involves the inhibition of DNA gyrase enzyme. In susceptible organisms, this inhibition effect distorts the structure of the DNA and halts cell replication of the microorganism.

PHARMACOKINETICS

Ciprofloxacin has excellent bioavailability and is well absorbed from the GI tract. About 50–70% of the oral dosage is excreted unchanged in the urine and the remainder recovered in the feces or as urinary metabolites. Bile concentration may be several-fold higher than serum levels.

INDICATIONS

Experimental models show that ciprofloxacin is comparable to rifampin in the treatment of *Legionella* pneumonia. In humans, there are reports of severe cases treated with ciprofloxacin with favorable results.

SIDE EFFECTS AND CONTRAINDICATIONS

Side effects are usually minor and include CNS stimulation — headache, dizziness, insomnia, and restlessness — after several days of therapy. Nausea, vomiting, diarrhea, and mild transaminase elevations have been reported.

Ciprofloxacin is contraindicated in pregnancy, during breast-feeding, and in children under age 18 years due to arthropathy reported during use in immature animals.

The optimal ciprofloxacin dosage for *Legionella* pneumonia is 400 mg IV q12h, but clinical reports demonstrate favorable results with 200 mg IV q12h. In severe cases of pneumonia, combination therapy using erythromycin is indicated. Rifampin should be used if erythromycin is contraindicated. Treatment should be continued for a minimum of 3 weeks, since relapses are common.

DOSAGE AND ADMINISTRATION

Tablets are available in 250-, 500-, and 750-mg sizes. The IV form of ciprofloxacin as a premixed unit dose of 200 or 400 mg is available. Infusion time should be 60 minutes.

The usual dosage for other respiratory tract, skin, or joint infections is 500 mg or 750 mg q12h for severe infections for 7–14 days. Dosage should be reduced in patients with severe renal impairment.

Summary

1. *Legionella* pneumonia is primarily a clinical diagnosis with complement fixation as confirmatory evidence.
2. Primary therapy is erythromycin 1 g IV q6h for 3 weeks. Oral therapy can be used to complete the course once the patient has become afebrile with decreasing white blood cell count.
3. In several cases, ciprofloxacin or rifampin may be added. Both agents should be used together if erythromycin is contraindicated.
4. Oral erythromycin's side effects are mostly related to GI tract and are dosage related. Dosing the drug with a large amount of water has been reported to decrease the side effects.
5. Intravenous erythromycin often causes thrombophlebitis; this side effect can be reduced by slowing the infusion rate.
6. Erythromycin increases theophylline levels.
7. Rifampin has a low side effect profile, with rash, fever, nausea, and vomiting each occurring in about 1% of cases. Fatal cases of hepatitis have been reported, but they are rare.
8. Ciprofloxacin side effects are minor and include CNS stimulation: headache, insomnia, restlessness, nausea, vomiting, diarrhea, and mild transaminase election.
9. Ciprofloxacin is contraindicated in pregnancy and during breast-feeding and for children under age 18 years.
10. Ciprofloxacin elevates theophyline and cimetidine levels. It has also altered dipheylhydration metabolism.
11. Ciprofloxacin has poor anaerobic coverage and should be avoided as a single agent when anaerobic coverage is indicated.
12. Antacids may interfere with ciprofloxacin's absorptions.

References

1. Brisson-Noel, A., et al. Mechanism of action of spiramycin and other macrolides. *J. Antimicrob. Chemother.* 22 (Suppl. B):13–23, 1988.

2. Grosset, J., and Leventis, D. Adverse affects of rifampin. *Rev. Infect. Dis.* 5 (Suppl. 3):440–446, 1983.

3. Havlichek D., et al. Comparison of ciprofloxacin and rifampin in experimental *Legionella pneumophila* pneumonia. *J. Antimicrob. Chemother.* 20, 6:875–881, 1987.

4. Hobby, G. L., and Lenert, T. F. Observations on the action of rifampin and ethambutol alone and in combination with other antituberculous antibiotics. *Am. Rev. Respir. Dis.* 105:292–295, 1972.

5. Kapusnik, J. E., et al. The use of rifampin is staphylococcal infections — a review. *J. Antimicrob. Chemother.* 13:61–66, 1984.

6. Levasseur-Rajagopalan, P. Comparison of the activity of three an-

tibiotic regimens in severe Legionnaires' disease. *J. Antimicrob. Chemother.* 26 (Suppl. B):129–39, 1990.

7. Lucas, R., Kazmowych, T., Spagnolo, S. V. Legionella pneumonia presenting as a bulging fissure on the chest radiograph. *Chest* 100: 567–568, 1991.
8. Sanders, C. C. Ciprofloxacin: In vitro activity, mechanism of action and resistance. *Rev. Infect. Dis.* 10:516–527, 1988.
9. Sippel, J. E., et al. Rifampin concentrations in cerebral fluid of patients with tuberculosis meningitis. *Am. Rev. Respir. Dis.* 109:579–580, 1974.
10. Spagnolo S. V., and Medinger, A. *Handbook of Pulmonary Emergencies.* New York: Plenum, 1986.
11. Thornsberry, C., et al. Rifampin: Spectrum of antibacterial activity. *Rev. Infect. Dis.* 5 (Suppl. 3):412–417, 1983.
12. Unertl, K. E., et al. Brief report: Ciprofloxacin in the treatment of legionellosis in the critically ill patients including those cases unresponsive to erythromycin. *Am. J. Med.* 87 (Suppl. 5A):128–131, 1989.
13. Wehrli, W. Rifampin: Mechanisms of action and resistance. *Rev. Infect. Dis.* 5 (Suppl. 3):407–411, 1983.

Anaerobic Lung Infections

Truvor V. Kuzmowych

Anaerobic lung infections are due to aspiration of material or secretions infected with anaerobic bacteria, most frequently originating in the oropharynx. Conditions causing compromised consciousness and/or dysphagia usually predispose patients to aspirate. Other contributory factors are periodontal disease, bronchiectasis, or bronchial obstruction.

The spectrum of anaerobic pulmonary infections includes pneumonitis, necrotizing pneumonia, lung abscess, and empyema. Each of these conditions should be considered as a stage in the continuum of anaerobic lung infection. In other words, the aspirated bacterial nidus penetrates the pulmonary defense mechanisms and produces a pneumonitis, which develops into a necrotizing pneumonia, which can progress to a lung abscess. An empyema may result from either a lung abscess or a necrotizing pneumonia.

The presence of anaerobic lung infections is readily demonstrated by chest roentgenogram or CT. Their location in the lung depends on gravity and the posture of the patient at the time of aspiration. The most frequently involved areas of the lung are the posterior segments of the upper lobes and superior segments of the lower lobes.

The clinical presentation of such lung infections is nonspecfic and often subacute. Usually there is also an indolent progression of symptoms. It may be weeks to months before the patient will present to the physician complaining of a persistent cough productive of foul-smelling sputum, low-grade fever, weight loss, pleuritic chest pain, and dyspnea.

Anaerobic pleuropulmonary infections are polymicrobial. They usually consist of three to six different species of anaerobic bacteria. About half of these infections also involve one or more aerobic bacteria. All these organisms live in varying degrees of symbiosis with each other. Most often, the severity of the lung infection and the amount of parenchymal destruction is not due to the virulence of a single species of anaerobic bacteria but is the end result of different interdependent synergisms that exist among all of the organisms present at a site of infection.

The anaerobic bacteria most commonly isolated from these infections are the gram-negative rods *Bacteroides* sp. and *Fusobacterium* sp., as well as the gram-positive *Peptostreptococci*. Less commonly isolated organisms are the gram-positive rods *Eubacterium* sp., *Clostridium* sp., *Lactobacillus* sp., *Propionibacterium* sp., and *Actinomyces*. Occasionally the gram-negative cocci *Veillonella* sp. can be found.

The most commonly advocated regimens for therapy of anaerobic pleuropulmonary infections are penicillin, clindamycin, and penicillin and metronidazole. Penicillin is still preferred by some as the gold standard. It is effective and quite useful in patients who are not very ill. Seriously ill patients should be treated with clindamycin or penicillin plus metronidazole, since the frequency of isolation of anaerobic bacteria producing beta-lactamase has been increasing in pleuropulmonary infections, and the seriously ill patient has little time for therapeutic trials. Whatever the antimicrobial regimen, therapy must be prolonged in order to prevent relapse.

Clindamycin

Clindamycin is a lincosamide antimicrobial. It is the 7-deoxy, 7-chloro derivative of lincomycin. Lincomycin was originally isolated from the organism *Streptomyces lincolnensis,* which came from the soil near Lincoln, Nebraska.

Clindamycin is a weak base that is readily water soluble. The hydrochloride salt of the base is used orally in the form of a capsule. The palmitate ester is used as a pediatric suspension, and the phosphate ester is used for IM or IV injection.

BACTERIOLOGY

Clindamycin's mechanism of action is through the inhibition of bacterial protein synthesis. The clindamycin molecule becomes attached to binding sites on the 50S subunit of susceptible bacterial ribosomes. At that location, it interferes with the transpeptidation reaction and thus inhibits early polypeptide chain elongation. Macrolides like erythromycin and chloramphenicol bind to the same sites. In fact, the binding of any one of these antimicrobials to the ribosome may inhibit the interaction of the others, and no clinical indication exists for their concurrent use.

Although clindamycin is chemically related to lincomycin, its biologic activity is similar to erythromycin. Like erythromycin it has bactericidal activity against the viridans group of streptococci, *S. pneumoniae, S. pyogenes,* and staphylococci, including *S. aureus.* Occasionally clinical isolates of *S. pneumoniae, S. pyogenes,* and the viridans group of streptococci have been found to be resistant to clindamycin, but they are usually also resistant to erythromycin. Currently, the majority of *S. aureus* strains are sensitive to clindamycin. Some erythromycin-resistant strains of *S. aureus* are still sensitive to clindamycin, but methicillin-resistant strains are not.

Clindamycin is more active than erythomycin against most clincally significant anaerobic bacteria, particularly *Bacteroides fragilis.* It is one of the most active antibiotics against *B. fragilis.* The rate of resistance of the *B. fragilis* group to clindamycin is approximately 5%, and this rate has remained stable over the years.

Among the other anaerobic bacteria, 10–20% of clostridia (with the exception of *Clostridium perfringens*) are resistant to clindamycin, as are 10% of the peptococci. Most strains of *Fusobacterium varium* are resistant to clindamycin. Strains of *Actinomyces israelii* are sensitive.

Mycoplasma pneumoniae, Haemophilus influenzae, Neisseria meningitidis, the enterococci, and all Enterobacteriacae are resistant to clindamycin.

There are three mechanisms by which bacteria can develop resistance to clindamycin:

1. By alteration in a single 50S ribosomal protein at the receptor site, thus preventing binding of the antimicrobial to the ribosome. This type of resistance is the result of a chromosomal mutation. It confers resistance not only to lincosamides like clindamycin but also to macrolides like erythromycin.
2. Alteration of the 23S ribosomal RNA of the 50S ribosomal subunit by methylation of adenine. This type of resistance also results in decreased binding of the antimicrobial to the ribosome and is usually mediated by a plasmid. It is associated with resistance not only to lincosamides but also macrolides and streptomycin.
3. Inactivation of clindamycin by particular strains of staphylococci that have the enzyme 4-lincosamide 0-nucleotidyltransferase, which catalyzes the nucleotidylation of the hydroxyl group in position 4 of the antimicrobial. The ability to produce this inactivating enzyme by the staphylococci is also plasmid mediated.

PHARMACOLOGY

About 90% of an oral dose of clindamycin is absorbed from the GI tract, and peak serum levels are reached in about 1 hour. GI tract absorption is slowed but not decreased by food. Both the palmitate ester used for the oral suspension and the phosphate ester used for parenteral administration are inactive but are readily hydrolyzed to the active base form in the blood. Intramuscular injections cause little pain, and peak serum levels are reached in about 3 hours.

Clindamycin has good tissue penetration except for the cerebrospinal fluid (CSF). Ninety percent of the antimicrobial is bound to plasma proteins. It is widely distributed in many fluids and tissues, including bone. Clindamycin readily crosses the placental barrier and is actively transported into polymorphonuclear leucocytes and macrophages. Relatively high levels of concentration have also been found in experimental subcutaneous abscesses [7].

The normal serum half-life of clindamycin is 2.4 hours. Most of this antimicrobial is metabolized to the *N*-demethyl-clindamycin and clindamycin sulfoxide, probably by the liver. Both of these metabolites are excreted in the bile and urine.

The *N*-demethyl-clindamycin is biologically more active than clindamycin. Most of the clindamycin found in the bile is as the *N*-demethyl metabolite, but bile represents only a minor route of elimination of this antimicrobial. This may account for the activity of clindamycin in the feces after parenteral administration. Common bile duct obstruction results in markedly decreased to absent clindamycin activity in the bile.

High clindamycin bioactivity is also found in the urine, but accurate data of the proportion of absorbed clindamycin excreted in the urine are unavailable. In patients with severe renal failure, the half-life of clindamycin is increased from 2.4 to about 6 hours. Peak blood levels after parenteral administration are about twice those in normals. Hemodialysis or peritoneal dialysis does not remove significant amounts of clindamycin.

Prolongation of clindamycin activity can also occur in patients with severe liver disease. In patients with both severe liver and renal disease, significant modifications of the dosage of clindamycin must be made.

ADVERSE REACTIONS

Adverse reactions to clindamycin include a variety of rashes and fever and, rarely, exudative erythema multiforme (Stevens-Johnson syndrome) and anaphylaxis. Diarrhea occurs in about 20% of patients treated with clindamycin, more commonly after oral administration.

Pseudomembranous colitis (also known as *Clostridium difficile* colitis or antimicrobial-associated colitis) is reported in up to 10% of clindamycin-treated patients, occurring after oral, parenteral, or topical use of the antimicrobial. It is not related to dosage and may begin during or several weeks after therapy. The course can be protracted, and it may be fatal. A similar clinical picture can be seen with many other broad-spectrum antimicrobials, but it occurs less frequently than with clindamycin.

The syndrome of pseudomembranous colitis consists of fever, abdominal cramps, and diarrhea with mucus, or blood, or both in the stool. Yellow to white plaques can be seen on the colonic mucosa during proctoscopic examination. The cause of this syndrome is a toxin secreted by *C. difficile,* which overgrows the normal bacterial flora of the colon as result of clindamycin therapy. The *C. difficile* toxin can be detected by a cytotoxicity assay using tissue culture cells. This toxin can be detected in nearly all patients with pseudomembranous colitis and also in about 20% of patients with just clindamycin-associated diarrhea.

Therapy of pseudomembranous colitis consists of prompt cessation of clindamycin, and oral vancomycin 125–500 mg 4 times a day for 7–10 days. Oral bacitracin and metronidazole can also be effective. In some instances, cholestyramine works well, but it should not be used with oral vancomycin. The use of antiperistaltic drugs should be avoided, since they can make the colitis worse or prolong its course. Relapse after treatment occasionally occurs.

Minor, reversible transaminase elevations without other liver abnormalities have been seen commonly, particularly after parenteral clindamycin. Rare cases of true hepatotoxicity with jaundice and hepatocellular damage have been reported. Isolated cases of neutropenia, thrombocytopenia, and agranulocytosis have also been observed. Parenteral clindamycin is generally well tolerated, and local irritation is rare.

Clindamycin can inhibit neuromuscular transmission, and it may potentiate the effect of concurrently administered neuromuscular blocking agents. Clindamycin phosphate in solution is also physically incompatible with ampicillin, diphenylhydantoin, barbiturates, aminophylline, calcium gluconate, and magnesium sulfate.

INDICATIONS

Since clindamycin has the potential for serious or possibly even fatal toxicity with pseudomembranous colitis and because there are other antimicrobials that can provide similar coverage, the use of clindamycin should be limited to specific, clear-cut indications. These are infections outside the CNS that are most likely to involve *B. fragilis* or other penicillin-resistant anaerobic bacteria. Specific examples of such infections are anaerobic pleuropulmonary infections and intraabdominal infections resulting from fecal spillage or pelvic abscesses.

Of anaerobic pleuropulmonary infections, 15–20% involve beta-lactamase-producing strains of *B. fragilis, B. melaninogenicus, B. ruminicola,* and *B. ureolyticus*, which are resistant to penicillin [8]. Clindamycin is therefore preferable to penicillin for the treatment of anaerobic pleuropulmonary infections in patients who are seriously ill or have not responded to penicillin therapy. It is the drug of choice for the treatment of anaerobic lung infections in patients allergic to penicillin.

ADMINISTRATION AND DOSAGE

The site and severity of the infection, as well as the condition of the patient, are important factors in determining dosage. In adults the oral dosage is usually 150–300 mg q6h. For severe infections, the oral dosage may be increased to 450 mg q6h. Clindamycin may be given IV q6–12h in the dosage range of 600–2700 mg/24 hours. Intravenous dosages as high as 4800 mg/24 hours have been given to adults.

Metronidazole

Metronidazole is a derivative of the drug azomycin. Cosar demonstrated its antitrichomonal activity in 1959. Since then, this drug has been shown to be very effective against anaerobic bacteria and other protozoa that infect humans.

BACTERIOLOGY

Metronidazole has bactericidal activity against most strains of anaerobic and microaerophilic bacteria. The exceptions are a few strains of gram-positive, nonsporeforming, anaerobic or microaerophilic bacilli, *Capnocytophagia* species, and *Propionbacterium acnes*. *Treponema pallidum*, oral spirochetes, *Campylobacter fetus*, and *Gardnerella vaginalis* are all sensitive to metronidazole. Even *E. coli* may be inhibited by metronidazole in the presence of *B. fragilis*. Resistance to metronidazole is rare.

Metronidazole readily enters microorganisms by passive diffusion. Once in the cell, it undergoes rapid reduction of the nitro group on C5 by the enzyme nitroreductase. The source of the electrons for this reaction is probably reduced nicotinamide adenine dinucleotides or sulfides. By using up these substrates, metronidazole thus deprives the cell of reducing equivalents.

The reduction of metronidazole decreases the intracellular concentration of the unchanged drug. This increases the transmembrane concentration gradient of the unchanged drug and promotes its uptake by the microorganism. Reduction of metronidazole also generates short-lived intermediate compounds and free radicals. These compounds cause single- and double-stranded breaks and disrupt the helical structure of cellular DNA, resulting in death of the cell.

PHARMACOLOGY

Metronidazole is almost completely absorbed when given by mouth. The oral dosage produces similar blood levels to the IV dosage. Blood levels are proportional to the administered dosage, and peak levels occur 1–2 hours after the oral dose. Absorption is not affected by food, but peak levels may be markedly delayed. The drug is well absorbed rectally and vaginally.

Metronidazole diffuses freely into total body water. About 10% is protein bound in the plasma. Levels in the CSF, saliva, bile, bone, and breast are equivalent to serum levels. The drug readily crosses the placenta, and fetal serum levels are equivalent to maternal levels. Therapeutic levels are achieved in alveolar bone, saliva, all mucosal surfaces, middle ear discharge, CSF, brain abscess contents, pleural empyema fluid, hepatic abscess, the unobstructed biliary tract, breast milk, amniotic fluid, cord blood, myometrium, fallopian tubes, vaginal secretions, and seminal fluid.

Metronidazole is primarily metabolized by the liver through oxidation of the side chains or conjugation with glucuronide. Most of the drug and its metabolites are eliminated in the urine. Small amounts of the drug are also excreted in the feces. The serum half-life of metronidazole is about 8 hours. Its plasma clearance is delayed in patients with liver disease, and dosage of the drug should be reduced in patients with severe obstructive hepatic disease, alcoholic cirrhosis, or severe renal disease. The drug is readily removed by dialysis.

ADVERSE REACTIONS

Metronidazole is generally well tolerated, and adverse reactions are uncommon. When side effects do occur, they are most often gastrointestinal. These include glossitis, stomatitis, furry tongue, metallic taste, dry mouth, nausea, vomiting, epigastric discomfort, abdominal cramps, pancreatitis, and rarely pseudomembranous colitis. Neurologic side effects include headaches, incoordination, ataxia, dizziness, vertigo, cerebellar dysfunction, seizures, and a peripheral neuropathy.

The peripheral neuropathy is usually sensory and most often results in numbness or paresthesias in the lower extremities. Symptoms are more pronounced in winter and are usually associated with high dosages and prolonged use of the drug. After 6 months of therapy with metronidazole, about 50% of the patients develop a peripheral neuropathy. Early recognition and cessation of drug usually results in prompt resolution of symptoms.

Dermatologic side effects include uriticaria, flushing, pruritus, or a maculopapular rash. Vaginal dryness and burning, cystitis, dysuria, a sense of pelvic pressure, and a reddish-brown discoloration of the urine can occur. Fever and gynecomastia have been reported, as well as reversible neutropenia, after long-term use. With the use of buffered preparations for IV infusions, thrombophlebitis is a rare complication.

Metronidazole and its metabolites have been shown to be mutagenic in bacteria. The drug has also been shown to be carcinogenic in rodents. No mutagenic or oncogenic effects have been demonstrated in humans to date. However, as a precaution, **metronidazole should not be used in the first trimester of pregnancy or in lactating women.**

DRUG INTERACTIONS

Metronidazole can produce a disulfiramlike reaction when taken with alcohol. When taken with disulfiram it can produce confusional and psychotic states. It potentiates warfarin and prolongs the prothrombin time. Cimetidine decreases metronidazole clearance, but this interaction is not significant in patients with normal liver and kidney function. Metronidazole decreases dilantin clearance, and both dilantin and phenobarbital increase metronidazole clearance. The drug also interferes with certain chemical analyses for SGOT and produces falsely low or negative values.

The only absolute contraindication to the use of metronidazole is a specific sensitivity to the drug. Relative contraindications to its use are during the first trimester of pregnancy, in lactating women who breast-feed, a history of blood dyscrasias, and active neurologic disease, such as a seizure disorder or neuropathy.

INDICATIONS AND CLINICAL USES

As a single agent, metronidazole is ineffective for the treatment of anaerobic pleuropulmonary infections [4]. Most of these infections are polymicrobial, frequently containing aerobic, facultative, and microaerophilic, as well as anaerobic, bacteria. Metronidazole is bactericidal only for the anaerobic organisms; it has no effect on the aerobic, facultative, or microaerophilic bacteria. However, when metronidazole is combined with penicillin, ampicillin, or erythromycin in patients allergic to penicillin, it provides excellent coverage for anaerobic pleuropulmonary infections.

The *B. fragilis* group are probably the most common bacteria encountered in anaerobic infections. Only three drugs are consistently active against this group of organisms: metronidazole, chloramphenicol, and clindamycin. Recently a small degree of resistance of the *B. fragilis* group to clindamycin was reported [6]. If this becomes a trend, metronidazole with either a penicillin or erythromycin may have an even greater role in the treatment of pulmonary infections involving this organism.

Metronidazole is also clinically effective in the treatment of protozoal diseases such as *Trichomonas vaginitis,* amebic liver abscess, intestinal amebiasis, and giardiasis. Due to its excellent bactericidal activity and almost complete distribution throughout the body, metronidazole is an excellent antimicrobial for the treatment of a number of serious anaerobic infections, such as brain abscess or other CNS infection, endocarditis, and any serious anaerobic infection in an immunocompromised host. This drug is also useful in the treatment of anaerobic bone, joint and soft tissue infections, head and neck infections, oral and dental infections, and nonspecific vaginitis. Metronidazole is as effective as vancomycin in the treatment of pseudomembranous colitis. It has been successfully used in the treatment of bowel bacterial overgrowth syndromes and has been shown to have some beneficial effect in Crohn's disease. Topical metronidazole can be used to treat acne rosacea.

ADMINISTRATION AND DOSAGE

Metronidazole is available for parenteral infusion as a 500-mg/100-ml ready-to-use isotonic solution, or as a 500-mg vial of lyophylized powder that requires reconstitution, dilution, and neutralization to a pH between 6 and 7 prior to IV administration. Metronidazole is also available in 250-mg and 500-mg tablets and as a topical gel.

Intravenous therapy is recommended in all seriously ill patients, especially those with infections due to susceptible anaerobic bacteria or those who cannot take medication by mouth. When metronidazole is given IV, an initial loading dosage of 15 mg/kg is recommended. This dosage is then reduced to 7.5 mg/kg IV q6h. The infusion time should be about 1 hour, and the maximum daily dosage is 4 g.

Since serum levels after an oral dose are comparable to those following an IV infusion, patients can receive oral metronidazole as soon as they can tolerate it. The oral dosage is 1–2 g/day in 2–4 divided doses q6–12h. Metronidazole should not be used alone in the treatment of anaerobic pleuropulmonary infections.

References

1. Bartlett, J. G. Anaerobic bacterial infections of the lung. *Chest* 91:901–909, 1987.
2. Bartlett, J. G. Anaerobic Bacteria: General Concepts. In G. L. Mandell et al. (eds.), *Principles and Practice of Infectious Diseases* (3d ed.). New York: Churchill Livingstone, 1990.
3. Bartlett, J. G., and Gorbach, S. L. Treatment of aspiration pneumonia and primary lung abscess — penicillin G vs clindamycin. *JAMA* 234: 935–937, 1975.
4. Eykyn, S. J. The therapeutic use of metronidazole in anaerobic infection: Six years' experience in a London hospital. *Surgery* 93:209–214, 1983.
5. Finegold, S. M. Aspiration pneumonia. *Rev. Infect. Dis.* 13 (Suppl. 9):737–742, 1991.
6. Finegold, S. M., and Mathisen, G. E. Metronidazole. In G. L. Mandell et al. (eds.), *Principles and Practice of Infectious Diseases* (3d ed.). New York: Churchill Livingstone, 1990.
7. Joiner, K. A., et al. Antibiotic levels in infected and sterile subcutaneous abscesses in mice. *J. Infect. Dis.* 143(3):487–494, 1981.
8. Kirby, B. D., et al. Gram-negative anaerobic bacilli: Their role in infection and patterns of susceptibility to antimicrobial agents. I. Little Known *Bacteroides* species. *Rev. Infect. Dis.* 2:914–951, 1980.
9. Levison, M. E., et al. Clindamycin compared with penicillin for the treatment of anaerobic lung abscess. *Ann. Intern. Med.* 98:466–471, 1983.
10. Perlino, C. A. Metronidazole vs clindamycin treatment of anaerobic pulmonary infection–failure of metronidazole therapy. *Arch. Intern. Med.* 141:1424–1427, 1981.
11. Sande, M. A., and Mandell, G. L. Antimicrobial Agents: Tetracyclines, Chloramphenicol, Erythromycin and Miscellaneous Antibacterial Agents — Clindamycin. In A. G. Gilman et al. (eds.), *Goodman and Gilman's the Pharmacological Basis of Therapeutics (8th ed.). New York: Pergamon Press, 1990.*
12. Sanders, C. V., et al. Metronidazole in the treatment of anaerobic infections. *Am. Rev. Respir. Dis.* 120:337–343, 1979.
13. Smilack, J. D., et al. Tetracyclines, chloramphenicol, erythromycin, clindamycin, and metronidazole. *Mayo Clin. Proc.* 66:1270–1280, 1991.
14. Steigbigel, N. H. Erythromycin, Lincymocin, and Clindamycin. In G. I. Mandell et al., (eds.), *Principles and Practice of Infectious Diseases* (3d ed.). New York: Churchill Livingstone, 1990.
15. Webster, L. T. Drugs Used in the Chemotherapy of Protozoal Infections: Amebiasis, Giardiasis, and Trichomoniasis-Metronidazole. In A. G. Gilman et al., (eds.), *Goodman and Gilman's the Pharmacological Basis of Therapeutics* (8th ed.). New York: Pergamon Press, 1990.

Fungal

Samuel V. Spagnolo
Donn Quinn

Fungi are a distinct class of microorganisms, a few of which can produce disease in humans. These mycoses vary greatly in their manifestations but tend to be subacute to chronic diseases with indolent relapsing features. Pulmonary and disseminated fungal infections generally occur in immunosuppressed hosts and in that situation can have a fulminant and fatal course.

Coccidioidomyocosis, histoplasmosis, and blastomycosis may occur in immunocompetent hosts. Coccidioidomycosis is endemic to the western United States and varies from a benign respiratory infection to a disseminated fatal disease. Histoplasmosis is prevalent in the Mississippi and Ohio Valleys in the United States. Aspergillosis, Candidiasis, mucormycosis, and cryptococcus generally occur in immunosuppressed hosts. Cryptococcus can cause lung infection in healthy individuals, but the disease is self-limited, and treatment is not indicated. Antifungal therapy is always indicated in the immunosuppressed.

Amphotericin

Amphotericin B is an antimycotic polyene antimicrobial obtained from a strain of *Streptomyces nodosus*. It binds to sterols in the cell membrane of fungi, altering membrane permeability and allowing leakage of intracellular components.

PHARMACOKINETICS

Plasma half-life is approximately 24 hours. Amphotericin B appears to bind to plasma proteins and tissues, with subsequent slow release. It can be detected in urine up to 7 weeks after therapy has been discontinued. The routes of elimination in humans are unknown.

CLINICAL INDICATIONS

Amphotericin is indicated in systemic mycoses. The most common systemic mycoses are due to opportunistic infections in patients with impaired defense mechanisms. Candida, Aspergillus Cryptococcus, and Mucor are the main causative organisms.

SIDE EFFECTS AND CONTRAINDICATIONS

Adverse reactions to amphotericin are common. Fever and chills occur commonly. Headache, anorexia, and vomiting all occur. Phlebitis at injection site may occur, as well as myalgias, malaise, and abdominal pain. Renal impairment is an almost inevitable consequence, associated with hypokalemia, azotemia, and renal tubular acidosis. Less common adverse reactions are thrombocytopenia, tinnitus, hearing loss, arrhythmias, hypotension, and seizures.

DOSAGE AND ADMINISTRATION

A test dose of 1 mg amphotericin B in 250 ml of 5% dextrose in water (DSW) should be followed with 5 mg in 500 ml D_5W over 4–6 hours, then 5–10 mg over a 6-hour period, but not exceeding 50 mg in the first 24 hours. Daily infusion of 0.6 mg/kg body weight should then be maintained, provided that toxic effects are not observed. Side effects can usually be controlled by using a large vein, by giving hydrocortisone 25–50 mg just prior to infusion, and by using antipyretics and antihistamines. Heparin has been used to control local phlebitis.

Fluconazole

Fluconazole (Diflucan) is a fluorinated bis-triazole structurally related to the imidazoles. Like the imidazoles, it alters cell membrane permeability by interacting with the formation of membrane sterols. Fluconazole has less effect on human sterol synthesis than the imidazoles and is thus less toxic.

PHARMACOKINETICS

Fluconazole is almost completely absorbed from the GI tract. Concentrations in plasma are essentially the same when the drug is given orally or IV. Gastric acidity does not affect bioavailability. The elimination half-time is 25 hours, and the drug is 90% renally excreted. Fluconazole diffuses readily into body fluids, including sputum and saliva.

CLINICAL INDICATIONS

Fluconazole is indicated for systemic candida infections, including candida pneumonia. It has been particularly useful for therapy of cryptococcal disease among patients with acquired immunodeficiency syndrome (AIDS). However, there is limited experience with the use of fluconazole to treat cryptococcal pneumonia.

SIDE EFFECTS AND CONTRAINDICATIONS

The most common side effect is GI distress. Rash, eosinophilia, Stevens-Johnson syndrome, transient abnormalities of hepatic function, and thrombocytopenia have been reported. Fluconazole can increase plasma concentrations of phenytoin, sulfonylureas, and, to a lesser extent, warfarin and cyclosporine.

DOSAGE AND ADMINISTRATION

Fluconazole is available PO and IV. The usual dosage is 200 mg on day 1, followed by 100 mg daily. In cases of severe infection, the dosage is 400 mg on day 1, followed by 200–400 mg daily.

Ketoconazole

Ketoconazole (Nizoral) is an orally absorbed imidazole, active against a broad spectrum of pathologic fungi. It alters the permeability of yeast and fungal cell membranes by interfering with the formation of membrane sterols.

PHARMACOKINETICS

Ketoconazole readily but incompletely absorbs after oral dosing. Peak serum concentrations of ketoconazole occur within 3 hours of administration and are proportional to the dosage. Ketoconazole is extensively metabolized in the liver. It has been suggested that the elimination of ketoconazole is impaired in liver disease. Renal impairment has little effect on the kinetics of the drug. Plasma elimination is biphasic, with initial serum half-life of 1.5–2 hours and beta phase half-life about 8 hours after a 200-mg dose.

INDICATIONS

Ketoconazole can be used in the treatment of coccidioidomycosis and histoplasmosis.

SIDE EFFECTS AND CONTRAINDICATIONS

Asymptomatic elevation of hepatic enzymes to 50% above normal levels was found in 14% of over 1000 patients. Jaundice has been reported. A small number of fatalities have been reported, but the majority of these probably are in patients in whom therapy was continued despite clinical evidence of heptatic damage. Nausea, vomiting, pruritis, and abdominal pain have been reported. Diarrhea, urticaria, and dizziness occur uncommonly.

Ketoconazole causes rapid depression of serum testosterone. In a few patients, gynecomastia has been reported with therapeutic dosages. Higher or more frequent dosages may cause oligospermia and adrenal suppression, which appears to be dosage-related.

DOSAGE AND ADMINISTRATION

The usual adult dosage is 200–400 mg, once daily for 2 weeks. Since gastric acidity is required for absorption, the drug should not be taken with antacids or histamine antagonists. Use of ketaconazole may alter the metabolism of phenytoin, and drug levels should be monitored. The anticoagulant effect of coumadin may be enhanced, and prothrombin times should be monitored. Serum levels of cyclosporine may increase with use of ketoconazole.

Itraconazole

Itraconazole (Sporanox), a triazole compound recently approved (1993) by the Food and Drug Administration, acts by interfering with the formation of membrane sterols.

PHARMACOKINETICS

Itraconazole requires an acid environment for absorption. It is nearly insoluble in water, is highly lipophilic, and is protein bound. Although levels in serum are low, tissue levels are higher. Itraconazole is metabolized solely by the liver; there is no renal excretion. The drug has a half-life of about 15 hours.

INDICATIONS

Itraconazole has activity against a wide variety of mycoses. It is indicated in the treatment of pulmonary histoplasmosis, blastomycosis, and coccidioidomycosis. A number of studies have shown that itraconazole is effective in treating aspergillus infections. Patients with acute invasive aspergillosis, chronic necrotizing aspergillosis, and asperilloma have been treated with it.

SIDE EFFECTS AND CONTRAINDICATIONS

Adverse reactions include headache, nausea, heartburn, edema, and rash. Symptoms are usually mild. Reversible alterations in liver function tests have been documented in less than 5% of patients. Hypokalemia has been noted uncommonly. Unlike ketaconazole, testosterone and cortisol synthesis is unaffected. The use of itraconazole with terfenadine and astemizole is contraindicated because of an increased risk of arrythmias.

DOSAGE AND ADMINISTRATION

Itraconazole is available in 100-mg capsules. A dosage of 200 mg daily is recommended for the treatment of histoplasmosis and blastomycosis. Various studies have used from 100 to 400 mg daily for different mycoses. If dosages larger than 200 mg are used, it is recommended to divide the dosage to twice daily. Because gastric acidity is required for absorption, the drug should not be given with antacids or histamine antagonists. Because hypochlorhydria has been reported in HIV-infected patients, the absorption of itraconazole may be decreased in these patients.

References

1. Borgers, M. Mechanism of action of antifungal drugs, with special reference to the imidazole derivatives. *Rev. Infect. Dis.* 2:520, 1980.
2. De Souza, R. F., MacKinnon, S., Spagnolo, S. V., et al. Treatment of localized pulmonary phycomycosis *South. Med. J.* 72:609–612, 1979.
3. Drutz, D. J. Newer antifungal agents and their use, including an update on amphotericin B and flucytosine. *Curr. Clin. Topics Infect. Dis.* 3:97, 1982.
4. Kauffman, C. Use of the new oral azole antifungal drugs. *Infect. Med.* 9(12): 13–18, 1992.

5. Smith, C. M., and Reynard, A. M. *Textbook of Pharmacology*. Philadelphia: W. B. Saunders, 1992.

6. Stern, J. J., et al. Oral fluconazole therapy for patients with AIDS and cryptococcosis. Experience with 22 patients. *Am. J. Med.* 85:477–480, 1988.

Pneumocystis Pneumonia

Cynthia L. Gibert
Fred M. Gordin

Pneumocystis carinii was first recognized as a human pathogen in 1909 and classified as a protozoan. Prior to the 1980s, most cases of *carinii* pneumonia (PCP) occurred in organ transplant recipients and in persons receiving immunosuppressive drugs and irradiation for the treatment of malignancies. In the 1980s *carinii* was the most common pulmonary pathogen in persons with the acquired immunodeficiency syndrome (AIDS). Integral to the care of persons infected with HIV is appropriate prophylaxis and treatment of PCP. The Public Health Service (PHS) issued guidelines in 1992 for the prophylaxis of PCP.

The typical clinical presentation of PCP in an HIV-infected person includes chest tightness, followed by exercise intolerance, cough, and fever. The disease may progress slowly over weeks to months or abruptly over several days. Dyspnea at rest may occur; the cough is frequently nonproductive. Fever may be absent, low grade or high and spiking. Physical examination may reveal little other than fever and tachypnea. The chest radiograph most commonly reveals bilateral perihilar or diffuse interstitial infiltrates. The definitive diagnosis of pneumocystosis rests on the demonstration of the organisms in the lung tissue or material obtained from the lungs.

Pneumocystis Prophylaxis

PRIMARY PROPHYLAXIS

HIV-infected persons with a $CD4^+$ T-cell count of less than 200 cells/mm^3 should receive lifelong PCP prophylaxis. Persons with constitutional symptoms, including oral thrush or unexplained fever over 100°F for 2 or more weeks regardless of $CD4^+$ T-cell count should receive prophylaxis.

SECONDARY PROPHYLAXIS

After recovery from a documented episode of PCP, any HIV-infected person should receive lifelong prophylaxis.

PROPHYLACTIC AGENTS

Trimethoprim-sulfamethoxazole (TMP/SMX) and aerosolized pentamidine are the two drugs currently recommended, but dapsone is also used as a prophylactic agent.

Pneumocystis Pneumonia: Treatment

The following drugs are currently recommended for the treatment of PCP: TMP/SMX; intravenous pentamidine; trimethoprim and dapsone; clindamycin and primaquine; and atovaquone. Adjunctive corticosteroids are recommended for certain patients.

Trimethoprim-Sulfamethoxazole

Trimethoprim-sulfamethoxazole (Bactrim, Septra) is a synthetic antimicrobial combination product that has a fixed dosage ratio of 1 part TMS to 5 parts SMX. The drug may be given orally to treat acute PCP and as prophylaxis or IV to treat acute PCP.

PHARMACOKINETICS

TMP/SMX is an antifolate that blocks folate metabolism at two sites. TMP inhibits dihydrofolate reductase, while SMX interferes with dihydrofolic synthetase. TMS/SMX is well absorbed from the GI tract. The peak serum levels are reached in 1–3 hours, and the serum half-life is 12–13 hours. The maximal synergistic inhibition occurs at a serum TMP/SMX ratio of 1 : 20, which is achieved by administering the drugs in a fixed 1 : 5 ratio. TMP/SMX is excreted by glomerular filtration and tubular secretion in the kidneys. Because TMP/SMX is excreted primarily by the kidneys, dosages must be decreased in severe renal insufficiency.

CLINICAL INDICATIONS

For both the prophylaxis and treatment of PCP, TMP/SMX is the therapy of choice for HIV-infected patients who are able to tolerate this agent. The initial drug regimen for an HIV-infected patient or patient at risk for HIV presenting with pneumonia should include TMP/SMX. Induced sputum or bronchiolar lavage fluid should be obtained promptly and stained for *P. carinii.*

SIDE EFFECTS AND CONTRAINDICATIONS

There is a high incidence of adverse reactions to TMP/SMX in HIV-infected persons. Side effects include rash, fever, leukopenia, thrombocytopenia, hepatotoxicity, mucositis, and GI disturbances. More rarely, Stevens-Johnson syndrome and antimicrobial-associated colitis are reported. Hypersensitivity to TMP/SMX occurs in 50–80% of HIV-infected patients. Oral outpatient desensitization is an option for patients whose adverse reaction was morbilliform rash, pruritus, or malaise and myalgia.

TMP/SMX is teratogenic and should not be prescribed to pregnant women. Serum levels of phenytoin and warfarin may be increased. TMP/SMX may potentiate the action of oral hypoglycemics. The myelotoxicity of TMP/SMX may increase that of azidothymidine (AZT) with concurrent usage.

DOSAGE AND ADMINISTRATION

For PCP prophylaxis, the preferred regimen is TMP/SMX (160/800 mg) 1 double-strength (DS) tablet daily. Alternative doses are TMP/SMX DS 1 tablet twice daily 2 or 3 days/week, or 1 tablet daily 3 days/week. For the treatment of acute pneumocystis pneumonia, oral or IV TMP/SMX may be given at a total daily adult dosage of TMP 15–20 mg/kg with SMX 70–100 mg/kg in divided doses q6–8h. The usual length of therapy is 21 days. For patients with acute respiratory failure, worsening respiratory status, or GI intolerance to the oral drug, IV therapy is indicated.

SUMMARY

1. When treating acute PCP, hypoxia may worsen over the initial 3–4 days of therapy.
2. Initial therapy may usually be continued for 5–10 days before changing the regimen because of poor clinical response.
3. Hyponatremia is not uncommon while being treated with IV TMP/SMX because of the large IV volume of 5% dextrose in water.
4. Failure to improve in 5–10 days should be considered treatment failure and alternative therapies administered. In one study, over 40% of patients treated for PCP who had respiratory failure survived, so aggressive treatment is appropriate.
5. TMP/SMX has efficacy in preventing toxoplasmosis.

Pentamidine Isethionate

Pentamidine isethionate, an aromatic diamidine, has known activity against *carinii*. The mode of action is not fully understood, but there is in vitro evidence that pentamidine interferes with folate metabolism, anaerobic glycolysis, oxidative phosphorylation, and nucleic acid replication.

PHARMACOKINETICS

The pharmacokinetics are not well understood. Gastrointestinal absorption is poor. When this agent is administered parenterally peak serum levels are obtained in 1 hour, and the elimination half-life is between 6 and 10 hours. It may, however, take several days to achieve adequate levels in the lung tissue. The half-life of pentamidine in lung tissue is more than 30 days. Aerosolized pentamidine has a long half-life in the lungs with low systemic drug levels and toxicity.

CLINICAL INDICATIONS

Intravenous pentamidine (Pentam 300) is the second most commonly used drug to treat acute PCP. It is generally as effective as TMP/SMX. Aerosolized pentamidine (Nebu Pent) was the first drug approved by the Food and Drug Administration for PCP prophylaxis. Aerosolized pentamidine (AP) is now used as PCP prophylaxis primarily for those intolerant to TMP/SMX. AP does not have a role in the treatment of active PCP.

SIDE EFFECTS AND CONTRAINDICATIONS

The development of extrapulmonary or pulmonary pneumocystis while receiving AP as prophylaxis is a major concern. Patients who develop acute PCP while receiving AP prophylaxis often have atypical radiographic findings, including predominately upper lobe disease. Other side events associated with AP include bronchospasm, cough, a metallic taste, fatigue, dizziness, and rash. Less frequent side effects reported with AP include hypoglycemia, pancreatitis, hypotension, and arrhythmias.

Side effects are more frequently associated with IV pentamidine and include hypotension, hypoglycemia, hyperglycemia, cardiac arrhythmias (e.g., torsade de pointes), acute renal failure, leukopenia, thrombocytopenia, and Stevens-Johnson syndrome.

All patients should be evaluated for tuberculosis before AP is initiated. A medical history, tuberculin skin test (Mantoux method), chest radiograph, and, if cough or pulmonary infiltrate is present, smears and cultures of sputum for acid-fast bacilli should be obtained. Before each subsequent AP treatment, patients must be evaluated for symptoms of possible active tuberculosis.

Aerosolized pentamidine must be administered in a private room or booth with negative-pressure ventilation relative to nearby areas. The air in the treatment room or booth should be exhausted directly to the outside. The treatment room or booth should not be used again for at least 20–30 minutes, and any other person entering it should wear a particulate respirator.

Any patient who develops cough, wheezing, or chest pain while using an AP nebulizer should be given an inhaled $beta_2$ agonist and be premedicated 10 minutes prior to receiving AP in the future.

The nephrotoxicity of IV pentamidine is increased when administered with concomitant amphotericin B, with acute and rapidly progressive renal failure reported. The renal failure is reversible when the pentamidine is discontinued.

While a patient is receiving IV pentamidine, the antiretroviral agent ddI (Videx) must be discontinued because there are reports of severe pancreatitis occurring in patients receiving both drugs concurrently. There is a risk of developing severe, sometimes fatal, hypocalcemia when parenteral pentamidine is given to a patient also receiving foscarnet sodium.

DOSAGE AND ADMINISTRATION

For PCP prophylaxis, AP may be administrated by one of two nebulizers, the Respigard II jet nebulizer or the Fisoneb ultrasonic hand-held nebulizer. With the Respigard II nebulizer, the pentamidine dosage is 300 mg, dissolved in 6 ml of water, administered every 4 weeks. With the Fisoneb nebulizer, the pentamidine dosage is 60 mg dissolved in 3 ml of water. There is an initial loading dosage with the Fisoneb nebulizer of 5 60-mg doses 24–72 hours apart given over a 2-week period, followed by a maintenance dosage of 60 mg every 2 weeks. AP prophylaxis is lifelong if tolerated.

For the treatment of *P. carinii* pneumonia, IV pentamidine is administered over a 1-hour period at a dosage of 4.0 mg/kg q24h. The IV medication must be infused slowly to decrease the risk of profound hypotension and cardiac arrhythmias. Therapy should be continued for 21 days.

SUMMARY

1. Aerosolized pentamidine is less effective than TMP/SMX as primary and secondary prophylaxis. Up to 20% of patients given AP as secondary prophylaxis had recurrence of PCP within 1 year.
2. Spontaneous pneumothorax and extrapulmonary pneumocystosis involving liver, bone marrow, spleen, and other sites are reported while receiving AP.

Dapsone

Dapsone, effective in the treatment of leprosy, has also been used as pneumocystis prophylaxis and for treatment.

PHARMACOKINETICS

Dapsone (Aivosulfon) is a sulfone that interferes with folic acid synthesis. Oral absorption is good, and peak serum concentration occurs in 4–8 hours. The half-life is from 10 to 50 hours (average 28 hours). Dapsone is eliminated from the body primarily by acetylation and oxidative metabolism. Overall, 70–80% of dapsone is excreted as metabolites in the urine.

CLINICAL INDICATIONS

Only limited data are available on the efficacy of dapsone to prevent or treat pneumocystis in HIV-infected persons. Dapsone is recommended as PCP prophylaxis only in those intolerant of TMP/SMX or AP. Dapsone, in combination with trimethoprim, may be used as the initial treatment of mild pneumocystis pneumonia in those intolerant to TMP/SMX and able to take an oral regimen or to complete the usual 21-day treatment of acute PCP for those who respond well to initial treatment with IV TMP/SMX or pentamidine.

SIDE EFFECTS AND CONTRAINDICATIONS

All patients must be screened for glucose-6-phosphate dehydrogenase *(G6PD)* deficiency prior to taking dapsone. Dapsone should not be prescribed to patients with *G6PD* deficiency as severe hemolysis may occur. Methemoglobinemia is reported and appears to be related to the dosage and dosing interval. Other adverse events include peripheral neuropathy and motor weakness, anemia, rash, hyperkalemia, male infertility, and a mononucleosislike illness.

Rifampin lowers dapsone levels 7- to 10-fold by accelerating its metabolism. To improve the absorption of ddI, buffers contained in ddI neutralize gastric acid, which significantly reduces the absorption of dapsone. Patients taking both ddI and dapsone should take the medications several hours apart.

DOSAGE AND ADMINISTRATION

The dosage of dapsone for PCP prophylaxis is not established, and a wide range has been used. At this time, the dosage ranges from 50–100 mg orally daily to 100 mg 2 to 3 times/week. The drug may be given as 1 dose or in 2–4 divided doses.

In the treatment of acute PCP, dapsone 100 mg orally daily is given with trimethoprim 15–20 mg/kg orally q24h in 3 divided doses.

SUMMARY

1. Higher levels of trimethoprim and dapsone are achieved when both are given together, which may increase efficacy but also toxicity.
2. When a patient receiving dapsone becomes hypoxic, methemoglobin levels must be obtained.

Atovaquone

Atovaquone (Mepron) is an antiprotozoal agent approved in 1992 for the treatment of mild to moderate PCP in patients intolerant to TMP/SMX.

PHARMACOKINETICS

Atovaquone is a hydroxy-1,4-naphthoquinone, an analogue of ubiquinone, with activity against pneumocystis. The mechanism of action is not fully elucidated. Atovaquone is a highly lipophilic compound with low aqueous solubility. The bioavailability of the drug is increased three-fold when administered with meals, especially fatty foods. Atovaquone has a long half-life (approximately 30 hours). The drug is protein bound, has presumed enterohepatic cycling with fecal elimination, and is not metabolized in humans.

CLINICAL INDICATIONS

Atovaquone is indicated for the oral treatment of acute mild to moderate *P. carinii* pneumonia [(A-a) $DO_2 \leq 45$ mm Hg] in patients intolerant to TMP/SMX. Atovaquone has not been studied for the treatment of more severe PCP or as an agent for PCP prophylaxis.

SIDE EFFECTS AND CONTRAINDICATIONS

In the preliminary studies of atovaquone, many adverse side effects were reported: rash, fever, nausea, diarrhea, headache, vomiting, insomnia, and pruritus. Laboratory abnormalities included anemia, neutropenia, elevated hepatic transaminases, alkaline phosphatase, and amylase, as well as hyponatremia.

If atovaquone is not given with food, absorption may be decreased. The lower plasma concentration may limit response to therapy. Atovaquone should be used with caution in pregnant or nursing women. Atovaquone is highly bound to plasma proteins and therefore should be used with caution when given with other highly protein-bound drugs with narrow therapeutic indices. Atovaquone does not affect the therapeutic effects of phenytoin nor phenytoin that of atovaquone.

DOSAGE AND ADMINISTRATION

The recommended dosage is 750 mg (three 250-mg tablets) given with food 3 times a day for 21 days. Meals with a fat content of more than 23 grams improve absorption significantly, increasing the bioavailability approximately threefold.

Adjunctive Corticosteroids

The addition of corticosteroids during the treatment of moderate to severe PCP improves outcome. When corticosteroids are administered within 72 hours of the initiation of antipneumocystis therapy, the frequent initial decline in oxygenation is diminished or prevented. The recommended dosage of adjunctive corticosteroids is as follows: (1) prednisone 40 mg PO q12h for 5 days, (2) followed by prednisone 40 mg PO q2h for 5 days, and (3) prednisone 20 mg PO q24h for 11 days. Prior to the institution of corticosteroid therapy, the patient must be evaluated for possible infectious tuberculosis, as well as any serious fungal or other opportunistic infection. Oral thrush, genital or rectal herpes simplex infection, and hyperglycemia may occur while on prednisone.

Alternative Treatments

For persons unable to tolerate the above therapies for the treatment of acute PCP, two alternative regimens should be considered. Clindamycin (600 mg orally q8h) given with primaquine (15 mg orally q24h) for 21 days is an alternative regimen for patients with mild disease unable to tolerate sulfa drugs. Intravenous trimetrexate may be used to treat patients unable to tolerate or failing to respond to parenteral pentamidine or TMP/SMX who require a parenteral agent. Eflornithine and piritrexim have been used to treat acute PCP.

Pneumocystis Prophylaxis and Treatment in Pregnancy

TMP/SMX should be used with caution only if no suitable alternative is available. TMP/SMX is contraindicated at term since it increases the risk of kernicterus in newborns and may cause hemolysis in newborns with *G6PD* deficiency.

The safety of pentamidine, atovaquone, and dapsone in pregnancy is not established, and these drugs should be used with caution. For pregnant women able to tolerate AP, it is the preferred prophylaxis.

References

1. Allegra, C. J., et al. Trimetrexate for the treatment of *Pneumocystis carinii* pneumonia in patients with the acquired immunodeficiency syndrome. *N. Engl. J. Med.* 317:978–985, 1987.
2. Consensus statement on the use of corticosteroids as adjunctive therapy for pneumocystis pneumonia in the acquired immunodeficiency syndrome. *N. Engl. J. Med.* 323:1500–1504, 1990.
3. Falloon, J., et al. A preliminary evaluation of 566C80 for the treatment of pneumocystis pneumonia in patients with the acquired immunodeficiency syndrome. *N. Engl. J. Med.* 325:1534–1538, 1991.
4. Fossieck, Jr., B. E., Spagnolo, S. V. Pneumocystis carinii pneumonitis in patients with lung cancer. *Chest* 78:721–722, 1980.
5. Hardy, W. D., et al. A controlled trial of trimethoprim-sulfamethoxazole or aerosolized pentamidine for secondary prophylaxis of *Pneumocystis carinii* pneumonia in patients with the acquired immunodeficiency syndrome. *N. Engl. J. Med.* 327:1842–1848, 1992.
6. Hughes W. T., et al. Prevention of *Pneumocystis carinii* pneumonia in AIDS patients with weekly dapsone. *Lancet* 336:1066, 1990.
7. Hughes, W. T., et al. Successful chemoprophylaxis for *Pneumocystis carinii* pneumonitis. *N. Engl. J. Med.* 297:1419–1426, 1977.
8. Leoung, G. S., et al. Dapsone-trimethoprim for *Pneumocystis carinii* pneumonia in the acquired immunodeficiency syndrome. *Ann. Intern. Med.* 105:45–48, 1986.
9. Masur, H. Prevention and treatment of pneumocystis pneumonia. *N. Engl. J. Med.* 327:1853–1860, 1992.
10. Noskin, G. A., et al. Salvage therapy with clindamycin/primaquine for *Pneumocystis carinii* pneumonia. *Clin. Infect. Dis.* 14:183–188, 1992.
11. Recommendations for prophylaxis against *Pneumocystis carinii* pneumonia for adults and adolescents infected with human immunodeficiency virus. *MMWR* 41 (RR-4):1–11, 1992.
12. Schneider, M. N., et al. A controlled trial of aerosolized pentamidine or trimethoprim-sulfamethoxazole as primary prophylaxis against *Pneumocystis carinii* pneumonia in patients with human immunodeficiency virus. *N. Engl. J. Med.* 327:1836–1841, 1992.
13. Suttler, F. R., et al. Trimethoprim-sulfamethaxazole compared with pentamidine for treatment of *Pneumocystis carinii* pneumonia in the acquired immunodeficiency syndrome: A prospective crossover study. *Ann. Intern. Med.* 109:280–287, 1988.

Chlamydia

Samuel V. Spagnolo
Donn Quinn

Members of the genus chlamydia are obligate intracellular parasites that were once believed to be large viruses. They are bacteria, however, because they have a true bacterial cell wall. Three species cause disease in humans: *Chlamydia psittaci, C. trachomatis,* and *C. TWAR*. *C. psittaci* causes psittacosis, which is contracted through inhalation of respiratory secretions or dust from droppings of infected birds. Clinically, psittacosis is an acute infection of the lower respiratory tract, usually presenting with acute onset of fever, headache, malaise, dry, hacking cough, and x-ray evidence of bilateral interstitial pneumonia. *C. trachomatis* causes a pneumonic illness generally seen in infants. The organism has been recovered from the lower respiratory tracts of immunosuppressed patients who had interstitial pneumonia. *C. TWAR* has been associated with mild pneumonia, pharyngitis, laryngitis, and bronchitis in young adults.

Minocycline

Minocycline (Minocin) is a semisynthetic tetracycline antimicrobial. Like other tetracyclines, it has a wide spectrum of activity. Its main mechanism of action is on protein synthesis.

PHARMACOKINETICS

Minocycline is almost completely absorbed after oral administration. After a single 200-mg dose, peak serum levels of 2–3 μg/ml are attained in 2 hours. Plasma half-life is 12–16 hours in patients with normal renal or hepatic functions. In severe renal impairment, the plasma half-life increases to approximately 32 hours.

Minocycline is widely distributed in human body tissue and fluids. In most instances, tissue levels exceed serum levels with highest concentrations in bile, thyroid, lung, and liver but also good penetration into breast, skin, and sinuses.

INDICATIONS

Minocycline can be used to treat respiratory infections. It has the advantage of requiring twice daily dosing and may be active against some organisms that are resistant to the older tetracycline [2]. A vestibular toxicity unique to minocycline may limit its use.

SIDE EFFECTS AND CONTRAINDICATIONS

No potentially life-threatening adverse reactions have been reported. Minocycline should be used with caution in patients with severe renal failure. Gastrointestinal disturbances including nausea and vomiting have been reported. Dermatological reactions are rare. Erythema multiforme, Stevens-Johnson syndrome, and photosensitivity have been reported. It may cause reversible dizziness, vertigo, nausea, and tinnitus. Minocycline should not be used in pregnant women after the first trimester, because tetracyclines may cause staining of the deciduous teeth. Tetracyclines also have been found to cause permanent tooth discloration, enamel hypoplasia, and depressed bone growth in children under age 12 years. Tetracyclines may also exacerbate systemic lupus erythematosis.

DOSAGE AND ADMINISTRATION

The most commonly used dosage is 50–100 mg bid, but up to 400 mg has been given. Tablets of 100 mg and 50 mg are available.

Doxycycline

PHARMACOKINETICS

Doxycycline (Doryx, Vibramycin) is a semisynthetic tetracycline antimicrobial. Like other tetracyclines, it has a wide spectrum of activity. Doxycycline has its main mechanism of action on protein synthesis. It is more lipid soluble than other tetracyclines (except minocycline) and passes directly through the lipid bilayer of the bacterial cell wall. In addition, an energy-dependent transport system pumps the drug through the inner cytoplasmic membrane. Once inside the bacterial cell, doxycycline inhibits protein synthesis by binding specifically to the 30s ribosomes.

CLINICAL PHARMACOLOGY

Doxycycline is primarily a bacteriostatic antimicrobial. It has a similar spectrum of activity to other tetracyclines and is active against Chlamydia, Mycoplasma, and a wide range of rickettsiae.

PHARMACOKINETICS

Like minocycline, doxycycline has the advantage of once to twice daily dosing. A dosage of 100 mg q24h, following an initial loading dosage of 200 mg gave serum concentrations in 12 normal volunteers of 3.1–3.5 mg/liter 3 hours after each dose and 1.4–1.9 mg/liter 24 hours after each dose. The drug is cleared by renal and biliary mechanisms.

SIDE EFFECTS AND CONTRAINDICATIONS

Like all other tetracyclines, doxycyclines may cause permanent staining of developing teeth and hypoplasia of enamel, so it should not be used in pregnant women or children. Nausea occurs in less than 4% of patients. Rash occurs in less than 3% of patients. Hypersensitivity reactions may occur, and photosensitivity is reported.

DOSAGE AND ADMINISTRATION

The usual adult dosage of doxycycline is 200 mg on day 1, followed by a maintenance dosage of 100 mg daily. In severe infections, the dosage should be 200 mg daily.

References

1. Bennet, D. R. *AMA Drug Evaluations*. Philadelphia: W. B. Saunders, 1992.
2. Dollery, C. *Therapeutic Drugs*. New York: Churchill Livingstone, 1991.
3. Grayston, J. T. Chlamydia pneumoniae strain TWAR. *Chest* 95(3):664–669, 1989.
4. Massen, F. P., et al. Doxycycline and minocycline in the treatment of respiratory infections: A double-blind comparative, clinical, microbiological and pharmacokinetic study. *J. Antimicrobial Chemother.* 23(1):123–129, 1989.
5. Saiven, S., and Howin, G. Clinical pharmacokinetics of doxycycline and minocrycline. *Clin. Pharmacokinetics* 15(6):355–366, 1988.

Viral Pneumonia

Richard Carl Bernstein
Samuel V. Spagnolo

Cytomegalovirus Pneumonia

Pulmonary infection with cytomegalovirus (CMV) is a major concern in immunocompromised and transplant patients since it is often fatal if untreated [4]. In the acquired immunodeficiency (AIDS) population, eventually 90% will develop an infection caused by CMV, including pneumonitis [5]. Cytomegalovirus pneumonia is a difficult infection to diagnose and may be seen concurrently with other opportunistic lung infections.

Cytomegalovirus is a member of the herpes virus group and includes the common herpes structure of linear double-stranded DNA, an icosadeltahedral capsid with 162 capsomers, and an envelope derived from host cell nuclear membrane. The major difference between CMV and herpes simplex virus (HSV) is that CMV is larger in both absolute size and the size of its genome [7].

Cytomegalovirus can be found in the urine, stool, saliva, semen, and vaginal secretions of infected and asymptomatic carriers for prolonged periods — up to several years. The major reservoir for the virus is asymptomatic individuals. In transplant patients, the virus may be acquired from the donated organ or blood transfusions [7].

Clinically CMV pneumonia presents with symptoms consistent with any other viral or atypical pneumonia, including fever, nonproductive cough, and shortness of breath. Rales are sometimes present on chest auscultation. The arterial blood gas analysis may reveal mild to profound hypoxemia. The chest roentgenogram will usually demonstrate a diffuse, usually bilateral infiltrate with accentuation of the infiltrate in the lower lobes [2].

The diagnosis of CMV pneumonia depends on obtaining positive viral cultures in the setting of typical lung histology [1].

Gancyclovir

Gancyclovir (Cytovene) is a synthetic nucleoside analogue of 2-deoxygunaosine that inhibits in vitro and in vivo replication of herpes virus by interfering with viral DNA polymerase. Sensitive human viruses include CMV, herpes simplex virus (HSV) 1 and 2, Epstein-Barr virus (EBV), and varicella-zoster virus (VZV).

PHARMACOKINETICS

With a slow IV infusion over 1 hour, gancyclovir shows dosage-dependent kinetics. The plasma half-life of gancyclovir is 2.9 +/− 1.3 hours. The major route of excretion is renal, with most of drug being excreted unmetabolized. Therefore, the dosage must be adjusted based on creatinine clearance.

CLINICAL INDICATIONS

Gancyclovir is approved in the United States by the Food and Drug Administration (FDA) only for CMV retinitis in immunocompromised patients. Clinical studies show that it clears CMV from respiratory secretions [6, 10] and is useful in treatment of CMV pneumonia [6].

SIDE EFFECTS AND CONTRAINDICATIONS

Granulocytopenia (neutrophils < 1000) develops in as many as 40% of immunocompromised patients on gancyclovir for serous CMV infections. Approximately 20% develop thrombocytopenia (platelet < 50,000). Other side effects include possible infertility in males by inhibition of spermatogenesis, nausea, and skin rash. Gancyclovir is contraindicated in patients with hypersensitivity to gancyclovir or acyclovir.

DOSAGE AND ADMINISTRATION

The package insert should be reviewed prior to using gancyclovir. Gancyclovir is available only as sterile powder in a 10-ml vial with the sodium equivalent of 500 mg of gancyclovir. For CMV retinitis the treatment is 5 mg/kg bid for 14–21 days followed by maintenance treatment of 5 mg/kg/once per day.

When the creatinine clearance is <80 ml/minute/dose the dosing intervals of gancyclovir need to be adjusted:

Creatinine clearance (ml/minute)	Gancyclovir dosage (mg/kg)	Interval (h)
50–79	2.5	12

Creatinine clearance (ml/minute)	Gancyclovir dosage (mg/kg)	Interval (h)
25–49	2.5	24
<25	1.25	24

Gancyclovir dosage for pneumonia ranges from 2.5–7.5 mg/kg q12h for a 14–21-day course. The higher the dosage is, the better is the clinical outcome, but the higher the incidence of side effects [12].

Treatment with gancyclovir with high-dosage IV immune globulin in CMV infection after bone marrow transplant may give greater efficacy than gancyclovir alone.

Herpes Simplex Pneumonia

Herpes simplex virus has two major serologic types: HSV-1, associated most commonly with infections of the perioral mucosa, upper airway mucous membrane, trachea, and occasional pneumonia [7], and HSV-2, usually associated with disease of the genitourinary tract. HSV has a structure similar to that described for CMV but is a smaller virus.

The virus is found in fluid of active vesicular herpetic lesions and has a point prevalence of shedding in respiratory secretions of 1–2% of asymptomatic adults previously infected. Portal of entry of upper and lower airway HSV is through the eye and oropharynx mucous membrane. After a primary infection, the virus is latent in the nerve ganglia in the distribution of the original infection and may reactivate later in the same location.

Clinical illness of HSV-1 can include acute gingivostomatitis, exudative pharyngitis, and, in the AIDS population, esophagitis.

HSV pneumonia is associated with malignancy, burns, and organ transplantation. The lung infection is either secondary to hematogenous dissemination from a localized source or from direct extension from the upper airway [8]. Symptoms of HSV pneumonia include dyspnea, cough, and hypoxemia. When the infection is due to direct extension, then localized or multifocal infiltrates are present on chest roentgenogram, whereas pneumonia secondary to hematogenous dissemination appears as a more diffuse infiltrate [8].

Diagnosis of pneumonia requires a sample of involved lung for viral culture and testing for HSV antigen.

Acyclovir

Acyclovir (Zovirax) is a synthetic purine nucleoside analogue with in vitro and in vivo inhibition against HSV-1 and HSV-2, VZV, EBV, and CMV. Acyclovir is preferentially taken up by virus-infected cells leading to less toxicity for noninfected cells.

PHARMACOKINETICS

After a single dose of slow IV infusion, acyclovir demonstrates dosage-independent kinetics. Plasma half-life is 2.5 ± 0.6 hours in patients with normal renal function and 19.6 hours in anuric patients. It is excreted through the kidneys with 60–90% unchanged. The acyclovir dosage must be adjusted based on the creatinine clearance. Acyclovir is incompletely absorbed after oral administration, with approximately 15–30% oral availability.

CLINICAL INDICATIONS

Acyclovir is indicated for herpes simplex infections in immunocompromised host, initial episodes of herpes genitalis, herpes simplex encephalitis, and varicella-zoster infections in immunocompromised patients, including herpes tracheobronchitis [11].

SIDE EFFECTS AND CONTRAINDICATIONS

With IV infusion, acyclovir causes phlebitis at injection site in 9% of patients and transient elevation of serum BUN and creatinine in 5–10%. With oral administration, nausea and vomiting are seen in 7%. Other side effects, which occur less than 2%, include rash or hives, elevation of liver enzymes, and encephalopathic changes. Acyclovir is contraindicated in anyone who develops hypersensitivity to the drug.

DOSAGE AND ADMINISTRATION

Acyclovir is available in 10-ml sterile vials with 500 mg of acyclovir sodium equivalent or 20-ml vials with 1000 mg. It is also available as 5% ointment in 3- and 15-tubes, or 200- or 800-mg tablets. A suspension with 200 mg/5 cc is also available for those who are unable to swallow tablets. **The package insert should be reviewed prior to using acyclovir.**

Acyclovir is not FDA approved for herpetic tracheobronchitis or pneumonia, but it has been given in a dosage of 8–10 mg/kg q8h for 10 days [11].

For patients with renal insufficiency the dosage and dosing interval should be adjusted as follows:

Creatine clearance (ml/minute)	% of recommended dosage	Dosing interval (h)
>50	100	8
25–50	100	12
10–25	100	24
0–10	50	24

Varicella-Zoster Virus

The VZV causes a primary infection (varicella or chicken pox) consisting of a vesiculopustular rash that appears after a prodrome of mild upper respiratory symptoms accompanied by fever and general malaise. The reactivation form of VZV results in a singular dermatomal eruption (herpes zoster or shingles).

Varicella-zoster virus is a member of the human herpes virus family, sharing the basic structural characteristics as described for cytomegalovirus.

Varicella is usually a disease of childhood. It is highly contagious and spreads through respiratory secretions. Although the progressive rash is very pruritic, the clinical outcome in children is usually good. On the other hand, adults who contract varicella have up to a one-third incidence of VZV pneumonia. Typically pneumonia associated with VZV occurs 1–6 days after the onset of the rash. Symptoms include cough, dyspnea, pleuritic chest pain, and hemoptysis. Severe VZV pneumonia can lead to death.

Radiologically there is a diffuse nodular infiltrate often associated with hilar adenopathy and pleural effusions. Most patients recover in a few days without any sequela.

Acyclovir

Acyclovir (Zovirax) may improve the clinical outcome in patients with varicella pneumonia given in IV dosages similar to what is given for herpes tracheobronchitis. **Refer to the package insert, and see the previous section for a review of this drug.**

References

1. Abdallah, P. S., et al. Diagnosis of cytomegalovirus pneumonia in compromised hosts. *Am. J. Med.* 61:326, 1976.
2. Beschorner, W. E., et al. Cytomegalovirus pneumonia in bone marrow transplant recipients: Miliary and diffuse patterns. *Amer. Rev. Respir. Dis.* 122:107, 1980.
3. Emanuel, D., et al. Cytomegalovirus pneumonia after bone marrow transplantation successfully treated with the combination of gancyclovir and high-dose intravenous immune globulin. *Ann. Intern. Med.* 109:777, 1988.
4. Erice, A., et al. Gancyclovir treatment of cytomegalovirus disease in transplant recipients and other immunocompromised hosts. *JAMA* 257:3082, 1987.
5. Laskin, O. L., and Stahl-Baylis, C. M. Use of gancyclovir to treat serious cytomegalovirus infections in patients with AIDS. *J. Infect. Dis.* 155:323, 1987.
6. Macher, A. M., and Reichert, C. M. Use of gancyclovir to treat serious cytomegalovirus infections in patients with AIDS. J. *Infect. Dis.* 155:323, 1987.
7. Murray, J. F., and Nadel, J. A. *Textbook of Respiratory Medicine.* Philadelphia: W. B. Saunders, 1988.
8. Ramsey, P. G., et al. Herpes simplex virus pneumonia: Clinical, virologic, and pathologic features in 20 patients. *Ann. Intern. Med.* 97:813, 1982.
9. Reed, E. C., et al. Treatment of cytomegalovirus pneumonia with

gancyclovir and intravenous cytomegalovirus immunoglobulin in patients with bone marrow transplants. *Ann. Int. Med.* 109:783, 1988.

10. Shepp, D. H., et al. Activity of 9-[2-hydroxy-1-hydroxy-1-(hydroxymethyl) ethoxymethyl] guanine in the treatment of cytomegalovirus pneumonia. *Ann. Intern. Med.* 103:368, 1985.
11. Sherry, M. K., et al. Herpetic tracheobronchitis. *Ann. Intern. Med.* 109:229, 1988.
12. Wade, J. C., and McGuffin, R. W. Treatment of cytomegaloviral pneumonia with high-dose acyclovir and human leukocyte interferon. *J. Infect. Dis.* 148:557, 1983.
13. Whitley, R. J., and Gnann, J. W. Acyclovir: A decade later. *NJM* 327:782, 1992.

4

Tuberculosis

Samuel V. Spagnolo
John F. Wiley
David P. Remy

From 1953 to 1984, the number of tuberculosis cases each year in the United States gradually decreased. In 1985, there were 22,200 cases of tuberculosis reported in the United States. In 1991, 26,283 cases were reported to the Centers for Disease Control (CDC), an increase of 18.4% over 1985. The largest increases in the reported cases of tuberculosis appear to have occurred in areas that have the most cases of acquired immunodeficiency syndrome (AIDS) [26].

Most cases of tuberculosis occur in individuals who have developed clinical tuberculosis for the first time. The drugs currently used to treat tuberculosis are rapidly effective and, when used appropriately, cure nearly all patients with pulmonary tuberculosis.

Clinical Aspects

There are no specific symptoms of pulmonary tuberculosis; however, the majority of patients develop a productive cough and frequently have such accompanying complaints as weakness, weight loss, and fever. Although hemoptysis does occur, it is usually a later manifestation of more serious disease.

Pulmonary tuberculosis associated with HIV infection may deviate somewhat from the classic presentation but will vary considerably depending on the stage of HIV infection and the degree of immunosuppression. Tuberculosis appears to develop in many HIV-seropositive patients earlier in the course of immunosuppression than was previously realized. Between 24% and 70% of patients with HIV-associated tuberculosis have an extrapulmonary site of disease [11].

Obtaining a positive acid-fast stain of microorganisms present in the sputum is presumptive evidence for the clinical diagnosis of pulmonary tuberculosis and is sufficient for the initiation of drug treatment. A definitive diagnosis rests on the growth of the tubercle bacillus from clinical specimens.

When patients are unable to produce sputum, other procedures for obtaining secretions, tissue, or both can be undertaken, including bronchoscopy with bronchial biopsy and washings, transbronchial lung biopsy, percutaneous thin-needle (23/25 gauge) aspiration, and open lung biopsy.

The chest roentgenogram of patients with pulmonary tuberculosis may reveal almost any picture, from small, segmental infiltrates to lobar or multilobar areas of involvement with or without cavitation of the lung. Although x-ray abnormalities secondary to tuberculosis are most commonly seen in the upper lobes, virtually any part of the lung may be involved, and the clinician should always maintain a high degree of clinical suspicion for this disease.

Perspectives on Therapy

During the early years of chemotherapy for pulmonary tuberculosis, prolonged treatment with multiple drugs was necessary for the success of initial therapy and the achievement of low relapse rates. However, a new era in the treatment of pulmonary tuberculosis began in the 1970s when the combination of rifampin and isoniazid was first used.

During the past 15 years, numerous chemotherapeutic regimens of isoniazid and rifampin, sometimes in combination with other agents, were evaluated in extensive prospective, controlled studies. Almost without exception, the experience with these regimens in pulmonary tuberculosis was favorable. The length of treatment reported in these studies varied from as little as 6 months to as much as 16 months of therapy. Early studies demonstrated that daily administration of isoniazid and rifampin for 9 months, supplemented with ethambutol for the first 2 months, was highly effective in treating advanced pulmonary tuberculosis [9]. Our own study supported these results [39, 42].

Modern drug regimens have been based on several characteristics of the tubercle bacillus responsible for the infection, such as the likely presence of resistant bacterial mutants and the variable growth rates of the organisms. Given these characteristics, it is apparent that even with the excellent drugs available for the treatment of pulmonary tuberculosis, treatment must continue for months, not weeks, in order to keep relapse rates at less than 3%. It is probable that this period of prolonged therapy is necessary for the drugs to reduce the population of slowly growing tubercle bacillus or “persisters.”

With few exceptions, patients who have tuberculosis and HIV infection have a good response to antituberculosis therapy [11, 38, 41].

Therapy

The initial drug therapy will vary depending on the clinical situation. In patients with drug-susceptible infection, standard therapy with isoniazid, rifampin, and pyrazinamide is appropriate until drug-susceptibility tests are available (Table 4-1). The recommended initial regimen for managing drug-susceptible tuberculosis in HIV-infected adults includes isoniazid, 300 mg/day; rifampin, 600 mg/day; and pyrazinamide, 20–30 mg/kg/day, up to a maximum of 2.5 g/day (Table 4-2).

For patients in whom there is a strong suspicion or clear-cut drug-resistant infection, two other agents should be added to isoniazid, rifampin, and pyrazinamide (see Table 4-1). These drugs can be selected on the basis of surveillance data of local drug-resistant

Table 4-1. Recommended initial therapy for tuberculosis with and without associated HIV infection

Clinical situation	Concurrent HIV	No HIV
Drug-susceptible infection	Isoniazid (300 mg/day), rifampin (600 mg/day), and pyrazinamide (20–30 mg/kg/day*) until drug-susceptibility test results are available	Same as for concurrent HIV
Probable drug-resistant infection	Isoniazid (300 mg/day), rifampin (600 mg/day), and pyrazinamide (20–30 mg/kg/day*) plus at least two other drugs to which the infecting *Mycobacterium tuberculosis* strain is likely to be susceptible (based on surveillance of local drug-resistance patterns). The two other drugs can be selected from Table 4-3.	Same as for concurrent HIV

*Maximum dosage, 2.5 g/day.
Recommendations are based on those of Centers for Disease Control; *MMWR* 38:236–248, 1989, and 40:586–691, 1991: American Thoracic Society. Treatment of tuberculosis and tuberculosis infection in adults and children. *Am. Rev. Respir. Dis.* 134:355–363, 1986. P. T. Davidison. Drug resistance and the selection of therapy for tuberculosis. *Am. Rev. Respir. Dis.* 134:355–363, 1986.

patterns. The two additional drugs can be selected from Table 4-3.

When single drug-resistant disease is suspected based on epidemiologic information, the CDC and the American Thoracic Society (ATS) recommend that patients with probable or proved tuberculosis — regardless of HIV antibody status — be started on a regimen of isoniazid, 300 mg/day; rifampin, 600 mg/day; ethambutol, 15–25 mg/kg/day; and pyrazinamide 20–30 mg/kg/day, up to a maximum of 2.5 g/day. When drug-susceptibility test results are known, the regimen should be adjusted accordingly.

In HIV-positive patients with multidrug-resistant tuberculosis, some experts recommend treating patients initially and promptly with a regimen of isoniazid, 300 mg/day; rifampin, 600 mg/day; and pyrazinamide, 20–30 mg/kg/day, up to a maximum of 2.5 g/day; plus at least two other drugs to which the infecting *Mycobacterium tuberculosis* strain is likely to be susceptible, based on surveillance of local drug-resistant patterns [32]. The regimen should be adjusted as necessary once drug-susceptibility test results are available. No data are available from controlled clinical trials regarding management of multidrug-resistant tuberculosis. As a result, therapy for multidrug-resistant tuberculosis must be individualized. In the

Table 4-2. Recommended long-term therapy for tuberculosis with and without associated HIV infection

Clinical situation	Concurrent HIV	No HIV
Drug-susceptible infection	After 2 months of the initial regimen, continue with isoniazid (300 mg/day) and rifampin (600 mg/day) for 7 months or more, or for 6 months after culture conversion to negative, whichever is longer. (If drug-susceptibility test results suggest another course, follow accordingly.)	After 2 months of the initial regimen, continue with isoniazid (300 mg/day) and rifampin (600 mg/day) for 4 months more. (If drug-susceptibility test results suggest another course, follow accordingly.)
Drug-resistant infection	Adjust the regimen accordingly to drug-susceptibility test results. Duration of therapy depends on clinical, roentgenographic, and bacteriologic response.	Same as for concurrent HIV.
Isoniazid resistance or intolerance	Rifampin (600 mg/day) and ethambutol (15–25 mg/kg/day) for 18 months, or for 12 months after culture conversion to negative, whichever is longer. Many experts also suggest giving pyrazinamide (20–30 mg/kg/day[a]).	Rifampin (600 mg/day) and ethambutol (15–25 mg/kg/day) for 12 months. Many experts also suggest giving pyrazinamide (20–30 mg/kg/day[a]).
Rifampin intolerance[b]	Isoniazid (300 mg/day), pyrazinamide (20–30 mg/kg/day[a]), and ethambutol (15–25 mg/kg/day) for 18 months, or for 12 months after culture conversion to negative, whichever is longer.	Isoniazid (300 mg/day), pyrazinamide (20–30 mg/kg/day[a]), and ethambutol (15–25 mg/kg/day) for 18 months.

[a]Maximum dosage, 2.5g/day.
[b]There are no accepted recommendations in cases of rifampin intolerance. Regimens shown are based on recommendations of P. F. Barnes et al. Tuberculosis in patients with human immunodeficiency virus. *N. Engl. J. Med.* 324:1644–1650, 1991.
Recommendations are based on those of Centers for Disease Control; *MMWR* 38:236–248, 1989. American Thoracic Society. Treatment of tuberculosis and tuberculosis infection in adults and children. *Am. Rev. Respir. Dis.* 134:355–363, 1986.

Table 4-3. Currently available second-line drugs for managing multidrug-resistant tuberculosis in HIV-infected patients

Agent	Recommended dosage
Ethionamide	250 mg, 2–4 times daily
Cycloserine	250–1000 mg/day in divided doses
Paraaminosalicylate[a]	12–16 g/day in divided doses
Amikacin	15 mg/kg/day, 5 days/week IV or IM
Kanamycin	15mg/kg/day, 5 days/week IM
Capreomycin	15 mg/kg/day, 5 days/week IM
Ciprofloxacin	500–750 mg twice daily
Ofloxacin	400 mg twice daily
Clofazimine	200–300 mg/day
Rifabutin (ansamycin LM-427)[b]	150–300 mg/day

[a]Recently made available again in the United States through the Centers for Disease Control under an investigational new drug agreement.
[b]Investigational drug available through the Centers for Disease Control.

presence of documented secondary drug resistance, the ATS suggests that patients be treated for a minimum of 12 months [3].

These drug recommendations will likely be modified as information about tuberculosis and multidrug-resistant tuberculosis in this country continues to accumulate.

The CDC and the ATS recommend that therapy for tuberculosis in HIV-infected patients be continued for at least 6 months beyond conversion of sputum cultures to negative, or for a total of 9 months, whichever is longer.

For disseminated tuberculosis with CNS involvement, we recommend adding ethambutol to the initial regimen of isoniazid, rifampin, and pyrazinamide and adjusting the drugs after drug-susceptibility test results are known.

In the extreme and undesirable instance when patients cannot be given isoniazid, use a regimen of rifampin (600 mg/day) and ethambutol (15–25 mg/kg/day) for at least 18 months, or for 12 months after cultures become negative, whichever is longer. We also suggest administering pyrazinamide (20–30 mg/kg/day; maximum, 2.5 g/day) (see Table 4-3).

For patients with rifampin resistance or intolerance, we recommend a regimen of isoniazid (300 mg/day), pyrazinamide (20–30 mg/kg/day; maximum, 2.5 g/day), and ethambutol (15–25 mg/kg/day) for 18 months or for 12 months after culture conversion to negative, whichever is longer (see Table 4-2).

Emperic antituberculous therapy may be indicated in some HIV-infected patients with respiratory symptoms and chest roentgenographic abnormalities that suggest tuberculosis but in whom no other pathologic evidence is identified.

ADVERSE EFFECTS

The rate of adverse effects for antituberculous drugs seems to be higher in HIV-positive patients. In these patients, there is an 18–20% incidence of adverse drug reactions of sufficient severity to cause a change in therapy. In contrast, the incidence of adverse-drug reactions was 3.7% in HIV-seronegative patients.

Some investigators have also recently noted an increased frequency of adverse effects from rifampin. Most of these (90%) reactions were noted during the first 2 months of treatment.

DRUG INTERACTIONS

Pharmacokinetic interactions of isoniazid and rifampin with ketoconazole and fluconazole can result in subtherapeutic levels of rifampin, ketaconazole, and fluconazole.

NEW AGENTS

New drugs with in vitro activity against *M. tuberculosis* include the fluoroquinolones, rifabutin (formerly known as anasamycin LM-427), and clofazimine (see Table 4-3). Among the fluoroquinolones, ciprofloxacin and ofloxacin appear to be most active against *M. tuberculosis* in vitro. Only limited data are available regarding the activity of lomefloxacin against *M. tuberculosis*. A recent study compared the in vitro antituberculous activity of three newly developed fluoroquinolones — fleroxacin, lomefloxacin, and sparfloxacin — with that of ofloxacin [29]. Sparfloxacin was apparently more active than ofloxacin, but both fleroxacin and lomefloxacin were less active than ofloxacin. Sparfloxacin and fleroxacin are not available for clinical use. Clinical experience with these new agents is very limited, and their potential role in managing tuberculosis (including multidrug-resistant tuberculosis) remains unclear and unproven.

Rifampin

Rifampin is one of the four first-line agents for the treatment of *M. tuberculosis*. Like isoniazid and pyrazinamide, rifampin is bactericidal. Rifampin's mycobactericidal action is the disruption of transcription. Specifically, rifampin inhibits the synthesis of RNA by inactivating DNA-dependent RNA polymerase. Rifampin, at standard dosages, has no effect on human RNA polymerase. Rifampin resistance is caused by a mutation of the mycobacterial RNA polymerase so that the drug can no longer bind to it.

ANTIMICROBIAL ACTIVITY AND INDICATIONS

Standard antituberculous regimens include rifampin and isoniazid daily for 9 months; rifampin, isoniazid, and pyrazinamide daily for 2 months; followed by isoniazid and rifampin daily for 4 months (see Table 4-2). Rifampin seems to be the most effective drug in killing organisms within caseous material. Rifampin is active in vitro against most mycobacterial organisms that cause disease. Rifampin is also indicated for the treatment of asymptomatic nasopharyngeal carriers of *Neisseria meningitidis*, to prevent clinical meningitis. Rifampin is not indicated for the treatment of meningococcal infection. Other potential but as yet unapproved uses of rifampin include the treatments of staphylococcal infections, gram-negative bacteremia of infancy, leprosy, and prophylaxis of meningitis after exposure to patients with *Haemophilus influenzae* meningitis.

PHARMACOKINETICS

Rifampin is well absorbed from the GI tract, with peak plasma concentrations occurring in 1–4 hours. Food interferes with the absorption of the drug. Thus, rifampin should be given 1 hour before or 2 hours after meals. The drug is 80% protein bound and very lipid soluble. It distributes widely and penetrates well into lung tissue, tuberculous cavities, and the cerebrospinal fluid (CSF). Rifampin concentrations in sputum and CSF exceed serum concentrations. Rifampin is metabolized in the liver by deacetylation. The metabolite retains antimycobacterial activity. Of each dose of rifampin, 40–70% is excreted in the bile, with approximately one-half in the deacetylated form. Rifampin and its metabolite undergo enterohepatic circulation, but the metabolite is poorly absorbed. The remainder of each dose is excreted in the urine, again with approximately one-half in the deacetylated form. Dosage adjustment of rifampin is necessary with hepatic failure but not with renal failure. Rifampin is not removed from the blood by hemodialysis or peritoneal dialysis.

ADVERSE EFFECTS

Rifampin usually discolors all body fluids, producing a reddish-orange tint. Permanent staining of contact lenses may occur. Between 1 and 5% of patients may report a rash, which is sometimes pruritic. Rifampin causes significant GI distress in 1–2% of patients. The most serious potential adverse effect of rifampin is hepatotoxicity, especially when used with other hepatoxic agents or if underlying liver disease is present. Asymptomatic elevations of liver enzymes, including alkaline phosphatase and bilirubin, occur in approximately 15% of patients, with frank hepatitis occurring in less than 1%. Asymptomatic elevations of liver enzymes and bilirubin should not necessarily prompt discontinuation of the drug. Asymptomatic elevation of aminotransferases greater than three times normal in a patient receiving both isoniazid and rifampin should prompt discontinuation of both drugs. Autoimmune thrombocytopenic purpura has been reported with rifampin and should also prompt discontinuation of the drug. When given intermittently, rifampin can produce a febrile, flulike syndrome, hemolysis, and renal failure. Rifampin is teratogenic in animals, but no data are available in humans. Rifampin should be used in pregnancy only when clearly indicated. Rifampin is excreted in breast milk. Rifampin may be used by children at a dosage of 10–20 mg/kg, not to exceed 600 mg/day. Overdosage of rifampin usually produces nausea, vomiting, lethargy, and hepatitis. Treatment includes gastric lavage, ingestion of activated charcoal, and forced diuresis. Rifampin is a potent inducer of drug metabolism. Rapid clearance of warfarin, corticosteroids, methadone, oral hypoglycemic agents, and oral contraceptives may occur. Appropriate adjustments in drug dosages may be necessary both when initiating and discontinuing rifampin.

DOSAGE

The usual adult dosage of rifampin is 600 mg/day. It is available in both oral and IV preparations.

CONCLUSION

Since its introduction in 1966, rifampin has become first-line therapy for mycobacterial disease. it remains one of the few bactericidal drugs that is generally well tolerated. As with all other antimycobacterial drugs, susceptibility of rifampin should be confirmed.

Ethambutol

Ethambutol remains a first-line agent for tuberculosis when drug resistance is suspected. Because it is bacteriostatic and not bactericidal, it is not included in initial regimens when drug susceptibility is expected (see Table 4-1). Ethambutol diffuses into Mycobacteria and inhibits the nucleic acid metabolism of growing organisms. It has no effect on nonproliferating Mycobacteria.

ANTIMICROBIAL ACTIVITY/INDICATIONS

Ethambutol is indicated for the treatment of pulmonary tuberculosis. Its most common role is as a replacement for isoniazid, rifampin, or pyrazinamide when one of these drugs cannot be tolerated or resistance to the drug is documented (see Table 4-2). Ethambutol may be used with other agents for the treatment of tuberculous meningitis even though it diffuses into the CSF poorly, even in the presence of inflammation. Ethambutol has no activity against fungi, viruses, or other bacteria.

PHARMACOKINETICS

Ethambutol is rapidly absorbed from the GI tract, with peak serum concentrations occurring 2–4 hours after administration. Ethambutol absorption is not influenced by food. Aluminum hydroxide containing antacids may delay and diminish the absorption of ethambutol. The drug is minimally metabolized by the liver and excreted in the urine, mostly in original form. Dosage adjustment with renal insufficiency is indicated.

ADVERSE EFFECTS AND CONTRAINDICATIONS

The most important toxic effect of ethambutol is retrobulbar neuritis, a dosage-related phenomenon. When ethambutol is used at the standard dosage of 15 mg/kg/day, the incidence is less than 1%.

A baseline ophthalmologic examination is indicated for all patients receiving ethambutol, but follow-up examinations are not indicated when the standard dosage is employed. Rather, because ocular symptoms often precede changes in visual acuity, patients should be warned to stop ethambutol if a change in vision occurs. The most common symptoms are blurry vision, central scotoma, and red-green color blindness. Constriction of peripheral fields has also been reported. Symptoms most commonly occur after 2 months of therapy and reverse after stopping the drug. When retrobulbar neuritis occurs, there are no discernible changes on ophthalmoscopy. In patients in whom there is some degree of visual impairment at baseline and evaluation of visual changes is difficult, ethambutol may not be the best drug if others are available. Similarly, because renal insufficiency can lead to high serum concentrations of ethambutol even when dosage is decreased, other agents should be considered in patients with impaired renal function. In retreatment regimens in which ethambutol is used at a dosage of 25 mg/kg/day, the incidence of optic neuritis increases to 5%. At the higher dosage, routine eye examinations are recommended.

The only other adverse reaction commonly reported with ethambutol is elevation of serum uric acid and precipitation of gout. Rarely, abdominal pain and nausea occur with the oral administration of ethambutol. Taking the drug with food usually relieves this problem. Ethambutol has no known drug interactions except for a decrease in absorption when taken with aluminum hydroxide antacids. Ethambutol is teratogenic in animals but has no known toxicity in pregnancy. Ethambutol is not recommended for children under age 13 years.

DOSAGE

For initial therapy, the recommended dosage of ethambutol is 15 mg/kg/day administered as a single oral dose. In retreatment regimens, the recommended dosage increases to 25 mg/kg/day during the first 2 months of therapy.

CONCLUSION

Ethambutol, although not a first-line drug for tuberculosis in routine cases, remains a first-line agent when resistant organisms are suspected, and it is considered the optimal replacement drug when isoniazid, rifampin, or pyrazinamide cannot be used. Ethambutol, at standard dosages, is very safe, with visual changes being the only symptom for which patients should be routinely questioned.

Ethionamide

Ethionamide is a second-line bacteriostatic drug for the treatment of *M. tuberculosis*. Its mechanism of action is the inhibition of mycolic acid synthesis. Patient intolerance often limits the drug's usefulness.

ANTIMICROBIAL ACTIVITY AND INDICATIONS

Ethionamide is indicated for all types of *M. tuberculosis* infections where first-line drugs have failed. It is also useful for empiric therapy when multiple drug-resistant organisms are probable (see Table 4-1).

PHARMACOKINETICS

Ethionamide is administered orally and yields peak plasma concentrations in 3 hours. It distributes well into the CSF. The medication is usually given with food to minimize GI intolerance, but it is unknown whether food or antacids decrease absorption of the drug. Ethionamide is extensively metabolized in the liver. The primary sulfoxide metabolite retains antituberculous activity. Less than 1% of unchanged drug is excreted in the urine.

ADVERSE EFFECTS AND CONTRAINDICATIONS

Nausea, vomiting, anorexia, and abdominal pain following an orally administered dose of ethionamide often limit its clinical usefulness. Sometimes these adverse effects can be decreased if the drug is given with food. Ethionamide can produce hepatitis similar to that seen with other antituberculous drugs. In fact, ethionamide may intensify the adverse effects of other antituberculous drugs, especially cycloserine. Hepatitis seems to occur more commonly in diabetics, and this drug may make management of diabetes more difficult.

Ethionamide is teratogenic in animals. It should probably not be used in pregnancy unless other alternative drugs are unavailable. Ethionamide may be used in children.

DOSAGE

The usual adult dosage is 500–1000 mg/day. Gastrointestinal intolerance may be decreased by giving up to 4 250-mg oral doses per day with food (see Table 4-3). The pediatric dosage is 10–20 mg/kg/day in divided doses, up to 750 mg/day.

CONCLUSION

Ethionamide is a second-line antituberculous drug that is usually very effective but often poorly tolerated. Its use will likely increase as more cases of multidrug-resistant organisms occur.

Kanamycin

Kanamycin is the aminoglycoside least often used for tuberculosis secondary to its significant toxicity. Like amikacin, streptomycin, and capreomycin, kanamycin is bactericidal. All aminoglycosides irreversibly bind to bacterial ribosomes, causing misreading of the genetic code, altered protein synthesis, and cell death.

ANTIMICROBIAL ACTIVITY AND INDICATIONS

Kanamycin has significant antimicrobial activity against many gram-negative organisms and some strains of staphylococci, as well as *M. tuberculosis*. The drug's primary indication is in the treatment of organisms resistant to multiple drugs, including other aminoglycosides. Cross-resistance between kanamycin and other aminoglycosides is variable, although all share a common mechanism of action. This phenomenon has not been explained.

PHARMACOKINETICS

Aminoglycosides as a group have similar pharmacokinetics. All are poorly absorbed orally. Systemic infections require parenteral administration. All distribute widely in the extracellular space and are minimally protein bound. Aminoglycosides are excreted almost completely in the urine in unchanged form. No aminoglycoside metabolites have ever been identified. Major dosage adjustment is necessary in renal failure.

ADVERSE EFFECTS AND CONTRAINDICATIONS

Kanamycin appears to have more ototoxicity than the other aminoglycosides. Monthly audiometry is recommended for patients receiving this drug. Vestibular toxicity is rare with kanamycin. The nephrotoxicity of aminoglycosides is caused by acute tubular necrosis. Streptomycin appears to have less renal toxicity than the other aminoglycosides. The renal toxicity of kanamycin, capreomycin, and amikacin is probably equivalent. Serum creatinine should be monitored in patients receiving these drugs. An aminoglycoside may not be the best drug for patients with preexisting renal or auditory impairment. Similarly, aminoglycosides can potentiate muscle weakness in patients with neuromuscular disorders and should be used with caution in this patient population. They may potentiate the adverse effects of other nephrotoxic, ototoxic, and neuromuscular blocking drugs. Aminoglycosides are removed by both peritoneal dialysis and hemodialysis. The drugs should probably not be used in pregnancy because cases of total bilateral irreversible congenital deafness have been reported in newborns whose mothers received streptomycin. Aminoglycosides may be used in children. The elderly appear to be at increased risk for the adverse effects of kanamycin and the other aminoglycosides.

DOSAGE

The dosage of kanamycin is 15 mg/kg to a maximum of 1 g, administered IM, 5 days/week.

CONCLUSION

Kanamycin is an aminoglycoside whose use in treating tuberculosis is limited by its significant ototoxicity and nephrotoxicity. The drug should be reserved for patients with organisms in whom sensitivity to kanamycin and resistance to the other aminoglycosides have been documented.

Clofazimine

Clofazimine, also known as lamprene, is a second-line bactericidal antituberculous drug. Its main use is in the treatment of leprosy and *Mycobacterium avium-intracellulare* (MAI) infections. The drug binds to myobacterial DNA and inhibits cell growth.

ANTIMICROBIAL ACTIVITY AND INDICATIONS

Clofazimine has no known activity against nonmycobacterial organisms. It has the most activity against *Mycobacterium leprae*. The drug also exerts antiinflammatory properties in leprosy patients through an unknown mechanism. Clofazimine has limited activity against *M. tuberculosis*. It should be used to treat tuberculosis only when drug-resistant organisms are probable and local drug-resistance patterns indicate that organisms will be sensitive to it (see Table 4-1). Recently, clofazimine has been used in regimens to treat disseminated MAI infections in AIDS patients. In this setting, it has shown efficacy in reducing the symptoms of MAI bacteremia, mainly fever and weight loss. Clofazimine should never be used as monotherapy for any mycobacterial infection.

PHARMACOKINETICS

Clofazimine is not well absorbed from the GI tract. Absorption is improved if the drug is taken with food. Clofazimine is highly lipophilic and taken up avidly by the tissues, especially adipose and the reticuloendothelial system. Its half-life is several weeks. The precise metabolism and excretion of clofazimine are not known.

SIDE EFFECTS AND CONTRAINDICATIONS

Clofazimine discolors skin and body fluids from pink to black in most patients. Skin discoloration may take years to resolve after the conclusion of therapy. Severe abdominal symptoms may occur after an oral dose. Splenic infarction, bowel obstruction, and GI bleeding have been reported. Clofazimine has not been shown to be teratogenic but does discolor the skin of the fetus. It is excreted in breast milk. Clofazimine has been given successfully to children, but safety and efficacy in this population have not been established.

DOSAGE

The usual adult dosage of clofazimine is 100–300 mg PO, once per day.

CONCLUSION

Clofazimine, a drug used primarily in the past to treat leprosy, is now part of a standard regimen to treat disseminated MAI infections in patients with AIDS. Its use in the treatment of drug-resistant tuberculosis will likely increase as more virulent organisms are encountered.

Ofloxacin

Ofloxacin (Floxin) was the third fluoroquinolone marketed in the United States. Since its release in 1991, it has become a second-line agent for the treatment of *M. tuberculosis*. The drug's mechanism of action is the inhibition of bacterial DNA gyrase.

ANTIMICROBIAL ACTIVITY AND INDICATIONS

Ofloxacin has various clinically approved uses against many gram-positive and gram-negative bacteria. In vitro studies have shown it to be quite active against *M. tuberculosis* [29]. Ofloxacin's in vitro activity against other species of *Mycobacteria* has not been as good [39]. Ofloxacin has not been approved for use against *Mycobacteria*. Like the other drugs in Table 4-3, however, ofloxacin is indicated for the treatment of tuberculosis when first-line drugs have failed or when multiple-drug-resistant organisms are probable (see Table 4-1).

PHARMACOKINETICS

Oral ofloxacin is almost completely absorbed. It is minimally metabolized, with approximately 75% of each dose being excreted unchanged in the urine. Ofloxacin has a large volume of distribution. High tissue levels are found in lung, liver, kidney, and prostate. Cerebrospinal fluid levels have not been adequately studied. Ofloxacin appears to penetrate well into tuberculous pleural effusions [45] and atelectatic lung [31].

CLINICAL TRIALS

Ofloxacin's in vitro activity against *M. tuberculosis* has been established. In vivo studies have concentrated on the use of ofloxacin in treatment failures. Ofloxacin has been found to be useful in some patients who initially failed conventional therapy [14, 23, 31]. One study showed that a regimen including ofloxacin produced sputum conversion in 13 of 22 patients with multidrug-resistant tuberculosis [45].

ADVERSE EFFECTS AND CONTRAINDICATIONS

Nausea, diarrhea, headache, dizziness, and insomnia are the most common adverse reactions to ofloxacin, but all are rare (less than 5% incidence). All quinolones, including ofloxacin, cause cartilage erosion in young experimental animals. For this reason, use of this drug is contraindicated in children, pregnant women, and lactating mothers. Ofloxacin has been reported to potentiate the anticoagulant affects of warfarin. Unlike ciprofloxacin, it does not appear to increase serum theophylline concentrations. Calcium, aluminum, magnesium, iron, and zinc containing compounds may interfere with the absorption of ofloxacin.

DOSAGE

The usual adult dosage of ofloxacin is 400 mg bid. It is available in oral and IV forms.

CONCLUSION

While not yet approved for the treatment of mycobacterial disease, ofloxacin may be a potentially useful second-line drug in the treatment of multidrug-resistant tuberculosis. It appears to be very safe and well tolerated.

Rifabutin

Rifabutin, formerly known as ansamycin, in an investigational antimycobacterial drug available through the CDC. This compound, chemically related to rifampin, has mainly been used for the treatment of MAI infections in AIDS patients. Recent work suggests that rifabutin is a promising second-line drug for the treatment of tuberculosis.

ANTIMICROBIAL ACTIVITY AND INDICATIONS

Rifabutin has a broad spectrum of activity in vitro against many gram-positive, gram-negative, and acid-fast organisms. Rifabutin appears to be more active in vitro against *M. tuberculosis* than rifampin. Moreover, many rifampin-resistant strains of *M. tuberculosis* are sensitive to rifabutin. Rifabutin appears to have even greater activity in vitro against nontuberculous acid-fast bacilli, particularly MAI. Finally, rifabutin has been shown to inhibit replication of the HIV virus in tissue culture.

PHARMACOKINETICS

Rifabutin is rapidly absorbed from the GI tract. Its absorption does not appear to be affected by food. Peak serum levels occur 4 hours after oral administration of a 300-mg dose, with measurable amounts of the drug present in serum 24 hours after ingestion. Rifabutin is taken up by all tissues and appears to concentrate in the lung, where levels are 5–10 times higher than those in the plasma. Like rifampin, the drug is metabolized by deacetylation. Two primary metabolites have been identified, one of which retains antimicrobial activity. The drug is excreted in both the urine and the bile. Whether dosage adjustment is necessary in patients with kidney or liver failure is unknown, but most patients with significant abnormalities of hepatic or renal function have received half the usual dosage.

CLINICAL TRIALS

Between October 1983 and September 1985, the CDC provided rifabutin to 811 patients with life-threatening mycobacterial diseases — the majority MAI infections associated with AIDS. Forty-seven patients had multidrug-resistant tuberculosis with organisms sensitive to rifabutin in vitro. Although definitive statements concerning drug efficacy are not possible from this trial because there was no control group, the authors demonstrated improved trends in survival in patients receiving 300 mg of rifabutin versus patients receiving 150 mg of the drug. No separate survival statistics are given for the group of patients with tuberculosis. The sputum conversion rate for patients with tuberculosis was 35%, with no difference found between the two doses of rifabutin [34]. A study in Hong Kong of patients with multidrug-resistant tuberculosis found rifabutin to be of limited value [13]. Only two of the patients in the study had rifabutin-sensitive organisms. Both initially responded to therapy, but resistance to rifabutin rapidly emerged. A recent study in France found rifabutin to be more promising [37]. In this study, all patients had rifampin- and isoniazid-resistant organisms that were susceptible to rifabutin. Of the patients who received a regimen containing rifabutin for at least 12 months, over 50% had sputum conversion. Many of the patients in this group were also receiving a quinolone.

Between October 1983 and January 1988, the CDC also provided rifabutin to 406 patients with severe pulmonary MAI infections who had failed standard therapy. These patients did not have disseminated disease. The majority did have underlying lung disease but no other chronic medical condition, though no specific information on HIV status is provided. The remaining drugs used to treat each patient were left to the discretion of the treating physician. Although high-dosage rifabutin was found to correlate with sputum conversion as opposed to a lower dosage of the drug, no survival benefit was found. The authors concluded that the use of rifabutin does not have a significant effect on the outcome of pulmonary MAI infections [34].

The treatment of MAI infections in patients with AIDS is discouraging. The goal of therapy usually is not cure but an improvement in symptoms, particularly weight loss and fever, and prolonged survival. In this regard, rifabutin appears to be a useful drug. A regimen containing rifabutin, clofazimine, ethambutol, and isoniazid has been shown to improve symptoms and sterilize blood cultures in AIDS patients with disseminated and respiratory MAI infections [1]. A recent study in France using the same regimen had similar results [15].

ADVERSE EFFECTS AND CONTRAINDICATIONS

Rifabutin, like rifampin, discolors all body fluids and may permanently stain contact lenses. Gastrointestinal upset following an oral dose may occur but is uncommon. Hypersensitivity reactions have also been reported. Bone marrow suppression causing neutropenia or thrombocytopenia and hepatotoxicity are the most serious, commonly seen adverse effects. Both usually resolve with cessation of therapy. Autoimmune hemolytic anemia has also been reported. Thus, CBC and liver enzymes should be monitored in patients receiving the drug. Rifabutin, unlike rifampin, does not significantly induce catabolic enzymes and alter the pharmacokinetics of other drugs, with the possible exception of an increase in the metabolism of corticosteroids. Adverse reactions of all types seem to be more common in AIDS patients with disseminated MAI infections [34].

DOSAGE

The usual adult dosage of rifabutin is 300 mg PO once per day. In patients with significantly abnormal renal, hepatic, or hematopoietic function, the dosage should be halved.

CONCLUSION

Rifabutin, a new antimycobacterial drug related to rifampin, shows promise as a second-line therapy for multidrug-resistant tuberculosis. It also may have a role in improving the symptoms of patients with disseminated MAI infections secondary to AIDS. Its usefulness for the treatment of severe pulmonary MAI infections in HIV-negative patients appears less hopeful. Controlled clinical trials using the drug in all three patient populations are needed.

Cycloserine

Cycloserine is a broad-spectrum bacteriostatic antimicrobial; it is produced by a strain of *Streptomyces orchidaceus* and can also be synthesized. It exists as a water-soluble white powder, which is stable at alkaline pH, and acts as an antagonist of D-alanine, thus inhibiting mycobacterial cell wall synthesis. Cycloserine is taken orally, and despite being produced by *Streptomyces*, is unrelated to the aminoglycosides and thus exhibits no cross-resistance with these agents.

ANTIMICROBIAL ACTIVITY AND INDICATIONS

Cycloserine, an effective antimycobacterial agent, is indicated for use against susceptible organisms causing active pulmonary or extrapulmonary tuberculosis only after initial therapy has failed. Cycloserine should be used with other antituberculous drugs, not as the sole agent.

PHARMACOKINETICS

After oral administration, cycloserine is rapidly absorbed from the GI tract, achieving peak blood concentrations in 4–8 hours. The drug is widely distributed in all body fluids and tissues, including the CSF. Approximately 65% of a given dose is excreted unchanged in the urine by 72 hours; thus, urinary tract tuberculosis can be treated with normal dosages. The remainder of a given dose is metabolized to unknown substances.

ADVERSE EFFECTS AND CONTRAINDICATIONS

Abnormalities of the CNS are the most important adverse effects of the use of cycloserine; both neurological and psychic disturbances are seen. Neurologic reactions include seizures, headache, tremor, dysarthria, vertigo, paresis, or even coma; the use of ethionamide or isoniazid with cycloserine can potentiate these effects. To prevent these neurologic complications, large dosages of pyridoxine (100 mg 3 times daily) can be given with cycloserine.

Psychic abnormalities are also quite common with administration of cycloserine, ranging from irritability and nervousness to actual psychotic episodes, seen in about 10% of treated individuals. These abnormalities are occasionally related to supertherapeutic serum drug levels (seen with dosages in excess of 500 mg daily) but usually are unpredictable. In a patient who develops a psychotic reaction, the drug should be stopped immediately and the patient watched closely; suicide has been reported in occasional cases. Most psychotic reactions resolve within 2 weeks; recovery can be hastened by giving large dosages of chlorpromazine.

Other less common side effects include congestive heart failure, reported in patients receiving 1–1.5g/daily; allergy, not dosage related; skin rash; and elevated serum transaminases.

Cycloserine is thus contraindicated in patients with hypersensitivity to cycloserine; known seizure disorders; alcohol use; depression, anxiety, or psychosis; or renal insufficiency. Also, in patients with reduced renal function, blood levels should be checked at least weekly.

DOSAGE

Patients should be started on a dosage of 250 mg q12h for the first 2 weeks. If tolerated, the dosage can be increased every few days by 250 mg, to obtain a final dosage of 500 mg–1g daily, in divided doses. During therapy, the blood levels should be monitored weekly if the patient has renal insufficiency, is receiving greater than 500 mg daily, or shows signs of toxicity; a level greater than 30 μg/ml is associated with higher toxicity.

The recommended dosage for children is 10–20 mg/kg/day, the total daily dosage also not to exceed 1 g.

CONCLUSIONS

Cycloserine is an effective antituberculous drug used in combination with other agents in the treatment of active pulmonary or extrapulmonary tuberculosis caused by susceptible organisms, after primary therapy has failed. Its use is limited, however, by its CNS toxicity.

Paraaminosalicylic Acid

Paraaminosalicylic acid (PAS) is available in its acidic form or as its sodium salt, aminosalicylate sodium. It is thought to be a selective inhibitor of the production of paraaminobenzoic acid in *M. tuberculosis*, secondary to the similar structures of PAS and paraaminobenzoic acid.

ANTIMICROBIAL ACTIVITY AND INDICATIONS

Paraaminosalicylic acid is weakly bacteriostatic against *M. tuberculosis* but is helpful in preventing the onset of resistance of the tubercle bacillus to isoniazid or streptomycin. It was widely used for this reason before ethambutol became available and is now used in combination with other antituberculous agents against susceptible organisms in the retreatment of tuberculosis, after initial therapy has failed. It is also used in children under age 2 years as a substitute for ethambutol.

PHARMACOKINETICS

Paraaminosalicylic acid is rapidly absorbed after oral administration, the free acid slightly slower than the sodium salt. The drug is widely distributed in the body, obtaining high concentrations in pleural and caseous tissue and low concentrations in the CSF. Greater than 50% of the drug is acetylated in the liver, and 80% is renally excreted as free acid or metabolites. The half-life of PAS is approximately 1 hour.

ADVERSE EFFECTS AND CONTRAINDICATIONS

The two major reasons that patients discontinue PAS are hypersensitivity to the drug and GI side effects. Approximately 4% of patients develop hypersensitivity to PAS, which can become severe. Symptoms of hypersensitivity include fever, skin rash, leukopenia, agranulocytosis, thrombocytopenia, hemolytic anemia, hepatitis, and vasculitis. Gastrointestinal side effects are more common, seen in 15% of patients taking PAS. They include nausea and vomiting, diarrhea, and abdominal pain. In addition, PAS can decrease the absorption of digoxin and vitamin B^{12}, possibly necessitating an increase of the digoxin dosage in patients taking digoxin, and parenteral adminstration of vitamin B^{12}.

DOSAGE

Paraaminosalicylic acid usually given as the sodium salt, is administered at a dosage of 150–200 mg/kg daily in 2 or 3 divided doses with meals. The maximum total daily dosage is 12–16 g. In children, dosages of 200–300 mg/kg/day can be given in 2 or 3 divided doses.

CONCLUSIONS

Paraaminosalicylic acid is a bacteriostatic antituberculous agent used in combination with other agents in the retreatment of tuberculosis that has failed primary treatment. In addition, PAS inhibits the development of resistance of the tubercle to isoniazid and streptomycin.

Capreomycin

Capreomycin, a polypeptide antimicrobial with four poorly characterized microbiologically active components, is isolated from

Streptomyces capreolus. It is water soluble, almost colorless in solution, and supplied as its disulfate salt.

ANTIMICROBIAL ACTIVITY AND INDICATIONS

Capreomycin is indicated for the retreatment of pulmonary tuberculosis caused by susceptible strains, if primary therapy has failed, or if the primary agents (isoniazid, rifampin, ethambutol, and pyrazinamide) cannot be used secondary to either toxicity or resistant strains. Capreomycin, which is effective against *M. tuberculosis*, *M. bovis*, and most strains of *M. kansasii*, should always be used in combination with other antituberculosis drugs. Frequent cross-resistance has been reported between capreomycin and kanamycin and neomycin; however, there is no known cross-resistance between capreomycin and isoniazid, PAS, cycloserine, streptomycin, ethionamide, or ethambutol.

PHARMACOKINETICS

Capreomycin must be adminstered parenterally because it has insignificant absorption after an oral dose. Peak serum concentrations occur 1–2 hours after an IM injection of 1 g, and approximately 50% of the drug is excreted unchanged in the urine in 12 hours in patients with normal renal function. Capreomycin is not significantly metabolized.

ADVERSE EFFECTS AND CONTRAINDICATIONS

Capreomycin can cause a number of side effects, including nephrotoxicity, ototoxicity, hepatic and hematologic abnormalities, and hypersensitivity reactions. The most important of these is the renal toxicity; patients can develop elevation of BUN levels, decreased creatinine clearance, and albuminuria. In 722 patients treated with capreomycin, 36% had an elevation of their BUN to greater than 20 mg/100 ml; however, less than 10% of patients need to stop therapy because of renal toxicity. Also, the renal abnormalities caused by taking capreomycin usually return to normal with cessation of the drug. Fatal toxic nephritis was seen in one patient with tuberculosis and portal cirrhosis who was treated with capreomycin (1g) and PAS daily for 1 month; autopsy revealed resolving acute tubular necrosis. Finally, hypokalemia is a relatively rare complication of using capreomycin, necessitating the monitoring of blood potassium levels.

Of patients treated with capreomycin, 11% developed subclinical hearing loss; in 3%, the loss was clinically apparent. In some of the patients, the hearing loss was reversible; in those with permanent deficits, the hearing loss was not progressive following the cessation of the drug. In addition, tinnitus and vertigo have been described. Therefore, it is suggested that patients have audiometric measurements and their vestibular function evaluated before and during therapy.

For these reasons, capreomycin use is rare in patients with renal insufficiency; in addition, the drug should not be used in combination with other nephrotoxic or ototoxic agents, such as gentamycin. Patients to be started on capreomycin should have baseline laboratory data checked before treatment begins and weekly checks of their serum chemistries, urinalysis, and CBC.

Additionally, patients on capreomycin in combination with other antituberculous agents can develop abnormal liver function tests, although to what extent this is due to the capreomycin is unknown. It is recommended that patients on capreomycin have their liver function bilirubin checked at regular intervals. Greater than 50% of patients taking daily capreomycin have eosinophilia, and leukocytosis and leukopenia have also been described. There are rare occurrences of thrombocytopenia. Finally, cases of hypersensitivity to capreomycin, causing fever and rash, are uncommon and not severe.

DOSAGE

Capreomycin is given only by deep IM injection; it is dissolved in 2 ml of sodium chloride or sterile water and allowed to sit for 2–3 minutes before injection until completely dissolved. The initial dosage is 15 mg/kg (approximately 1 g) daily for 2–4 weeks, followed by the same dosage 2 or 3 times a week for 6–12 months or even longer. The dosage has to be decreased in patients with a decreased creatinine clearance.

CONCLUSION

Capreomycin is an effective antituberculous agent used in the retreatment of pulmonary tuberculosis in combination with other agents. Its use is limited by its nephrotoxicity and ototoxicity and by the fact that it needs to be administered parenterally.

Pyrazinamide

Pyrazinamide (PZA), an amide derivative of pyrazine-2-carboxylic acid, is either bacteriostatic or bactericidal against *M. tuberculosis*, depending on the drug concentrations at the site of infection. In vitro, PZA exhibits antituberculous activity only at an acid pH. For the drug to become active in vivo, PZA has to be converted by the enzyme pyrazinamidase, made by susceptible strains of *M. tuberculosis*, to the active form of the drug, pyrazinoic acid. Therefore, the susceptibility of the tubercle bacillus to PZA correlates with the activity of the enzyme.

ANTIMICROBIAL ACTIVITY AND INDICATIONS

In the past, PZA was considered a second-line agent in the treatment of tuberculosis; it is now used in combination with other antituberculous agents in the initial therapy against active tuberculosis, caused by susceptible strains. The current CDC recommendations are to use 6 months of the isoniazid and rifampin, with the addition of PZA for the first 2 months, in the initial treatment of active, susceptible tuberculosis [3]. PZA can also be used against active tuberculosis after intitial treatment when other agents have failed.

PHARAMACOKINETICS

Peak serum concentrations of PZA are achieved about 2 hours after an oral dose, and the drug is widely distributed throughout the body, including the CSF. The peak levels of the active form of the drug, pyrazinoic acid, are higher than that of PZA and occur between 4 and 8 hours after the dose.

PZA is metabolized in the liver to its active form, pyrazinoic acid; this is then converted to hydroxypyrazinoic acid, its major excretory product. Most of the excretion occurs through the kidney; 70% of an oral dose is lost in the urine within 24 hours. Of the oral dose, 3% is excreted unchanged, and 40% is lost in the urine as pyrazinoic acid.

ADVERSE EFFECTS AND CONTRAINDICATIONS

The most important side effect of PZA is hepatotoxicity, which is probably dosage related. In the past, when PZA was used in combination with isoniazid at dosages of 40–70 mg/kg, the incidence of hepatotoxicity was about 14%. This led to PZA's being used only as a second-line drug in the treatment of tuberculosis. The current dosage of PZA, 20–30 mg/kg, is not associated with an increased incidence of hepatotoxicity when used with isoniazid and rifampin. Also, the hepatotoxicity caused by PZA is usually not serious, especially when the drug is used for only 2 months.

The most common side effect of PZA is a polyarthralgia, which occurs in up to 40% of patients on the drug. In addition, treatment with PZA often causes asymptomatic hyperuricemia by inhibiting the renal excretion of urates. If symptoms of gout accompany the hyperuricemia, allopurinol or probenicid can be given to the patient, or the PZA can be stopped.

Other adverse effects caused by PZA include hypersensitivity reactions such as fever, rash, pruritis, or urticaria; hematologic abnormalities, including thrombocytopenia and sideroblastic anemia; nausea and vomiting; and porphyria. It is suggested that patients have a CBC, urinalysis, and serum chemistry profile (including liver function tests) before starting therapy and at least monthly during therapy.

DOSAGE

The current recommendations are a daily dosage of 20–30 mg/kg, the total not to exceed 2 g daily. A newer regimen, designed to improve patient compliance, is to give 50–70 mg/kg twice weekly.

CONCLUSION

Pyrazinamide is an important antimycobacterial drug, used in the initial treatment of active tuberculosis, in combination with other first-line agents against susceptible organisms. Its use with isoniazid and rifampin has allowed shortening of the conventional 9-

month regimen to 6 months, with similar results. It is also used in the retreatment of tuberculosis after other first-line agents have failed.

Isoniazid

Isoniazid (isonicotinic acid hydrazide, INH) is a synthetic antimycobacterial agent that is bactericidal against both intracellular and extracellular actively growing tubercle bacillus. It works by interfering with lipid and nucleic acid synthesis. It is water soluble and exists either as colorless or white crystals or as a white crystalline powder.

ANTIMICROBIAL ACTIVITY AND INDICATIONS

Isoniazid is the mainstay of therapy against tuberculosis. It is active against all forms of tuberculosis caused by susceptible organisms and is used for both preventive therapy and treatment of active tuberculosis. Preventive therapy is used in two situations: to prevent new infection and to prevent already infected patients from progressing to active tuberculosis. In the first case, therapy is given to a patient with a negative skin test who had close contact with an active case of tuberculosis. In the second case, prophylaxis is used in a patient already infected with the tubercle bacillus, as evidenced by a positive skin test, without signs of active tuberculosis (i.e., no active disease on the chest x ray). The chance of developing active disease without prophylaxis in an infected patient is about 5% for normal patients, and up to 40% in immunocompromised patients. Therefore, preventive therapy is currently recommended for the following patients, in order of priority [3]:

1. HIV-positive patients with a positive skin test.
2. Close contacts of patients with active pulmonary tuberculosis.
3. Patients with recent skin test conversion (within 2 years).
4. Patients with a history of tuberculosis who were not adequately treated.
5. Patients with a positive skin test and chest x-ray changes comparable with old tuberculosis (need to rule out active disease with negative sputum cultures and unchanging chest x ray).
6. Patients with a positive skin test at increased risk of progressing to active tuberculosis — those with silicosis, diabetes mellitus, hematologic and reticuloendothelial diseases such as leukemia and Hodgkin's disease, end-stage renal disease, chronic undernutrition, and those on long-term corticosteroids or immunosuppressive therapy.
7. All patients under age 35 years with a positive skin test.

Isoniazid is also very important in the treatment of active tuberculosis. In the past, INH was used in combination with rifampin or ethambutol for 18 months or longer, with good results. However, there were problems of increased cost and drug toxicity and decreased patient compliance with this regimen. Much shorter courses are now used, including 9- and 6-month regimens. The 9-month regimen of INH and rifampin has achieved good results against susceptible pulmonary and nonpulmonary tuberculosis. If resistance is suspected against INH, ethambutol can be added to the regimen. The 6-month course has also achieved good results for pulmonary tuberculosis. It consists of INH, rifampin, and PZA for the first 2 months, followed by 4 additional months of INH and rifampin [3]. This regimen is modified for patients who are HIV positive; INH, rifampin, and PZA are given for the first 2 months followed by INH and rifampin for 7 additional months (6 months if three negative cultures are obtained). In addition, ethambutol is added to this regimen if there is CNS involvement, if the tuberculosis is disseminated, or if drug resistance to INH is suspected.

PHARMACOKINETICS

Isoniazid can be given orally or parenterally. The oral dosage is rapidly absorbed and achieves peak serum concentrations within 2 hours; levels fall to about 50% by 6 hours. Food decreases the amount and rate of absorption. The drug is widely distributed in all bodily tissues and fluids and also crosses the placental barrier and is found in breast milk. Of a given dose of INH, approximately 50–70% is excreted in the urine within 24 hours, either unchanged or as metabolites.

The metabolism of INH occurs by enzymatic acetylation and dehydrazination; its half-life depends on the rate of acetylation. This rate is genetically determined; about 50% of blacks and Caucasians are "slow acetylators" and the remainder are "rapid acetylators." Asians and Eskimos are rapid acetylators. The effectiveness of INH does not seem to depend on the rate of acetylation; however, there may be higher blood levels of the drug in slow acetylators, possibly causing an increase of toxic effects, especially if there is concurrent decrease in renal function.

ADVERSE EFFECTS AND CONTRAINDICATIONS

The two major side effects caused by INH are hepatotoxicity and peripheral neuropathy. Isoniazid hepatitis can be severe or even fatal, can occur at any time during treatment, and is age related. The risk of hepatitis is about 3 per 1000 between the ages of 20 and 34 years and is 8 per 1000 for patients over age 65 years. The risk is also increased with daily consumption of alcohol. Of patients on INH, 10–20% will have asymptomatic elevations of their serum transaminase, usually in the first 4–6 months of therapy, but this can occur at any time. Most of the time, the abnormalities return to normal without the need to discontinue the drug, although some physicians will stop the INH if the transaminase is elevated during prophylactic (preventive therapy).

Patients on INH should be taught to look for and report early symptoms of hepatitis, such as fatigue, malaise, nausea, or vomiting. By stopping the drug at this point, patients rarely progress to actual hepatitis; if hepatitis does occur, the mortality can approach 7%. Patients should be seen and have liver function (AST, ALT, B. I. Rubin, Alk-Phos.) tests checked monthly. If INH does need to be discontinued, it can be restarted after the abnormalities return to normal, beginning with a very small dosage and gradually increasing the dosage toward normal. If any recurrent liver abnormalities occur, discontinue the drug immediately.

The other major side effect seen with INH is peripheral neuropathy, thought secondary to pyridoxine deficiency, which is probably caused by competition with pyridoxal phosphate for the enzyme apotryptophanase. This side effect is dosage related and is seen more often in the malnourished, "slow acetylators," and in patients more likely to have peripheral neuropathy, such as alcoholics and diabetics. It can be treated with pyridoxine 50–100 mg PO daily; some clinicians give 10–25 mg daily as prophylaxis.

There are many other adverse effects of INH. Seizures are seen in less than 1% of patients taking INH; however, the drug is not contraindicated in patients with an underlying seizure disorder. Optic neuropathy and toxic psychosis have also been reported; it is recommended to have regular ophthalmologic examinations even in the absence of visual symptoms. In addition, INH can cause GI effects such as nausea and vomiting; hematological abnormalities, including agranulocytosis, hemolytic, aplastic, or sideroblastic anemia, and thrombocytopenia; hypersensitivity reactions; arthralgias and arthritis; and various endocrine and metabolic disorders. There are reports that INH can be embryocidal in rats, although there are no known congenital abnormalities caused by this drug. Therefore, INH should be used only when absolutely necessary in pregnancy.

INH has numerous drug interactions. Concurrent alcohol or rifampin intake causes an increased risk of hepatitis, while INH can enhance the action of phenytoin and oral anticoagulants. Cycloserine used in combination with INH can cause an increase of CNS side effects.

DOSAGE

INH is given at a dosage of 300 mg/day orally for chemoprophylaxis. In the treatment of active tuberculosis, INH is given with other antituberculous drugs at a dosage of 5 mg/kg, up to 300 mg daily. If less frequent dosing is desired, 15 mg/kg can be given twice a week, each dose not exceeding 900 mg. In rare cases when INH cannot be given orally, up to 300 mg can be given parenterally daily. In children, a dosage of 10 mg/kg/day is used for preventive therapy, and 10–20 mg/kg/day is used in the treatment of active tuberculosis. As in adults, the total daily dosage should not exceed 300 mg. Finally, pyridoxine, at dosages of 6–50mg/day, is recommended to be given to patients who are malnourished or have a greater risk of developing neuropathy.

CONCLUSION

Isoniazid is probably the most important drug in the treatment of tuberculosis, being active against all forms of the disease caused by susceptible organisms. It is used alone in preventive treatment or in combination with other antituberculous drugs in the treatment of active tuberculosis. The two major side effects of INH are hepatitis and neuropathy; however, the drug can be used safely with proper monitoring and patient education.

Amikacin

Amikacin sulfate, a derivative of kanamycin, is a semisynthetic aminoglycoside. It exists as a clear to light-straw-colored solution intended for parenteral administration.

ANTIMICROBIAL ACTIVITY AND INDICATIONS

In addition to its activity against gram-negative organisms, amikacin has similar antituberculous activity to that of streptomycin and kanamycin. It can be used in place of these agents in the retreatment of tuberculosis resistant to the primary agents. Amikacin has also been shown to have activity against *M. avium complex* (MAC) in vitro [19]. Recent studies suggest that amikacin-containing regimens also have activity against MAC in patients with AIDS [8, 12].

PHARMACOKINETICS

Amikacin can be given IM or IV; approximately 85–90% of the dose is excreted in the urine within the first 8 hours and 94%–98% by 24 hours. The mean serum half-life of amikacin is 2 hours, it is minimally protein bound, and its major route of excretion is through the kidney. Adequate amounts of the drug are found in the following after a normal dose: bone, heart, gallbladder, lung, urine, bile, sputum, and pleural and synovial fluids. The serum half-life is increased in patients with renal failure.

CLINICAL TRIALS

M. avium complex in AIDS patients is very difficult to treat; no studies have shown good long-term results. Most treatment regimens for this disease have been reported to give only a short-term clinical response [1, 12]. A recent study reports on five patients treated with a regimen of amikacin, clofazimine, rifampin, ethambutol, and ciprofloxacin [8]. Four of the five patients had only short-term responses and died of other complications of AIDS; the fifth patient had a complete response and was free of disease for a 25-month follow-up period.

ADVERSE EFFECTS AND CONTRAINDICATIONS

Like other aminoglycosides, the major side effects caused by amikacin are ototoxicity, nephrotoxicity, and neuromuscular blockade. The frequency of these effects is increased in patients with preexisting renal insufficiency, with the use of other nephrotoxic or ototoxic drugs, or with prolonged use or excessive dosages.

Amikacin can cause both hearing loss and loss of balance, although hearing loss is more common. High-frequency deafness is usually seen before clinical hearing loss is noticed. In the kidney, amikacin can cause an elevation of the serum creatinine, azotemia, oliguria, casts, and proteinuria, but these effects usually reverse when the drug is stopped. Also, amikacin has been reported to cause acute muscular paralysis and even apnea. Additionally, rash, fever, headache, nausea and vomiting, anemia, hypotension, arthralgia, eosinophilia, and tremor are rare side effects. Aminoglycosides have been reported to cause fetal damage; therefore, the benefit of this drug in pregnancy should be weighed against its potential risk to the fetus.

To prevent some of these adverse effects, patients should be well hydrated before beginning therapy, renal function should be monitored before and during therapy, and the correct dosing should be used. Serum drug levels (peak and trough) should be followed to ensure appropriate dosing. If there is a progressive increase in azotemia or a decrease in urinary output, the drug should be discontinued. Finally, amikacin should be used with care in patients with neuromuscular disorders, as the drug could cause an increase in muscle weakness.

DOSAGE

Patients with normal renal function can be treated with a daily dosage of 15 mg/kg in 2 or 3 divided doses at equally divided intervals. In patients with a decreased creatinine clearance, a loading dosage of 7.5 mg/kg can be given, followed by a decreased maintenance dosage. The maintenance dosage should be decreased in proportion to the decrease of the creatinine clearance (maintenance dosage q/12h = patient's creatinine clearance/normal creatinine clearance × loading dosage). This should be adjusted by changing the dosage or the time interval according to the serum peak and trough levels. The normal duration of treatment in bacterial infections is 7–10 days; this is increased in the treatment of mycobacterial infections. The duration of therapy in patients with MAC ranges from 30–90 days, the length usually limited by nephrotoxicity or ototoxicity.

Children receive the same dosage as adults; for neonates, a loading dosage of 10 mg/kg is given, followed by a maintenance dosage of 7.5 mg/kg q12h.

CONCLUSION

Amikacin can be used in combination with other agents in the retreatment of tuberculosis (in place of streptomycin or kanamycin, depending on local drug resistance patterns) when there is resistance to the primary agents. It has also been shown to be partially effective as part of a multidrug regimen in the treatment of MAC in AIDS patients. Its use is limited by its ototoxicity and nephrotoxicity and because it needs to be administered parenterally.

Streptomycin

Streptomycin, an aminoglycoside antimicrobial, is derived from *Streptomyces griseus*. Although not often used today, it was the first antimicrobial with proved efficacy against tuberculosis. Streptomycin has to be given IM and is thought to work by an action on the bacterial ribosome, inhibiting protein synthesis.

ANTIMICROBIAL ACTIVITY AND INDICATIONS

Streptomycin is a bactericidal antimycobacterial agent effective against extracellular tubercle bacillus. Although for many years thought of as a first-line agent, the drug is currently used as a second-line agent in the retreatment of tuberculosis caused by susceptible organisms, in combination with other antituberculous agents. It is especially useful when a parenteral agent is needed.

PHARMACOKINETICS

After IM administration, streptomycin is rapidly absorbed, reaching peak serum concentrations in 30–60 minutes. There are negligble drug levels after an oral dose. Streptomycin is about 35% protein bound and is found in all organs except the brain, obtaining high concentrations in pleural cavities and fluid. The drug does not penetrate into the CSF. There is virtually no metabolism of streptomycin; it is excreted unchanged through the kidneys by glomerular filtration. The half-life is approximately 5 hours.

ADVERSE EFFECTS AND CONTRAINDICATIONS

As is the case with other aminoglycosides, the major toxicities of streptomycin are ototoxicity and nephrotoxicity, ototoxicity being more serious. Both vestibular and cochlear functions are affected with streptomycin use, with the vestibular abnormalities occurring more frequently. The patient may experience nausea, vomiting, or vertigo. Hearing loss can also occur; occasionally if the deficit is extensive, it will be permanent.

Nephrotoxicity also occurs with the use of streptomycin, although much less commonly than with the other aminoglycosides. It is seen more often in patients with preexisting renal disease and when other nephrotic drugs are used concurrently.

Streptomycin also can cause neurologic side effects, including optic and peripheral neuritis and neuromuscular blockade. The latter can occasionally cause respiratory muscle paralysis, especially after anesthesia or the use of muscle relaxants.

Hypersensitivity reactions are occasionally seen, usually in the early weeks of treatment. These manifest as rash or, less commonly, exfoliative dermatitis or anaphylactic shock. Finally, hematologic abnormalities can occur; these include eosinophilia, neutropenia, agranulocytosis, aplastic anemia, and thrombocytopenia.

Streptomycin is teratogenic in laboratory animals; therefore, the drug should not be given in the first trimester of pregnancy, and the total dosage should not exceed 20 g in the second half of pregnancy.

DOSAGE

Streptomycin should be given IM at a dosage of 15 mg/kg daily 5 days/week, the total daily dosage not to exceed 1 g. In patients over age 60 years, the dosage should be reduced to 10 mg/kg daily. In children, the dosage is 20–40 kg daily, not to exceed 1 g.

CONCLUSION

Streptomycin, the first effective antituberculous agent, is currently used mainly in the retreatment of tuberculosis caused by susceptible organisms. Its use is limited by the need for IM injection and its toxicity on the eighth cranial nerve.

Ciprofloxacin

Ciprofloxacin, a synthetic fluoroquinolone, is a broad-spectrum antimicrobial that can be given PO or IV. It exists as a light yellow crystal and is bactericidal. It works by binding to and inhibiting DNA gyrase, thus, probably causing cleavage of the bacteria's DNA backbone.

ANTIMICROBIAL ACTIVITY AND INDICATIONS

Ciprofloxacin has in vitro antimicrobial activity against many gram-positive and -negative organisms [44]. Recently, it has been shown to have significant in vitro activity against *M. tuberculosis* [18]. However, if it is used alone, the development of resistance to ciprofloxacin is greater with *Mycobacteria* than other bacteria. The drug also has activity against MAC; however, the minimum inhibitory concentration (MIC) is usually higher than achievable serum drug levels. In one study, the MIC 90 for MAI was found to be 16 μg/ml, although the peak drug level of ciprofloxacin is only 2–3 μg/ml after a 500-mg dose [22]. A more recent study showed an MIC 90 for MAI of only 2 μg/ml [21].

Because of these data, ciprofloxacin is emerging as an important antimycobacterial drug. It can be used as a second-line agent in the treatment of *M. tuberculosis* in combination with other antituberculous drugs, after primary therapy has failed. It also has shown promise as part of a multidrug regimen in the treatment of disseminated MAC in AIDS patients.

PHARMACOKINETICS

Ciprofloxacin can be given PO or IV. After an oral dose, the drug is well absorbed, achieving peak serum concentrations in 1–2 hours. Its bioavailability is about 70%, and its half-life is 4 hours. Of the total dosage, at least 50% is excreted unchanged in the urine, 20–35% is recovered in the feces, and approximately 15% is metabolized. The rate of excretion in the kidney exceeds that of glomerular filtration, suggesting that secretion of the drug into the tubules plays a major role. Food will slightly delay the absorption of ciprofloxacin; therefore, it is recommended that the drug be taken 2 hours after a meal. The drug is widely distributed throughout the body, achieving high concentrations in virtually all tissues and fluids. The major exceptions are the CSF, which achieves drug levels of 10% that of peak serum levels, and the vitreous and aqueous humors of the eye.

CLINICAL TRIALS

Ciprofloxacin has good in vitro activity against *M. tuberculosis*; its activity against MAI is somewhat less marked. A recent study reported on 11 patients with *M. tuberculosis* who were treated with multidrug regimens including ciprofloxacin [28]. These patients, who had failed primary therapy because of drug resistance, intolerance to primary agents, or an underlying disease making treatment with standard therapy dangerous, all had good responses to the ciprofloxacin-containing regimen. One patient had a prolonged course because of a draining sinus, while two patients had to stop therapy secondary to adverse drug reactions, one with worsening liver function and one with leukopenia.

Several studies have looked at the effect of ciprofloxacin as part of a multidrug regimen on disseminated MAC in patients with AIDS. One described 31 AIDS patients treated with a four-drug regimen (rifampin, ethambutol, clofazimine, and ciprofloxacin) for MAC. They found a reduction in symptoms and bacteremia in the first 4 weeks of therapy, although the colony counts increased after therapy was stopped. Six of these patients had to discontinue ciprofloxacin secondary to adverse drug effects [30]. There are only rare reports of patients who have had long-term responses after treatment of MAC. One describes a patient who remained free of disease for a 25-month follow-up period after treatment for MAC with a five-drug regimen including ciprofloxacin [7].

ADVERSE EFFECTS AND CONTRAINDICATIONS

Ciprofloxacin is a relatively safe drug, needing to be discontinued because of an adverse reaction only 3.5% of the time. The most common side effects seen are GI (nausea, diarrhea, vomiting, and abdominal pain), followed by rash, headache, and restlessness. These were usually mild and quickly abated with the discontinuation of the drug. Many other side effects attributed to ciprofloxacin occur in less than 1% of the patients using the drug: painful oral mucosa, dysphagia, dizziness, insomnia, ataxia, hallucinations, irritability, tremor, lethargy, weakness, seizures, pruritis, urticaria, fever, chills, angioedema, blurred vision, joint pain, interstitial nephritis, crystalluria, hematuria, palpitations, syncope, myocardial infarction, cardiopulmonary arrest, pulmonary edema, hemoptysis, brochospasm, and many others. Ciprofloxacin can also cause abnormal laboratory values, including increased SGPT, SGOT, alkaline phosphatase, lactic dehydrogenase, bilirubin, creatinine, BUN, amylase, uric acid, and glucose.

There are also important drug interactions involving ciprofloxacin. The use of ciprofloxacin in a patient taking theophylline can cause an elevation of the serum theophylline level; therefore, close monitoring of the theophylline level is important. Ciprofloxacin also causes an enhanced response to oral anticoagulants; therefore, the prothrombin time should be monitored more closely in patients on these two agents. The use of antacids containing magnesium or aluminum can decrease the oral absorption of ciprofloxacin; if possible, these should be discontinued while on ciprofloxacin. Finally, probenicid causes a decrease in the tubular secretion of ciprofloxacin; thus, it may cause an increase in the serum level of this drug.

Ciprofloxacin should not be used in patients under age 18 years, in pregnant women, or in lactating women. In rat studies, no teratogenicity was seen with the use of ciprofloxacin; however, these studies have not yet been completed in humans.

DOSAGE

For the treatment of bacterial infections, the recommended dosage of ciprofloxacin is 250–750 mg q12h, depending on the location of the infection. In the case of *M. tuberculosis*, the current studies use a single daily dose of 500–750 mg, with a duration of therapy ranging from 6 to 20 months [26]. In AIDS patients with MAC, 750 mg q12h was used in the most recent studies [30].

CONCLUSIONS

Ciprofloxacin, a broad-spectrum fluoroquinolone antimicrobial, has been shown in vitro to have good activity against *M. tuberculosis* and slightly less activity against MAI. This drug, which is relatively safe, will become more important as a second-line agent in the retreatment of tuberculosis, after primary therapy has failed. It is also useful as part of a multidrug regimen in the treatment of MAC in AIDS patients, although complete resolution of this infection is rare.

References

1. Agins, B. D., et al. Effect of combined therapy with ansamycin, clofazimine, ethambutol, and isoniazid for *Mycobacterium avium* infection in Patients with AIDS. *J. Infect. Dis.* 159:784–787, 1989.
2. American Thoracic Society. Treatment of tuberculosis and tuberculosis infection in adults and children. *Am. Rev. Respir. Dis.* 134:355–363, 1986.
3. American Thoracic Society. Diagnostic standards and classification of tuberculosis. *Am. Rev. Respir. Dis.* 142:725–735, 1990.
4. Armstrong, D., et al. Treatment of infections in patients with the acquired immunodeficiency syndrome. *Ann. Intern. Med.* 103:738–743, 1985.
5. Barnes, P. F., et al. Tuberculosis in patients with human immunodeficiency virus infection. *New Engl. J. Med.* 324:1644–1650, 1991.
6. Baron, E. J., and Young, L. S. Amikacin, ethambutol and rifampin for treatment of disseminated Mycobacterium avium intracellulare infections in patients with acquired immunodeficiency syndrome. *Diag. Microbiol. Infect. Dis.* 5:215–220, 1986.
7. Benjamin, M., Spagnolo, S. V. Rifampin in initial therapy of M. Kansasii pulmonary disease. *Am. Rev. Resp. Dis.* 125:183(S), 1982.
8. Benson, C. A., et al. Successful treatment of acquired immunodeficiency syndrome–related Mycobacterium avium complex disease with a multiple drug regimen including amikacin. *Arch. Intern. Med.* 151:582–585, 1991.

9. British Thoracic and Tuberculosis Association: Short course chemotherapy in pulmonary tuberculosis. Third report at five years. *Lancet* 1:1182–1183, 1980.

10. Chadwick, M., et al. Brief report: Combination chemotherapy with ciprofloxacin for infection with Mycobacterium tuberculosis in mouse models. *Am. J. Med.* 87:5A-35S-36S, 1989.

11. Chaisson, R. E., and Slutkin, G. T. Tuberculosis and HIV infection. *J. Infect. Dis.* 159:96–100, 1989.

12. Chiu, J., et al. Treatment of disseminated *Mycobacterium avium* (MAI) with ciprofloxacin, ethambutol, rifampin, and amikacin. Abstracts of the Fifth International Conference on AIDS, Montreal, Canada. Ottawa, Canada: International Development Research Center, 1989.

13. Chan, S. L. et al. The early bactericidal activity of rifabutin measured by sputum viable counts in Hong Kong patients with pulmonary tuberculosis. *Tubercle Lung Dis.* 73(1):33–38, 1992.

14. Cynamon, M. H., and Klemens, S. P. New antimycobacterial agents. *Clin. Chest Med.* 10:355–364, 1989.

15. Dautzenberg, B. Rifabutin in combination with clotazamine, isoniazid and ethambutol in the treatment of AIDS patients with infections due to opportunist mycobacteria. *Tubercle.* 72:168–175, 1991.

16. Davidson, P. T. Drug resistance and the selection of therapy for tuberculosis. *Am. Rev. Respir. Dis.* 136:255–257, 1987.

17. Davidson, P. T. Treating tuberculosis: What drugs, for how long? *Ann. Intern. Med.* 112:393–395, 1990.

18. Davies, S., et al. Comparative in vitro activity of five fluoroquinolones against Mycobacteria. *J. Antimicrob. Chemother.* 19:605, 1987.

19. Davis, C. E., Jr., et al. In vitro susceptibility of *Mycobacterium avium complex* to antibacterial agents. *Diagn. Microbiol. Infect. Dis.* 8:149, 1987.

20. *Diagnostic Facts and Comparisons*. Philadelphia: J. B. Lippincott, 1992.

21. Fenlon, C. H., and Cynamon, M. H. Comparative in vitro activities of ciprofloxacin and other 4-quinolones against Mycobacterium tuberculosis and Mycobacterium intracellulare. *Antimicrob. Agents Chemother.* 29:386–388, 1986.

22. Gay, J. D. In vitro activities of norfloxacin and cipiofloxacin against Mycobacterium tuberculosis, M. avium complex, M. chelone, M. fortuitum, and M. kansasii. *Antimicrob. Agents Chemother.* 26:94–96, 1984.

23. Girling, J. A controlled study of sifabutin and an uncontrolled study of ofloxacin in the retreatment of patients with pulmonary tuberculosis resistant to isoniazid, streptomycin and rifampicin. *Tubercle Lung Dis.* 73:59–67, 1992.

24. Hawkins, C. C., et al. Mycobacterium avium complex infections in

patients with the acquired immunodeficiency syndrome. *Ann. Intern. Med.* 105:184–188, 1986.

25. Heifets, L. B., and Lindholm-Levy, P. J. Bacteriostatic and bactericidal activity of ciprofloxacin and ofloxacin against Mycobacterium tuberculosis and Mycobacterium avium complex. *Tubercle* 68:267–276, 1987.
26. Hopewell, P. C. Tuberculosis and human immunodeficiency virus infection. *Semin. Respir. Infect.* 4(2):111–122, 1989.
27. Iseman, M. D., and Madsen, L. A. Drug-resistant tuberculosis. *Clin. Chest Med.* 10:341–353, 1989.
28. Kahana, L. M., and Spino, M. Ciprofloxacin in patients with mycobacterial infections: Experience in 15 patients. *DICP Ann. Pharmacother.* 25:919–923, 1991.
29. Kawahsa S., et al. In vitro activities of newly developed fluoroquinolones fleroxacin, lomefloxacin and sparfloxacin against mycobacterium tuberculosis. *Kekkaku.* 66:429–431, 1991.
30. Kemper, C. A., et al. Treatment of Mycobacterium avium complex bacteremia in AIDS with a four-drug oral regimen. *Ann. Intern. Med.* 116:466–472, 1992.
31. Leysen, D. et al. Mycobacteria and the new quinolones. *Antimicrob. Agents Chemother.* 33:1–5, 1989.
32. Centers for Disease Control. Transmission of multidrug-resistant tuberculosis from an HIV–positive client in a residential substance-abuse treatment facility. *MMWR.* 40: 129–131, 1991.
33. Medinger, A., Spagnolo, S. V. Mycobacterium szulgai pulmonary infection. *South. Med. J.* 74:85–86, 1981.
34. O'Brien, R. Rifabutin (Ansamycin LM427): A new rifamycin-s derivative for the treatment of mycobacterial diseases. *Rev. Infect. Dis.* 9(3):519–530, 1987.
35. Perez-Stable, E. J. and Hopewell, P. C. Current tuberculosis treatment regimens. *Clin. Chest Med.* 10:323–339, 1989.
36. *Physician's Desk Reference.* Oradell, NJ: Medical Economics Company, 1992.
37. Pretet, S. Combined chemotherapy including rifabutin for rifampin and isoniazid resistant pulmonary tuberculosis. *Eur. Respir. J.* 5:680–684, 1992.
38. Small, P.M., et al. Treatment of tuberculosis in patients with advanced immunodeficiency virus infection. *N. Engl. J. Med.* 324:289–294, 1991.
39. Spagnolo, S. V., and Raver, J. M. Nine month chemotherapy for pulmonary tuberculosis. *South. Med.* 75:134–138, 1982.
40. Spagnolo, S. V., Pulmonary tuberculosis-clinical perspectives. *Treatment Drug Therapy.* 15:67–72, 1985.
41. Sunderam, G., et al. Tuberculosis as a manifestation of the acquired immunodeficiency syndrome. *JAMA* 256:362–366, 1986.

42. Torrisi, P., Spagnolo, S. V. Antituberculosis chemotherapy of pulmonary tuberculosis. Report at 10 years of a nine-month regimen (final report). *Am. Rev. Resp. Dis.* 135:459(A)(S), 1987.

43. Van Caekenberghe, D. Comparative in vitro activities of two fluoroquinolones and fusidic acid against mycobacterium. *J. Antimicob. Chemother.* 26:381–386, 1990.

44. Walker, R. C., and Wright, A. J. The fluoroquinolones. *Mayo Clin. Proc.* 66:1249–1259, 1991.

45. Yew, W. et al. Ofloxacin penetration into tuberculosis pleural effusion. *Antimicrob. Agents Chemother.* 35:2159–2160, 1991.

46. Young, L. S., *Mycobacterium avium complex* infection. *J. Infect. Dis.* 157:863–867, 1988.

47. Young, L. S., et al. Activity of ciprofloxacin and other fluorinated quinolones against Mycobacteria. *Am. J. Med.* 82:4A-23-26, 1987.

5

Bacterial Parapneumonic Pleural Effusions and Empyema

Prashant K. Rohatgi

Pleural empyema literally means "collection of pus in the pleural space"; however, because of difficulties in establishing exactly how many polymorphonuclear leukocytes in the pleural fluid define it to be pus, it is probably more practical to define it as "an infected pleural exudate," as evidenced by positive pleural fluid culture or Gram's stain.

Empyema is most commonly caused by an adjacent suppurative process in the lung parenchyma, most often bacterial pneumonia. However, it is important to recognize that empyema may also follow:

Penetrating thoracic injuries, either traumatic or iatrogenic.
Transdiaphragmatic spread of infection from a subphrenic abscess.
Contiguous spread from a paravertebral abscess, osteomyelitis of rib, or purulent mediastinitis.
Ruptured esophagus (generally this empyema is on the left side).
Hematogenous seeding of the pleural space from a distant suppurative site.

The subsequent comments that follow are aimed primarily at parapneumonic pleural effusions and empyemas associated with bacterial pneumonia.

Stages of Bacterial Parapneumonic Effusion

The evolution of a pleural space infection from an adjacent bacterial pneumonia, i.e., bacterial parapneumonic effusion, can be divided into three pathologic stages, which merge imperceptibly into each other. Stage 1, the exudative phase, is characterized by rapid outpouring of thin, serous, exudative, and sterile pleural fluid, with relatively low white cell count and normal pleural fluid glucose, pH, and a lactate dehydrogenase (LDH) level. At this stage, the patient responds to antimicrobial therapy, either alone or combined with needle aspirations.

Stage 2, the fibrinopurulent phase, is characterized by invasion of pleural fluid by bacteria and transformation of fluid to fibrin-rich purulent exudate, with loculation. There is a progressive decrease in pleural fluid glucose and pH and a rise in pleural fluid LDH. At this stage, it is usually not feasible to drain the pleural space with needle aspiration alone, and generally thorcostomy tube drainage with breaking of the loculations or rib resection with large thoracostomy tubes is required for effective drainage of pus.

Stage 3 is the organization phase, in which fibroblasts grow into the exudate from both the visceral and parietal pleurae and envelop the lung in an inelastic membrane, "the peel." At this final stage, thoracotomy with decortication may be required to free the entrapped lung. If untreated, the empyema may drain spontaneously through the chest wall (empyema necessitans) or into the lung and produce a bronchopleural fistula.

Bacteriology

Table 5-1 lists the common bacterial pneumonias associated with parapneumonic pleural effusions, as well as the incidence of parapneumonic effusions associated with these bacterial pneumonias, along with the frequency with which these effusions are found to be infected.

Clinical Signs and Symptoms

The clinical signs and symptoms of empyema are not diagnostic except to direct attention to the chest and to suggest an infectious process. Almost all patients have fever (100.4°F). Some patients are critically ill with high fever and obvious signs of sepsis. Clinical signs and symptoms that specifically suggest pleural space disease include pleuritic chest pain, pleural friction rub, and physical findings of a pleural effusion.

Table 5-1. Common bacteria producing pneumonia, the incidence of associated parapneumonic effusions, and the frequency of finding positive cultures in these effusions

Bacteria producing pneumonia	Incidence of associated parapneumonic effusion (%)	Parapneumonic effusions with positive cultures (complicated) (%)
Anaerobes [1]	35	90
Streptococcus pneumoniae [8]	40–60	5
Staphylococcus aureus [12]	40	20
Streptococcus pyogenes [11]	90	35
Haemophilus influenzae [4]	50	20
Escherichia coli [9]	50	90
Pseudomonas aeruoginosa [10]	50	90

Definitive Diagnosis

It is apparent from the discussion of the natural history of pleural space infections that the prognosis and therapeutic approach to parapneumonic effusion are largely determined by the stage in which the disease is recognized. Ideally, therefore, in patients with parapneumonic effusions, one must balance the need to avoid unnecessary tube thoracostomies in patients who can be managed conservatively with antimicrobials and needle aspiration as in the exudative stage, with the need to start tube drainage of the pleural space as early as possible in patients suspected to be in the fibrinopurulent stage of disease, because drainage becomes progressively more difficult the longer it is delayed. Thus, the aim in the diagnosis and management of parapneumonic effusions is the ability to predict which of the exudative effusions are likely to resolve with conservative treatment (i.e., uncomplicated parapneumonic pleural effusion) and which of the effusions are likely to progress to complicated stages of fibrinopurulent or fibrotic reaction (i.e., complicated parapneumonic pleural effusion), requiring complete evacuation of the pleural cavity.

Table 5-2 lists clinical features and pleural fluid characteristics that are helpful in identifying complicated bacterial parapneumonic effusions.

The pleural findings that suggest that no further diagnostic or therapeutic measures are needed for management of parapneumonic pleural effusion are (1) pleural fluid pH above 7.20 (note the *Proteus* exception), (2) pleural fluid glucose above 60 mg/dl, and (3) pleural fluid LDH below 1000 international units/liter.

The pleural fluid findings are considered to be indeterminate when (1) pleural fluid pH is between 7.00 and 7.20, (2) LDH level is above 1000 international units/liter, and (3) pleural fluid glucose is between 40 and 60 mg/dl. In these borderline cases, the need for thoracostomy tube drainage is determined by the size and rapidity of accumulation of fluid and the direction of change in serial pleural fluid samples obtained at 12- to 24-hour intervals.

Table 5-2. Clinical features and pleural fluid characteristics indicative of complicated bacterial parapneumonic features

Clinical features
- Presence of loculated fluid or air fluid levels within the pleural space
- Rapid reaccumulation of fluid after thoracentesis
- Failure of parapneumonic effusion to respond to antimicrobials

Pleural fluid characteristics
- Grossly purulent fluid
- Putrid odor
- Demonstration of bacteria on Gram's stain
- Glucose $<$ 40 mg/dl
- pH is less than 7.00 except in *Proteus* infection

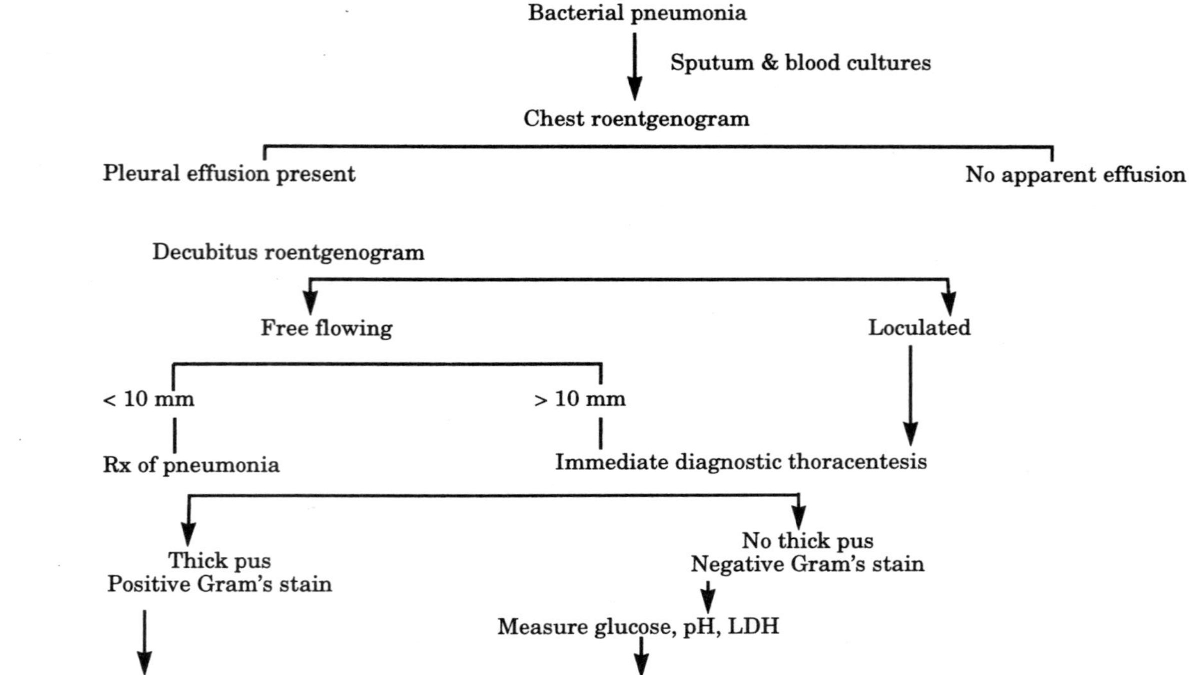
Bacterial pneumonia
Sputum & blood cultures
Chest roentgenogram
Pleural effusion present
No apparent effusion
Decubitus roentgenogram
Free flowing
Loculated
< 10 mm
> 10 mm
Rx of pneumonia
Immediate diagnostic thoracentesis
Thick pus
Positive Gram's stain
No thick pus
Negative Gram's stain
Measure glucose, pH, LDH

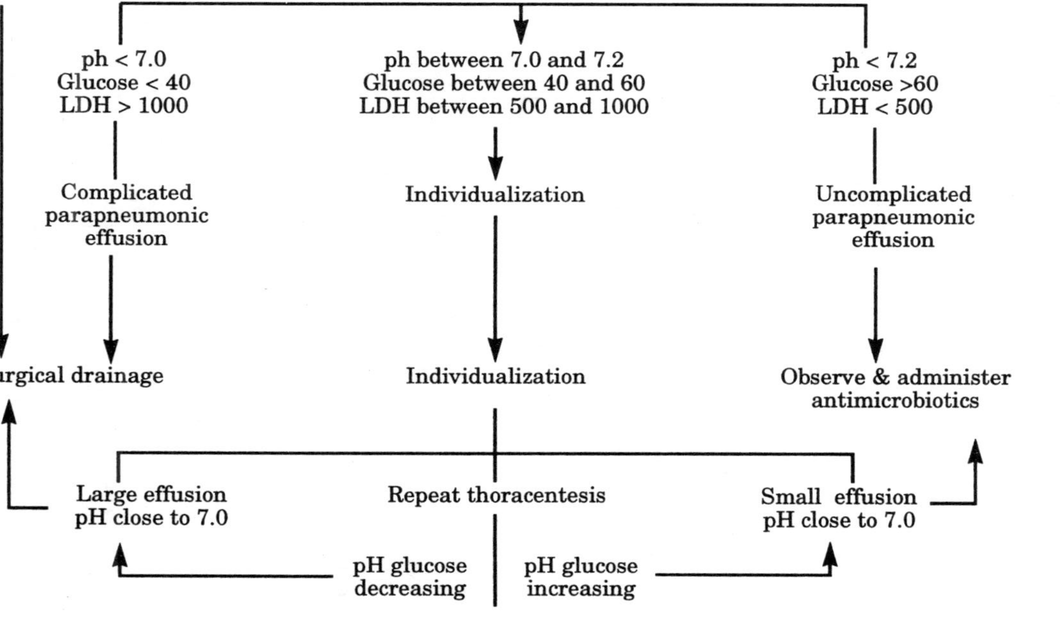

Fig. 5-1. Suggested decision tree for patients with bacterial pneumonia and pleural effusion.

Management

Figure 5-1 provides an outline for management of parapneumonic effusions — both uncomplicated and complicated. The management consists of appropriate antimicrobial therapy depending on the organisms identified on Gram's stain and culture of the pleural fluid or the organisms recovered from the contiguous or distant foci of infection thought to be responsible for empyema. For appropriate dosage and duration of antimicrobials, see Chapters 3 and 4.

Complicated parapneumonic pleural effusions or pleural empyema require expedient evacuation of pleural cavity.

CLOSED DRAINAGE

For the majority of the patients with complicated parapneumonic pleural effusion or pleural empyema, needle thoracentesis, even when done repeatedly and with either ultrasound guidance or CT direction, is unsuccessful in evacuating the pleural cavity. This is because the fluid in complicated parapneumonic pleural effusion or pleural empyema is viscous and loculated.

Closed drainage with thoracostomy tube should be attempted. A thoracostomy tube of as large a diameter as possible should be placed in the most dependent area of fluid accumulation. During tube insertion, an attempt should be made to break the loculations with a finger. In loculated effusions, more than one thoracostomy tube drainage may be necessary. The tube should be left in place until the purulent drainage disappears and the amount of serous drainage decreases to less than 75 ml/day, when it should be gradually withdrawn and removed.

FIBRINOLYTIC THERAPY

Fibrinolytic therapy has been attempted in a limited number of cases to lyse adhesions and promote complete evacuation of the pleural cavity. This is achieved by installation of 250,000 units of streptokinase dissolved in 50–100 ml of saline through the thoracostomy tube and clamping the tube for 4 hours. Patients for this intervention should be selected carefully, because it is effective only in early stages of complicated parapneumonic pleural effusions and before the mature collagen is laid down. The patient needs to be observed carefully for local bleeding (see Chap. 6). If it appears to be effective, then the treatment regimen can be repeated daily for 10–14 days.

OPEN DRAINAGE

If no clinical improvement is apparent within 24–48 hours after closed thoracostomy tube drainage or if it is ineffective in clearing the pleural cavity, then either a rib resection with thoracostomy drainage or formation of an Eloesser flap — pleural cutaneous fistula — may be required.

DECORTICATION

Occasionally after the empyema is controlled with closed or open drainage, there may be a residual organized peel enveloping the lung. In these circumstances, it may be necessary to decorticate and remove the organized peel so that the lung can expand and function normally.

References

1. Bartlett, J. G., et al. Bacteriology of empyema. *Lancet* 1:338–340, 1974.
2. Bergh, N. P., et al. Intrapleural streptokinase in the treatment of haemothorax and empyema. *Scand. J. Thorac. Cardiovasc. Surg.* 11:265–268, 1977.
3. Himelman, R. B., and Callen, P. W. The prognostic value of loculations in parapneumonic pleural effusions. *Chest* 90:852–856, 1986.
4. Levin, D. C., et al. Bacteremic hemophilus influenzae pneumonia in adults: A report of 24 cases and a review of the literature. *Am. J. Med.* 62:219–226, 1977.
5. Light, R. W. Management of parapneumonic effusions. *Arch. Intern. Med.* 141:1339–1341, 1981.
6. Moran, J. F. Surgical management of pleural space infections. *Semin. Respir. Infect.* 3:383–394, 1988.
7. Rohatgi, P. K. Catastrophic Pleural Disease. In S. V. Spagnolo and A. Medinger (eds.), *Handbook of Pulmonary Emergencies*. New York: Plenum, 1986.
8. Taryle, D. A., et al. The incidence and clinical correlates of parapneumonic effusions in pneumococcal pneumonia. *Chest* 74:170–174, 1978.
9. Tillotson, J. R., and Lerner, A. M. Characteristics of pneumonias caused by escherichia coli. *N. Engl. J. Med.* 277:115–119, 1967.
10. Tillotson, J. R., and Lerner, A. M. Characteristics of nonbacteremic pseudomonas pneumonia. *Ann. Int. Med.* 68:295–302, 1968.
11. Welch, C. C., et al. Beta-hemolytic streptococcal pneumonia: Report of an outbreak in a military population. *Am. J. Med. Sci.* 242:157–165, 1961.
12. Wiita, R. M., et al. Staphylococcal pneumonia in adults: A review of 102 cases. *Am. J. Roentgenol.* 86:1083–1091, 1961.

6

Pulmonary Thromboembolic Disease (Pulmonary Embolism) and Deep Venous Thrombosis (DVT)

Aram A. Arabian

Pulmonary thromboembolism (PE) occurs when an embolized thrombus, usually originating in a systemic vein, impact in the pulmonary artery. The most common site of origin is the iliofemoral venous system, but the smaller calf veins may be the site of origin, as may the veins of the upper extremity or the chambers of the right heart. This section will deal with thrombi that have embolized to the pulmonary artery, but other materials may impact here, such as tumor emboli, fat or amniotic fluid emboli, organisms (parasites, for example), foreign body emboli, or air emboli.

The consequences of an embolized thrombus impacting a pulmonary artery are several:

1. Mechanical problems result from occlusion of a substantial percentage of the pulmonary arterial system and the obstruction to blood flow [8,62].
2. The obstruction, if significant, results in increased right heart work, sometimes requiring a great increase that the heart cannot accommodate. The result is dilatation and failure of the right heart, leading to a reduction in cardiac output and arrhythmias [60].
3. There are hormonal consequences to the release of various vasoactive substances, often platelet derived, that can exacerbate the situation leading to worsening of ventilation/perfusion (V/Q) mismatch and bronchospasm [40].
4. There are neurologic consequences that may stress a failing system further [32,59].

The consequences of a pulmonary embolus relate to its size and the state of health of the person prior to embolization. A small embolus might be asymptomatic in an otherwise normal host but fatal in a person with pulmonary hypertension. It might pass with no detectable consequences to this otherwise normal person but might result in a pulmonary infarction in a person with concomitant congestive heart failure. The multiple possible presentations for this disorder result in the need for a high index of suspicion if pulmonary embolism is to be recognized.

Diagnosis

Definitive diagnosis of pulmonary embolism requires showing the thrombus in a pulmonary artery, but this is not always practical or possible. Given the proper clinical setting, it is often not necessary, and indirect studies may be substituted. Table 6-1 gives the incidences of symptoms and signs in angiographically proved pulmo-

Table 6-1. Symptoms and signs of patients with arteriographically proved pulmonary thromboembolism (percentage of patients with various findings)

Symptoms	
Chest pain	83
Pleuritic	74
Nonpleuritic	14
Dyspnea	84
Apprehension	59
Cough	53
Hemoptysis	30
Sweats	27
Syncope	13
Signs	
Respirations > 16	92
Rales	58
Inc. S_2P	53
Pulse > 100	44
Temperature > 37.8°C	43
Gallop	36
Phlebitis	32
Murmur	28
Edema	24
Cyanosis	19
Associated conditions	
Current venous disease	45
Immobilization	58
CHF and COPD	38
Malignancy	6

Inc. S_2P = increased intensity of the pulmonic component of the second heart sound; CHF = congestive heart failure; COPD = chronic obstructive pulmonary disease. Source: Adapted from W. R. Bell. Pulmonary embolism: Progress and problems. *Am. J. Med.* 72:181, 1982.

nary emboli [4]. The most common symptoms are dyspnea and pleuritic chest pain, with tachypnea being the most frequent sign. Although these findings are often present in acute PE, they are not specific for it, being found in many other unrelated conditions.

Pulmonary emboli may be simple or complicated. The complicating factors are the presence of a pulmonary infarct, hypotension, a significant pleural effusion, or a pneumonitis.

The gold standard for the diagnosis of pulmonary embolism is the pulmonary arteriogram [9,46]. A diagnostic test occurs when an intraluminal filling defect or an abrupt cutoff of a pulmonary artery is imaged. A less specific test is the $\dot{V}/\dot{Q}$ lung scan. Because of the ease of performance and the minimal invasive nature of the study, this test usually precedes a pulmonary arteriogram. The ventilation portion of the study uses various isotopic gases or radiolabeled particles less than 1 μm in diameter. It reflects the gas-occupying areas of the lung, including the conducting airways. The relative amount of gas exchange can be determined if a wash-in or wash-out study is included. To determine the relative amount of blood flow to regions of the lung, perfusion is measured by embolizing radiolabeled particulate matter, usually albumin, and scanning in six different positions (anterior, posterior, left lateral, right lateral, left posterior oblique, right posterior oblique). In experimental situations, the scan is always abnormal when a vessel of 3 mm or greater is obstructed. The injectate contains about 200,000 particles and in an otherwise normal pulmonary vascular tree would block less than 0.5% of the microvascular circulation. The half-life of these particles after impacting is 2–4 hours [49].

An indeterminate scan is one with a V/Q mismatch of fewer than two segments. Depending on the degree of the abnormality, these scans are often reported as low or intermediate probability for PE. A V/Q mismatch, usually reported as a high-probability scan, is defined as a defect of two segments or more in perfusion with a normal ventilation study in the area(s) of perfusion abnormality.

Because of the nonspecific nature of the symptoms and signs and the multiple causes for abnormalities in commonly acquired laboratory data for PE, the need for a definitive study to confirm the diagnosis is mandatory. The interpretation of that study is best done by integrating it with the clinical likelihood of the diagnosis of pulmonary embolism [20]. In a young woman on birth control pills just returned from a long automobile trip who experiences the sudden onset of dyspnea and pleuritic chest pain, a V/Q scan will usually suffice, especially if the chest radiograph is normal and the arterial blood gas analysis shows hypoxemia with a respiratory alkalosis. In an older person with obstructive pulmonary disease, an arteriogram may be necessary to establish the diagnosis, because the V/Q scan is expected to be indeterminate whether a PE has occurred or not.

Objective evaluation of the deep venous system of the legs may reveal the presence of clot, and therapy is justified on this basis. The gold standard for the deep venous thrombosis (DVT) is the dye contrast venogram. It is diagnostic of thrombosis when there is an intraluminal filling defect. As with the diagnosis of PE, there are less invasive and slightly less definitive tests for the presence of DVT of the lower extremity. The most commonly done studies are impedance plethysmography (IPG) (with or without a Doppler study), labeled fibrinogen leg scanning, and duplex scanning of the leg.

Figure 6-1 gives a flow diagram to diagnose PE. The sensitivity and specificity of these tests depend on the clinical likelihood of the PE's being present. Since the rest results are sometimes equivocal, other methods of interpreting or adding data must be used. When this happens, clinical judgment must be used, or indirect tests may be used to indicate the presence of recent clot. Fibrin or fibrinogen degradation products can be used to indicate the presence of recent clot lysis when the level is high, although exact indications for their use are not clear [6,54]. Impedence plethysmography and duplex scanning are usually done only to the lower extremities. As such, they miss thrombi from other sources and cannot reliably differentiate acute from chronic thrombi. On rare occasions, a complete clot may embolize, resulting in a normal IPG or duplex scan. If abnormal, an effort should be made to repeat these studies after the completion of therapy and/or the resolution of signs of DVT so a new baseline is established. If a prior study was abnormal, interpretation of an abnormal repeat study does not indicate a new thrombus. Studying the deep venous system is important because some treatments for DVT differ from those of PE. These include the use of thrombolytics when indicated, the need for vena cava interruption, and the need for surgical pulmonary embolectomy. Finally, it should be noted that equivocal pulmonary arteriograms are rare, and less definitive confirmatory tests may need to be substituted.

Heparin

Heparin is a polymer of alternating D-glucuronic acid and *N*-acetyl-*D*-glucosamine residues. Multiple modifications, many of which are incomplete, yield oligosaccharide structures within the glycosaminoglycan chain. Heparin, then, is a heterogeneous mixture of glycosaminoglycans.

HISTORY

Heparin was discovered in 1916 by a medical student investigating the nature of ether-soluble procoagulants and isolated a phospholipid antigcoagulant. The name *heparin* derives from its abundance in liver. It was used in vitro to prevent the clotting of blood removed from the body, and this led to its use in vivo to treat venous thrombosis.

Heparin is a mast cell–derived polysaccharide covalently bound to a core protein with a molecular weight of 60,000–100,000 daltons. The usual sources of heparin are porcine intestinal mucosa and bovine lung. During the isolation process, the protein is removed, and there is polysaccharide degradation yielding a heterogeneous mixture of 3000–60,000 daltons with small amounts of other aminoglycans. Although there is heterogeneity of different preparations, the biological properties remain similar.

Low-molecular-weight heparins (<7000 daltons) are produced by partial depolymerization chemically or by isolation from standard heparin by gel filtration or differential precipitation. To date, they have been used for DVT prophylaxis and recently became available in the United States.

MECHANISMS OF ACTION

The major mechanism of heparin-induced inhibition of blood coagulation is through its mechanism of reversibly binding to antithrombin III. Antithrombin III undergoes a conformational change and binds irreversibly to factors XIIa, XIa, Xa, IXa, and IIa, inactivating them. Heparin can then dissociate from the complex of antithrombin III and activated factor and bind to other antithrombin III molecules. Most of the anticoagulant effect of heparin is through its inhibition of thrombin (factor IIa) and factor Xa. Heparin molecules of molecular weight of 3000–4000 or less (i.e., low-molecular-weight heparins) do not inhibit thrombin. High concentrations of heparin (>5 units/ml) catalyze the inactivation of thrombin by

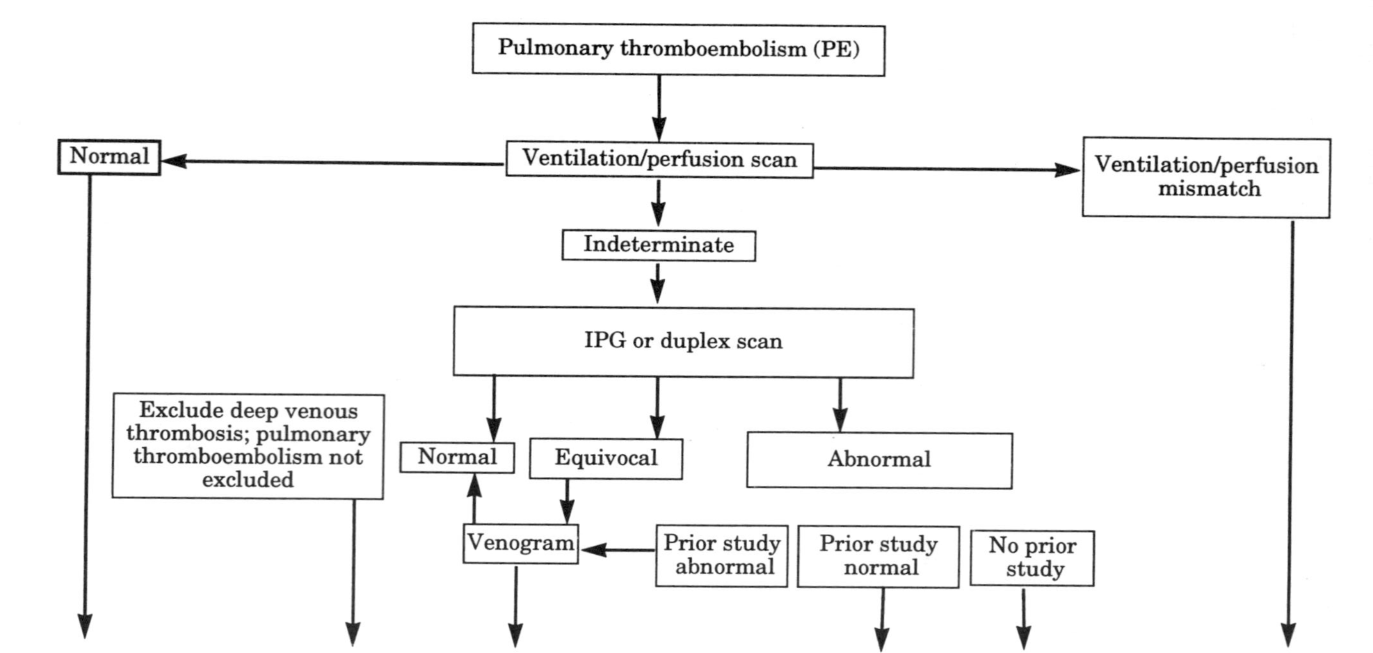

Pulmonary thromboembolism (PE)
Normal
Ventilation/perfusion scan
Ventilation/perfusion mismatch
Indeterminate
IPG or duplex scan
Exclude deep venous thrombosis; pulmonary thromboembolism not excluded
Normal
Equivocal
Abnormal
Venogram
Prior study abnormal
Prior study normal
No prior study

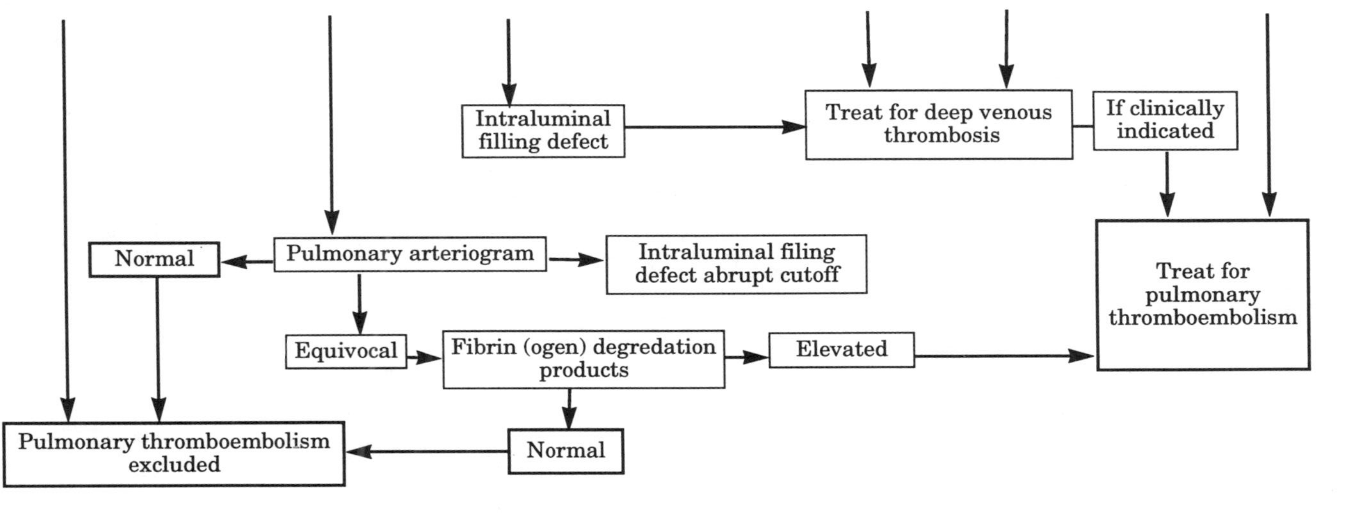

Fig. 6-1. Flow diagram for work-up of suspected pulmonary embolism.

heparin cofactor II. Although not usually measured directly, the concentration of heparin in plasma to inhibit thrombin and factor Xa is 0.1–1.0 unit/ml. Higher concentrations of heparin are required to inactivate thrombin than to inhibit thrombin formation from prothrombin. Heparin can also prevent the formation of a stable fibrin clot through its inhibition of the activation of fibrin-stabilizing factor by thrombin. The primary therapeutic action of heparin is to prevent thrombus formation and extension of existing clots; it is an anticoagulant.

Heparin, by releasing lipoprotein lipase from tissue, reduces the concentration of triglycerides in plasma. With the resultant hydrolysis of triglycerides, the concentration of free fatty acids increases in the blood.

Heparin does not cross the placenta and is not excreted in breast milk. Heparin is probably the therapy of choice for PE or DVT during pregnancy through the period of lactation, but osteoporosis and vertebral collapse have been reported to occur over 2–4 weeks during lactation.

ONSET OF ACTION, BINDING, METABOLISM, AND ELIMINATION

The onset of action of heparin is immediate when given by IV injection. It will be somewhat delayed if given by IV infusion without a bolus. When administered SC, the onset of action is 20–60 minutes. Heparin has a very high affinity for protein binding, primarily low-density lipoproteins, and less to globulins and fibrinogen. Removal from the circulation is by the reticuloendothelial system of the liver. The renal route of elimination is usually just for metabolites, but up to 50% may be excreted unchanged when high dosages are given IV. It is not removed by hemodialysis. The half-life is very variable, with an average of 1.5 hours and a range of 1–6 hours [68]. Increases in the half-life may be seen in patients with renal failure, hepatic dysfunction, and obesity. It may be decreased in patients with pulmonary embolism, infections, or malignancy.

USES AND ACTIONS

Full dosage heparin is the drug of choice for uncomplicated, acute PE and DVT. For preventive treatment (prophylactic), heparin is used in a different dosing schedule.

Prophylactic Use

Low-dosage (and, when available, low-molecular-weight) heparin is used for prophylaxis in patients with a significant risk of venous thrombosis. The list of patients at risk is extensive but may be broken down into three general categories: (1) patients with venous stasis (e.g., patients with congestive heart failure or those at bed rest for prolonged periods), (2) patients with venous disruption (as with trauma to an extremity resulting in venous injury), and (3) patients with a hypercoagulable state (as may occur in patients with certain carcinomas). It is also used to prevent blood clotting during hemodialysis and extracorporeal circulation. Some patients are at high risk for DVT, and heparin must be used in a greater dosage than is used with SC twice- or thrice-a-day dosing, as in patients with a recent hip fracture.

Heparin has been used with other agents for prophylaxis against DVT and PE. The use of SC heparin with dihydroergotamine has been used as prophylaxis in patients undergoing thoracic, abdominal, and pelvic surgery and as postoperative prophylaxis after total hip replacement. The combination significantly reduced the incidence of DVT over single therapy of heparin or dihydroergotamine and over placebo [44].

CONTRAINDICATIONS

Heparin is contraindicated in those known or suspected to be sensitive to it, in those with uncontrolled bleeding, and when suitable blood coagulation tests cannot be performed.

DOSAGES

Full therapeutic dosages for heparin have been given in several ways, the choice being made on the basis of rapidity to establish satisfactory prolongation of the activated partial thromboplastin time (APPT), convenience of delivery, and minimizing bleeding.

Continuous IV Infusion [23]

Loading dosage: 5000–10,000 units IV.

Maintenance dosage: 1000 units/hour, adjusted to keep the APTT in the therapeutic range of 1.5–2.0 times control. The usual dosage to establish this range is 700–2000 units/hour.

Heparin Therapy Adjusted to Body Weight [64]

Loading dosage: 75 units/kg body weight.

Maintenance dosage: 400 units/kg/day (range 250–600 units). Monitoring of the dosage is done twice daily. In one reference it was done by heparin assay to maintain a heparin level of 0.5 unit/ml.

Heparin Therapy Adjusted by Nomogram [14]

See Table 6-2. This method gives adjustment schedules for both subtherapeutic and supertherapeutic dosages of heparin as determined by the APTT.

Intermittent Infusion [28]

Subcutaneous administration: Loading dosage, 15,000 units; maintenance dosage, 15,000 units q12h.

Intravenous administration: Loading dosage, 5000 units; maintenance dosage: 5000–10,000 units, or 75–125 units kg q4h.

Adjusted Low-Dosage SC Heparin for Prophylaxis Against DVT After Total Hip Replacement [34]

The dosage of 3500 international units SC q8h is adjusted to keep the APTT between 31.5 and 36 seconds. Table 6-3 gives the dosage adjustment when the APTT was measured 6 hours after SC administration.

Table 6-2. Heparin nomogram

APTT (seconds)	Bolus (units)	Hold (minutes)	Rate change (ml/hour)[a]	Repeat APTT
<50[b]	5000	0	+3	6 hours
50–59	0	0	+3	6 hours
60–85	0	0	0	Next AM
86–95	0	0	−2	Next AM
96–120	0	30	−2	6 hours
>120	0	60	−4	6 hours

APTT = activated partial thromboplastin time.
[a]1 ml/hour = 40 units/hour.
[b]If the APTT was subtherapeutic despite a heparin dosage of 1440 units/hour or greater at any time during the first 48 hours of therapy, the response to an APTT of less than 50 seconds was a heparin bolus of 5000 units and a rate increase of 5 ml/hour.
Source: Adapted from M. K. Cruikshank et al. A standard nomogram for the management of heparin therapy. *Arch. Intern. Med.* 151:333, 1991.

Table 6-3. Adjustments for heparin 6 hours after subcutaneous administration according to the activated partial thromboplastin time (APTT)

APTT (seconds)	Heparin adjustment (IU)
<27.5	+1000
28–31	+500
31.5–36	0
36.5–39	−500
>39.5	−1000

Source: Adapted from P. F. Leyvraz et al. Adjusted versus fixed-dose subcutaneous heparin in the prevention of deep-venous thrombosis after total hip replacement. *N. Engl. J. Med.* 309:954, 1983.

Combination Therapy for Prophylaxis of DVT [16]

Heparin with dihydroergotamine
Subcutaneous administration
Heparin 5000 units bid or tid
Dihydroergotamine 0.5 mg bid or tid. A complication of dihydroergotamine is vasospasm, which occurs in less than 1% of patients. The incidence of vasospasm seems to be increased in patients with trauma, sepsis, hypotension, and peripheral ischemia.

When heparin is used prophylactically, physical measures may increase its antithrombotic effect. Elastic stockings or graduated compression stockings, intermittent pneumatic compression boots, or inferior vena caval interruption may be used with heparin to prevent DVT and reduce the incidence of PE [19].

LABORATORY MONITORING

Since the drug is standardized by its effect on the clotting time, it makes sense to monitor its effect by using a standardized test. The recommended test is the APTT adjusted to a level of 1.5–2.5 over control for continuous infusion [23] and 1.5–2.0 1 hour prior to the next dose for intermittent administration of heparin [57].

Other monitoring tests used are the Lee-White clotting time, measured at 3.5 hours after the last bolus when intermittent therapy is being used, and any time after steady state has been established during continous infusion. The technique for this test must be carefully standardized, and the therapeutic range is the same as that for the APTT above.

Several controversies exist about the monitoring of heparin therapy. First, it seems prudent to monitor therapy to ensure a therapeutic effect, although a level above therapeutic level may or may not be important in predicting the likelihood of untoward hemorrhage. Heparin affects many steps in the process of hemostasis, several of which are not monitored by the APTT, and these abnormalities may result in bleeding while the heparin level is in the therapeutic range. It has not been proved, however, that heparin's effects on the clotting time, on platelet function, or on increasing fibrinolytic effect increase the risk of bleeding when heparin is in the therapeutic range [10].

LENGTH OF THERAPY

When heparin is used at full anticoagulation, the usual time before conversion to oral anticoagulation is 5–10 days [24]. This time may be extended when a pregnant patient is near term, especially if breast-feeding is to be done since heparin does not cross the placenta and is not excreted in breast milk [17].

When used alone or as combination therapy for prophylaxis, the length of therapy is continued until the patient is ambulatory or the condition posing the increased risk has abated.

ADVERSE EFFECTS

The major side effect of heparin anticoagulation is bleeding. The method of administration of heparin may influence this [55], although not all studies have confirmed this. Several comorbid factors have been identified that lead to an increased incidence of bleeding: acute myocardial infarction, hypotension (systolic blood pressure less than 90 mm Hg), the need for an intraaortic balloon pump, a bilirubin greater than 1 mg/dl, macrocytosis, renal failure, a hematocrit less than 30% without recent bleeding, and cancer [24].

Heparin-induced thrombocytopenia is a serious adverse effect of heparin therapy [21]. It may occur with minimal amounts of heparin, even that of heparin-coated catheters. Reduced platelets may occur at various times after heparin administration. That which occurs on days 2–5 usually does not result in a significant platelet reduction or in evident bleeding. The platelet count rarely goes below 100,000 and often returns to normal even if heparin is continued. A more profound thrombocytopenia usually starts from day

6 to 14 after beginning heparin anticoagulation. It may be associated with bleeding or with arterial thrombosis due to platelet aggregation. The mechanism for the latter effect is immune mediated, and with subsequent dosage of heparin, the onset to significant thrombocytopenia may be only 1–2 days. The incidence of thrombocytopenia is reduced with porcine mucosal heparin and seems related to the high-molecular-weight fractions of heparin, but firm recommendations regarding the use of low-molecular-weight heparin, to prevent this are not yet available.

Skin necrosis has been described with the use of both low- and full-dosage heparin [35]. The cause may be from heparin-induced thrombocytopenia resulting in an arterial thrombus to the skin, or it may be due to an allergic vasospastic reaction. Protamine sulfate will not reverse this effect of heparin.

Allergic and anaphylactoid reactions have been described with the administration of heparin [2]. These reactions are usually serious enough to warrant the discontinuation of the drug.

Hyperkalemia from both low- and full-dosage heparin as well as from low-molecular-weight heparin has been described [15]. It is noted about 4 days after starting therapy with heparin and resolves about 6 days after stopping its use. The mechanism is thought to be an enzymatically induced aldosterone deficiency, resulting in a naturesis with potassium retention. But bleeding into the adrenal gland resulting in insufficiency must be excluded. Suspected predispositions for hyperkalemia are hypovolemia, congestive heart failure, cirrhosis, diabetes mellitus, renal failure, and medications that potentially increase serum potassium, such as potassium-sparing diuretics, angiotensin-converting enzyme inhibitors, nonsteroidal antiinflammatory agents, and beta-blockers.

Osteoporosis has been associated with the administration of heparin when the duration of therapy has been 6 months and the dosage has exceeded 15,000 units/day except in lactating females when the duration of therapy has been much shorter [1]. The cause has not been proved, but it has been associated with a subnormal level of vitamin D.

Other reactions of heparin are an elevation of aspartate transaminase and alanine transaminase without hepatic dysfunction [59]. There may be an interaction of heparin with IV nitroglycerin, resulting in resistance to the effects of heparin; although not all studies agree with this, it bears monitoring [21]. Unusual hair loss has also been noted with the long-term administration of heparin [68].

REVERSAL OF THE ANTICOAGULANT EFFECT: PROTAMINE SULFATE

Protamine sulfate is the specific antagonist to the anticoagulant effect of heparin. It is used only when life-threatening hemorrhage occurs since the anticoagulant effect of heparin disappears within hours of discontinuing the drug.

Protamines are low-molecular-weight proteins that bind tightly to heparin in vitro, neutralizing its anticoagulant effect. In vivo protamine has an anticoagulant effect by interacting with platelets and plasma proteins, so it should be given in minimal amount to neutralize heparin.

The usual amount of protamine is 1 mg for every 100 units of heparin remaining in the plasma [39]. The amount is estimated from the time of administration and the dosage of heparin given, knowing its half-life, which averages 1.5 hours. Protamine is administered by slow IV drip (not more than 50 mg over a 10-minute period).

Administration of protamine sulfate faster than recommended can result in anaphylaxis, hypotension, dyspnea, bradycardia, or flushing [39].

Vitamin K Antagonists

Oral anticoagulants of the vitamin K antagonist class are derivatives of 4-hydroxycoumarin or of the related compound indan-1, 3-dione.

Coumarins

HISTORY

At the turn of the last century, sweet clover was planted for silage in the northern United States and Canada because it was able to grow in nutrient-poor soil. Schofield reported a previously undescribed hemorrhagic disorder in cattle that had ingested this silage, and in 1939 the agent of the hemorrhagic disorder was found to be dicumarol. Warfarin (Coumadin) was introduced as a rodenticide in 1948 due to its increased potency over dicumarol. Suspected risk of toxicity prevented its use until 1951, when it was found to be acceptable for human use [39].

MECHANISM OF ACTION

This class of drugs antagonizes the effect of vitamin K–dependent factors II, VII, IX, and X. They also prevent the activation of anticoagulant proteins C and S. In the liver, reduced vitamin K is a cofactor in the carboxylation of certain glutamic acid residues of these proteins, a requirement for calcium binding. Oral anticoagulants block the regeneration of reduced vitamin K, producing a functional vitamin K deficiency. At therapeutic levels, warfarin decreases the amount of the vitamin K–dependent factors by 30–50%, and secreted undercarboxylated molecules have diminished activity.

These drugs have no effect on anticoagulant molecules that have been fully carboxylated; therefore, the anticoagulant effect of these drugs is not measurable until the fully carboxylated molecules are cleared. The half-lives of these factors are the following: for factor II, 50 hours; factor VII, 6 hours; factor IX, 24 hours; factor X, 36 hours; protein C, 8 hours; and protein S, 30 hours. Anticoagulation with warfarin is a balance between the dosage of oral anticoagulant and the amount of vitamin K in the diet [39].

ONSET OF ACTION, BINDING, METABOLISM, AND ELIMINATION

The time for oral anticoagulants to have a therapeutic effect is at least 3 days, the time necessary for a reduction in the fully carboxylated clotting factors. They are nearly completely absorbed when taken orally and can be detected in plasma within 1 hour of oral administration. Their bioavailability is nearly complete when taken IM, IV, or rectally.

Warfarin is nearly completely bound to plasma proteins, mainly albumin. Unlike other coumarins and indandiones, active warfarin is not found in milk. It is, however, found in fetal plasma [26].

The site of inactivation of warfarin is in the liver and kidneys, with excretion of metabolites in the urine and stool. Its half-life is 20–60 hours, and the duration of action is 2–5 days [39].

INDICATIONS FOR USE

Therapeutic Uses

Therapeutic dosages of warfarin are used for the long-term treatment of PE and DVT. Treatment should begin without a loading dosage and should overlap heparin therapy for 4–5 days while the vitamin K–dependent factors are depleted. Patients with recurrent DVT or a continuing risk factor for it, such as antithrombin III or protein C or S deficiency, should be anticoagulated for an indefinite period; otherwise, for DVT and PE, 3–4 months is usually sufficient [24,29,36].

Prophylactic Uses

For pretreatment of elective hip surgery as an alternative to adjusted-dosage heparin, warfarin is used as prophylaxis against DVT and PE; it is used in a range to prolong the PT to 1.3–1.5 times control. (This amounts to an international normalized ratio of 2.0–3.0 times control [26].

CONTRAINDICATIONS

Warfarin is contraindicated in pregnancy or those with recent or threatened obstetric complications, in those with bleeding tendencies, in those who are uncooperative, and in those who have had recent surgery or are about to have surgery [21]. Other contraindications are in patients with malignant hypertension, alcoholics, and psychotics and where there is not adequate monitoring available.

DOSAGES

Therapeutic

Oral therapy is initiated with warfarin 10–15 mg/day for 2–4 days followed by 2–15 mg/day as indicated by the prothrombin time (PT). Although not recommended, some have suggested starting warfarin at 40–60 mg followed by an adequate dosage to elevate the PT in the therapeutic range [39].

Warfarin is available for parenteral administration, either IM or IV. The dosage by either route is 10–15 mg/day followed by the above oral therapy of 2–15 mg/day. There is no decrease in the time to a therapeutic response when administered parenterally [39].

Prophylaxis

Warfarin 1 mg/day is used before and continued through and after surgery as fixed minidose prophylaxis against DVT. PT and APTT remain in the normal range during its use [50].

LABORATORY MONITORING

The one-stage PT is used to monitor the therapeutic effect of warfarin. Although the therapeutic range for anticoagulation in most situations is a PT of 1.3–1.5 times control, each thromboplastin reagent varies among laboratories. To resolve this, an international normalized ratio (INR) defined as the ratio of patient PT/control PT taken to the power of X, the ISI (international sensitivity index), which ranges from 1.9 to 2.6, is used. Therapeutic anticoagulation is achieved with an INR of 2–3. If high-intensity anticoagulation is needed, the INR would be in the range of 3–4.5. With fixed minidose warfarin, there is no need for laboratory monitoring [21,25].

LENGTH OF THERAPY

Warfarin is used for prophylaxis during the time the patient is at risk; this often means until the patient is ambulatory. Therapeutically, warfarin is used for anticoagulation after a single episode of PE or new onset DVT for 3–4 months. This therapy often follows treatment with heparin or thrombolytics, and the total time of lytic or anticoagulant therapy should be 3–4 months. If the patient has had more than one episode or is at risk of severe or fatal complications of PE, anticoagulants should be continued indefinitely [24,29,36].

ADVERSE EFFECTS

Hemorrhage is the most common adverse effect of warfarin. Major bleeding — defined as intracranial or retroperitoneal hemorrhage, or hemorrhage that results in transfusion, hospitalization, or death — occurs in 1–8% of patients. Studies have not consistently shown the failure of laboratory monitoring to be the cause of bleeding. In nearly half the cases, there is an underlying cause for the hemorrhage, the most common of which are carcinoma, hypertension, cerebrovascular disease, paraplegia, recent surgery, atrial fibrillation, or peptic ulcer disease. The most common sites of bleeding are gastrointestinal, soft tissue, intracranial, and genitourinary [21].

Skin necrosis is the most common dermatologic manifestation of warfarin treatment. It usually begins with a painful erythema 3–5 days after the start of therapy, which may progress to tissue necrosis. The cause is thrombosis of the subcutaneous vessels. The areas of involvement are sites with increased subcutaneous fat. Treatment is to start or restart heparin and administer vitamin K [45]. Another dermatologic manifestation of warfarin toxicity is the "purple toes syndrome." It is thought to be a consequence of embolization from atheromatous plaques and is manifest 3–8 weeks after the start of therapy. The purple color is most noted on the plantar surface of the feet and blanches with pressure. This discoloration fades when the feet are elevated. Treatment requires the discontinuance of warfarin [21,31].

Oral anticoagulation is not recommended during pregnancy because of birth defects in the first trimester and an increased incidence of abortion. Unlike other coumarins and indandiones, active warfarin is not found in milk [18,26].

Indandione Derivatives

Anisindione (Miradon) is similiar to warfarin in its actions and offers no clear advantage over it. Serious hypersensitivity reactions have been described, and the higher frequency of untoward effects prevents its recommendation [39].

REVERSAL OF ANTICOAGULANT EFFECT

Vitamin K was discovered after noting a bleeding disorder in chickens fed inadequate diets. Subsequent work showed that it was required for the synthesis of factors II, VII, IX, and X and of proteins C and S. Vitamin K exists naturally in two forms, vitamin K_1, or phytonadione, and vitamin K_2, or menaquinone; both are fat soluable. Vitamin K_3, or menadione (Synkayvite), is a vitamin precursor that in animals can be synthesized to menaquinone [41]. Vitamin K is essentially nontoxic to humans, but reactions have occurred when it was given intravenously; it is unknown whether the untoward reactions were due to the vitamin or to emulsifers in the preparation.

Phytonadione (Aquamephyton, Konakion, Mephyton) is marketed as 5-mg tablets and in a dispersion of 2- or 10-mg/ml solutions. Bleeding that occurs after oral anticoagulants may require the use of vitamin K and should be administered as vitamin K_1 rather than any of the synthetic derivatives since their consistency in reversing the effect of warfarin is erratic. The dosage required is usually 5–10 mg; it may have to be repeated if a large dosage of oral anticoagulant was taken or if it has a long half-life. If life-threatening bleeding occurs, fresh-frozen plasma (10–20 mg/kg) can restore the deficient factors [13,39].

Thrombolytic Drugs

The mechanism of action of the thrombolytic class of drugs is to convert plasminogen to plasmin, the enzyme that promotes fibrin dissolution. To be effective, all thrombolytic drugs must be administered at or very close to the time of clot formation, within 7 days.

Patients selected to receive thrombolytic therapy should not have invasive procedures during or near the time of therapy.

Streptokinase

Streptokinase is a plasminogen activator isolated from Lancefield group C strains of beta-hemolytic streptococci. It is a protein with a molecular weight of 47,000 daltons. Being a foreign protein, it has antigenic and immunologic properties.

Streptokinase was first isolated in 1933 by Tillet and Garner, who showed that a sterile filtrate from these streptococci could lyse fibrin clots and that clotted blood from patients with recent streptococcal infections was highly resistant to the lytic properties of the filtrate [66].

MECHANISM OF ACTION

Streptokinase is not an enzyme and does not directly act on plasminogen to form plasmin. It must first combine stochiometrically in a 1 : 1 ratio with plasminogen to form an activator complex; it is this complex that has proteolytic activity and can cleave a free molecule of plasminogen to form plasmin. If the dosage given is too great, all available plasminogen will be complexed to streptokinase, and little will remain to be activated to plasmin, reducing lytic activity. If too little is administered, the activator complex will convert the overabundant plasminogen to plasmin, resulting in excessive lysis [5]. Streptokinase combines with both circulating and fibrin-bound plasminogen to produce the activator complex and so is not fibrin specific. Proteins that are also degraded by this complex are fibrinogen, factor V, and factor VIII, among others [58]. It also induces an anticoagulant effect because of the elevated levels of fibrin and fibrinogen degradation products [27].

ONSET OF ACTION, METABOLISM, AND ELIMINATION

The onset of action of streptokinase is rapid, and it has a half-life of 80 minutes but only 16–18 minutes in the presence of antistreptococcal antibodies [63]. It is removed from the circulation by antibodies and by the reticuloendothelial system. It does not cross the placenta [42].

INDICATIONS FOR USE

Pulmonary Thromboembolism

Streptokinase is approved for use in patients with massive pulmonary emboli defined as those obstructing at least one lobar artery or the equivalent in segments. It is also used in acute PE accompanied by shock, regardless of the size of the embolus [4,65].

Venous Thrombosis

Streptokinase is approved for use in patients developing acute DVT in a vein of significant size.

CONTRAINDICATIONS

Absolute contraindications are active internal bleeding, recent (within 2 months) cerebrovascular process, acute pericarditis, and aortic dissection. The list of relative contraindications is extensive and involves conditions that require fibrin strands and plugs for hemostasis and conditions that might result in serious or uncontrolled hemorrhage. Table 6-4 gives specific processes that require close monitoring of the thrombolytic effect or consideration of alternative therapy. Because of its antigenic properties, streptokinase use should not be repeated within 6 months.

DOSAGES

The loading dosage is 250,000 international units administered over 30 minutes. The maintenance dosage is 100,000 international units/hour for 24 hours in PE and 72 hours in DVT (the regimen approved by the Food and Drug Administration).

Burst therapy for DVT consists of four steps, in the following order:

1. 250,000 international units over 1 hour.
2. 100,000 international units/hour for 5 hours.
3. No therapy for the next 12 hours.
4. 250,000 international units over 1 hour bid.

Table 6-4. Contraindications to thrombolytic therapy

Absolute contraindications
Active internal bleeding
Recent cerebrovascular process
Acute pericarditis
Aortic dissection

Relative contraindications
Conditions requiring fibrin plugs or strands (more than 10 days should pass before thrombolytic agents are used)
- Major surgery, organ biopsy, or puncture of a noncompressible blood vessel
- Postpartum period
- Cardiopulmonary resuscitation with rib fractures
- Thoracentesis, paracentesis, or lumbar puncture
- Recent serious trauma

Potentially serious bleeding
- Uncontrolled coagulation defects
- Severe hypertension
- Pregnancy

To prevent febrile reactions, acetaminophen, 650 mg, is administered 1 hour before a course of therapy. When necessary to continue anticoagulation, warfarin can be started without first heparinizing the patient. Twelve hours before the last dose of streptokinase, the patient is given 10 mg of warfarin. Twenty-four hours later, a PT is measured, and subsequent daily dosages of warfarin are adjusted to the therapeutic range for PT. (Refer to the section on warfarin.)

LABORATORY MONITORING

Tests that monitor the drug's effect are whole blood euglobin lysis time, thrombin time, partial thromboplastin or prothrombin time, and fibrin(ogen) degradation products.

Before therapy, check for normal coagulation; if it is abnormal, it must be corrected before thrombolytic therapy can be initiated. Then determine the baseline value for the monitoring test selected (it should be in the normal range). Repeat the test 3–4 hours after the initiation of therapy to ensure a fibrinolytic state has been achieved. If it has not, repeat the loading and maintenance dosages and again repeat the test. If the value of the test does not show lysis, use urokinase, recombinant tissue-type plasminogen activator (RTRA), or heparin.

Burst therapy usually does not require testing at regular intervals. Tests that have been described with this method are a significantly reduced fibrinogen level or a PTT at least twice normal at 10–12 hours after burst therapy.

LENGTH OF THERAPY

Using the standard regimen, streptokinase is administered for 12–24 hours for PE and 72–96 hours for DVT.

The usual length of burst therapy is 3–4 days, with a maximum of 6 days [47].

SIDE EFFECTS

The major types of adverse reactions are hemorrhagic, allergic, and febrile. Hemorrhagic reactions have occurred in a variable number of patients being treated with thrombolytics, with 1–30% requiring the discontinuation of therapy [5,21,37]. Allergic reactions are usually mild and occur in up to 15% of patients treated with streptokinase. The most commonly reported reactions are urticaria, itching, flushing, nausea, headaches, and muscular and skeletal pain. Rarely, bronchospasm, angioneurotic edema, and significant blood pressure changes have occurred. Finally, febrile reactions with a temperature elevation of about 0.5°C occur in about a third of patients. In these patients, the use of aspirin to treat the febrile episode should be avoided, because of the potential for increasing the risk of bleeding [5]. This reaction can be controlled with acetaminophen [52] or corticosteroids [57].

Less common reactions described to streptokinase are serum sickness, backaches, renal dysfunction, and reversible hepatic dysfunction (an acute hepatitislike reaction) [21]. Central nervous system reactions such as delirium, depression, and psychotic reactions have been described [5]. Cardiovascular complications are rare and have included arrhythmias, dyspnea, and tachycardia [5].

If a persistent bleeding state remains after stopping streptokinase [55], cryoprecipitate 10 units is administered until the fibrinogen level is 100 mg/dl or greater. Fresh-frozen plasma, 2–6 units, is given if the patient continues to bleed and the fibrinogen level is greater than 100 mg/dl. If bleeding persists, a bleeding time should be determined to assess platelet function; if it is greater than 9 minutes, administer 10 units of platelets. If the bleeding time is less than 9 minutes, consider the use of antifibrinolytic agents — aminocaproic acid or tranexamic acid. Tranexamic acid is more potent than aminocaproic acid by many times and has lower adverse effects.

The dosage of aminocaproic acid is 5 g slowly IV over 1 hour, followed by 1 g/hour over a period of 8 hours or until bleeding is controlled. Maximum dosage is 30 g in 24 hours. With renal impairment, the dosage must be reduced [51].

The dosage of tranexamic acid is 0.5–1.0 g given slowly intravenously over 5–10 minutes given 2–3 times a day. It may also be given PO in a dosage of 1–1.5g 2–3 times a day [51].

COMPARISON WITH ALTERNATIVES

Streptokinase is the drug of choice when thrombolytic therapy is indicated because of its low cost. Alternatives must be considered when the patient has had a recent streptococcal infection.

Urokinase

Urokinase is an enzyme produced by the kidneys and excreted in the urine. It is commercially available from isolates of human kidney cultures and contains both a high-molecular-weight form of 55,000 daltons and a low-molecular-weight form of 34,000 daltons.

MECHANISM OF ACTION

Urokinase acts directly on plasminogen, converting it to plasmin, which degrades fibrin, fibrinogen, and other proteins. Like streptokinase, it also induces an anticoagulant effect because of the elevated levels of fibrin and fibrinogen degradation products.

In studies with animals, urokinase has been combined with tissue-type plasminogen activator (TPA) with a synergistic effect on thrombolysis. The combination allows a lower dosage to be used, with the concomitant effect of reduced fibrinogen breakdown [11].

ONSET OF ACTION, METABOLISM, AND ELIMINATION

When urokinase is administered, the activation of plasminogen is immediate. In the circulation, urokinase has a half-life of about 16 minutes [5]. The clearance rate depends on plasminogen availability. The fibrinolytic activity of urokinase dissipates in a few hours after discontinuing the drug, but reduced levels of fibrinogen or elevated levels of fibrin and fibrinogen degradation products may persist for 12–24 hours [21]. Elimination is rapid, with most of labeled urokinase appearing in the liver and bladder in 15 minutes. Small amounts are excreted in the bile and urine [42]. It is not known if urokinase is excreted in milk or if it crosses the placenta.

INDICATIONS FOR USE

The indications for the use of urokinase are essentially the same as for streptokinase. The major differences are the cost of urokinase, which is much higher, and the many fewer allergic adverse effects.

CONTRAINDICATIONS

The contraindications for urokinase are not specific to the drug but rather to the class of drug–thrombolytics. Table 6-4 lists the conditions that require alternative therapy or very careful monitoring.

DOSAGES

For PE, the loading dosage is 4400 international units/kg IV over 10 minutes. The maintenance dosage is 4400 international units/kg/hour for 12–24 hours by continuous infusion (FDA-approved regimen). (See package insert.)

For intrapulmonary infusion [3], the initial dosage is 2700 international units/kg infused over 5–10 minutes. The maintenance dosage is 2700 international units/kg/hour for 12 hours.

Urokinase may be used when thrombolytics are indicated and streptokinase cannot be administered.

ADVERSE REACTIONS

Hemorrhagic reactions occur with the same or nearly the same frequency as with streptokinase. Because urokinase is a naturally occurring protein, allergic reactions are much less common than with streptokinase. Febrile reactions do occur with this medication, however. As with streptokinase, the use of aspirin to prevent or suppress a febrile reaction should be avoided.

COMPARISON WITH STREPTOKINASE

Hemorrhagic complications occur with about equal frequency in patients undergoing thrombolysis with urokinase or streptokinase. Allergic reactions are very infrequent with urokinase, and those that do occur are poorly documented. Febrile reactions can occur with urokinase but less frequently than with streptokinase.

Recombinant Tissue-Type Plasminogen Activator (Alteplase)

Endogenous human TPA is a single-chain, glycosylated, trypsinlike serine protease secreted mainly by vascular endothelial cells. Recombinant TPA (RTPA) is a biosynthetic form of the human TPA prepared from cultures of genetically modified mammalian cells. The commercially available form is a glycosolated, predominantly single-chain form of TPA (alteplase) [42].

MECHANISM OF ACTION

The binding of TPA and plasminogen to the fibrin clot is associated with a conformational change that increases the availability of plasminogen locally, resulting in a more efficient activation of plasminogen at the fibrin surface rather than in the circulation [63]. The ternary complex of TPA, plasminogen, and fibrin, facilitates the localization of fibrinolytic activity to the clot. The predominantly two-chain form of RTPA is associated with greater systemic fibrinogenolysis [42].

Tissue-type plasminogen activator has been used in combination with urokinase, and the effect has been found to be synergistic. The reduced amounts of thrombolytics used have resulted in reduced systemic activation of the fibrinolytic system [11].

ONSET OF ACTION, METABOLISM, AND ELIMINATION

The onset of action of RTPA is rapid because it occurs predominantly at the fibrin surface. Inactivation of clot-bound plasmin by alpha$_2$-antiplasmin occurs 100 times more slowly than circulating plasmin because the binding sites for alpha$_2$-antiplasmin are occupied by fibrin [33]. To obtain consistent and sufficient levels RTPA must be given IV. Clearance is principally by the liver, and more than 50% is cleared from the plasma within 5 minutes after discontinuing IV infusion, but the elimination half-life may be prolonged in patients with severe liver disease. It is not known whether alteplase crosses the placenta or is excreted in milk.

INDICATIONS FOR USE

Recombinant tissue-type plasminogen activator is indicated for therapy of acute PE that obstructs one or more lobes or multiple segments equivalent to one or more lobes, or when the PE is accompanied by hypotension [7,48]. Its use has also been described in patients with DVT of acute onset [68].

CONTRAINDICATIONS

Table 6-4 shows the contraindications for the use of thrombolytic agents. The main difference between this drug and others of this class is that invasive procedures can be performed 20–30 minutes after infusion is discontinued [21].

DOSAGES

In systemic therapy for PE, 100 mg is given IV over 2 hours. Begin heparin when APTT or TT returns to less than twice normal (FDA-approved regimen).

In pulmonary artery infusion, 30 or 50 mg is infused over 1.5–2 hours with or without concomitant heparin therapy [42,70], although some recommend heparin not be given concomitantly with any thrombolytic [30,38,43].

LABORATORY MONITORING

Routine monitoring is unnecessary since the duration of therapy is so short. Monitoring is recommended to assess bleeding status if the patient is at risk for significant hemorrhage before therapy or if hemorrhage occurs during or after therapy.

LENGTH OF THERAPY

The length of RTPA infusion is 2 hours followed by heparin. Refer to the section on heparin for the dosage and duration of heparin therapy.

ADVERSE EFFECTS

Hypersensitivity reactions with alteplase are unusual and when they occur are usually mild. Arrhythmias are usually related to rapid lysis of coronary artery thrombi, resulting in reperfusion-associated disturbances of rhythm. Embolization of intraventricular thrombi may result in systemic infarcts, so the benefits of therapy must be weighed against the harmful potential effects of lytic agents.

COMPARISON WITH ALTERNATIVES

The use of alteplase is of benefit when a patient needs thrombolysis and invasive procedures are planned. Compared to the use of urokinase for PE, alteplase results in more rapid lysis at 2 hours but is equivalent at 24 hours. In practical terms, there seem to be no real benefits of one thrombolytic over another.

Recombinant Single-Chain Urokinase-Type Plasminogen Activator (Pro-urokinase)

Single-chain urokinase-type plasminogen activator (scu-PA or pro-urokinase) is a direct activator of fibrin-bound plasminogen. In plasma it does not significantly activate plasminogen; therefore, fibrinolysis occurs, but there is some fibrinogenolysis [12,22].

INDICATIONS FOR USE AND DOSAGES

Currently scu-PA has been used for clot lysis in patients with acute coronary thrombosis. The dosage was 40–70 mg scu-PA IV over 1 hour [12]. The combination of TPA and scu-PA has been used in animals to reduce the systemic activation of the fibrinolytic system. The reduction is probably due to the decreased amounts of thrombolytic agents needed [12].

Anisoylated Plasminogen Streptokinase Activator Complex (Anistreplase)

Anisoylated plasminogen streptokinase activator complex (APSAC) is an inactive derivative of a plasminogen-streptokinase complex. It is activated in vivo by deacylation. Fibrin specificity has not been shown in all studies [12]. It can be given by bolus injection and has a plasma half-life of 70–90 minutes. [33]. Because of its long half-life, it can be given IV by bolus. Its antigenic and allergic adverse effects are much like those of streptokinase. This drug combination has been used primarily for coronary thrombolysis.

DOSAGE

The dosage in coronary thrombolysis is 30 units IV given by bolus over 2–5 minutes. [21].

Conclusions

For DVT and PE no drug or drug combination has been shown to be superior to streptokinase. Fibrin specificity is not 100% by any of these drugs, and bleeding complications are seen with each of them; the incidence of hemorrhage is nearly the same with all thrombolytics.

References

1. Aarskog, E. J., et al. Low 1, 25-dihydroxy vitamin D in heparin-induced hyperkalemia. *Lancet* 2:650, 1980.
2. Ainsley, E. J., et al. Adverse reaction to chlorocresol-preserved heparin. *Lancet* 1:705, 1977.
3. Barberena, J. Intraarterial infusion of urokinase in the treatment of acute thromboembolism: Preliminary report. *AJR* 140:883, 1983.
4. Bell, W. R. Pulmonary embolism: Progress and problems. *Am. J. Med.* 72:181, 1982.
5. Bell, W. R., and Meek, A. G. Guidelines for the use of thrombolytic agents. *N. Engl. J. Med.* 301(23):1266, 1979.
6. Bounameaux, H., et al. Measurement of D-dimer in plasma as diagnostic aid in suspected pulmonary embolism. *Lancet* 337:196, 1991.
7. Bounameaux, H., et al. Thrombolytic treatment with recombinant tissue-type plasminogen activator in a patient with massive pulmonary embolism. *Ann. Intern. Med.* 103:64, 1985.
8. Caldini, P. Pulmonary hemodynamics and arterial oxygen saturation in pulmonary embolism. *J. Appl. Physiol.* 20(2):184, 1965.

9. Cheely, R., et al. The role of noninvasive tests versus pulmonary angiography in the diagnosis of pulmonary embolism. *Am. J. Med.* 70:17, 1981.

10. Cines, D. B. Heparin: Do we understand its antithrombotic actions? *Chest* 89(3):420, 1986.

11. Collen, D. Synergism of thrombolytic agents in vivo. *Circulation* 74(4):838, 1986.

12. Collen, D. Molecular mechanism of action of newer thrombolytic agents. *J. Am. Coll. Cardiol.* 10:16B, 1987.

13. Consensus Conference. Fresh-frozen plasma. *JAMA* 253(4):551, 1985.

14. Cruickshank, M. K., et al. A standard nomogram for the management of heparin therapy. *Arch. Intern. Med.* 151:333, 1991.

15. Edes, T. E., and Sunderrajan, E. V. Heparin-induced hyperkalemia. *Arch. Intern. Med.* 145:1070, 1985.

16. Gent, M., and Roberts, R. S. A meta-analysis of the studies of dihydroergotamine plus heparin. *Chest* 89(5 Suppl.):396S, 1986.

17. Ginsberg, J. S., and Hirsh, J. Use of anticoagulants during pregnancy. *Chest* 92(2 Suppl.):156S, 1989.

18. Ginsberg, J. S., and Hirsh, J. Use of antithrombotic agents during pregnancy. *Chest* 102(4 Suppl.):385S, 1992.

19. Goldhaber, S. Z., et al. Diagnosis, treatment, and prevention of pulmonary embolism. *JAMA* 268(3):1727, 1992.

20. Griner, P. F., et al. Selection and interpretation of diagnostic tests and procedures. *Ann. Intern. Med.* 94 (4 part 2):553, 1981.

21. Guidry, J. R., et al. Anticoagulants and thrombolytics. *Crit. Care Med.* 7(3):533, 1991.

22. Gurewich, V. Experiences with pro-urokinase and potentiation of its fibrinolytic effect by urokinase and by tissue plasminogen activator. *J. Am. Coll. Cardiol.* 10:16B, 1987.

23. Hirsh, J. Heparin. *N. Engl. J. Med.* 324:1565, 1991.

24. Hirsh, J., and Hull, R. D. Treatment of venous thromboembolism. *Chest* 89(Suppl.5):426S, 1986.

25. Hirsh, J. Substandard monitoring of warfarin in North America. *Arch. Intern. Med.* 152:257, 1992.

26. Hirsh, J. Oral anticoagulant drugs. *N. Engl. J. Med.* 324(26):1865, 1991.

27. Hirsch, D. R., and Goldhaber, S. Z. Contemporary use of laboratory tests to monitor safety and efficacy of thrombolytic therapy. *Chest* 101(4 Suppl.):98S, 1992.

28. Hull, R., et al. Adjusted subcutaneous heparin versus warfarin sodium in the long-term treatment of venous thrombosis. *N. Engl. J. Med.* 306:189, 1982.

29. Hyers, T. M., et al. Antithrombotic therapy for venous thromboembolic disease. *Chest* 95(2 Suppl.):37S, 1989.

30. Hyers, T. M., et al. Antithrombotic therapy for venous thromboembolic disease. *Chest* 102(4 Suppl.):173S, 1990.

31. Hyman, B. T., et al. Warfarin-related purple toes syndrome and cholesterol microembolization. *Am. J. Med.* 82:1233, 1987.

32. Katz, S., and Horres, A. D. Medullary respiratory neuron response to pulmonary emboli and pneumothorax. *J. Appl. Physiol.* 33(3):488, 1972.

33. Kessler, C. M. The pharmacology of aspirin, heparin, coumarin, and thrombolytic agents. *Chest* 99(4 Suppl.):97S, 1991.

34. Leyvraz, P. F., et al. Adjusted versus fixed-dose subcutaneous heparin in the prevention of deep-venous thrombosis after total hip replacement. *N. Engl. J. Med.* 309:954, 1983.

35. Levine, E. L., et al. Heparin-induced cutaneous necrosis unrelated to injection sites. *Arch. Dermatol.* 119:400, 1983.

36. Levine, M. N., et al. Hemorrhagic complications of long-term anticoagulant therapy. *Chest* 95(2 Suppl.):26S, 1989.

37. Levine, M. N., et al. Hemorrhagic complications of thrombolytic therapy in the treatment of myocardial infarction and venous thromboembolism. *Chest* 102(2 Suppl.):364S, 1992.

38. Levine, M., et al. A randomized trial of a single-bolus dosage regimen of recombinant tissue plasminogen activator in patients with acute massive pulmonary embolism. *Chest* 98(6):1473, 1990.

39. Majerus, P. W., et al. Anticoagulants, Thrombolytic, and Antiplatelet Drugs. In A. G. Gilman et al. (eds.), *Goodman and Gilman's The Pharmacological Basis of Therapeutics* (8th ed.). New York: Pergamon Press, 1990.

40. Malik, A. B., and van der Zee, H. Time course of pulmonary vascular response to microembolism. *J. Appl. Physiol.* 43(1):51, 1977.

41. Marcus, R., and Coulston, A. M. Fat Soluble Vitamins. In A. G. Gilman et al. (eds.), *Goodman and Gilman's The Pharmacological Basis of Therapeutics* (8th ed.). New York: Pergamon Press, 1990.

42. McEvoy, G. K. (ed.). *AHFS Drug Information 1991*. Bethesda, MD: American Society of Hospital Pharmacists, 1991.

43. Mitchell, J. P., and Trulock, E. P. Tissue-plasminogen activator for pulmonary embolism resulting in shock: Two case reports and discussion of the literature. *Am. J. Med.* 90:255, 1991.

44. The Multicenter Trial Committee. Dihydroergotamine-heparin prophylaxis of postoperative deep vein thrombosis. *JAMA* 251(22):2960, 1984.

45. Nalbandian, R. M., et al. Coumarin necrosis of skin treated successfully with heparin. *Obstet. Gynecol.* 38:1233, 1987.

46. Novelline, R. A., et al. The clinical course of patients with suspected pulmonary embolism and a negative pulmonary arteriogram. *Radiology* 126:561, 1978.

47. Persson, A. V., et al. Burst therapy. *Am. J. Surg.* 147:531, 1984.

48. PIOPED Investigators. Tissue plasminogen activator for the treatment of acute pulmonary embolism. *Chest* 97(3):528, 1990.

49. Polak, J. F., and McNeil, B. J. Pulmonary scintigraphy and the diagnosis of pulmonary embolism. *Cl. Chest Med.* 5(3):457, 1984.

50. Poller, L., et al. Fixed minidose warfarin: A new approach to prophylaxis against venous thrombosis after major surgery. *Br. J. Med.* 295:1309, 1987.

51. Reynolds, J. E. F. (ed.). *Martindale: The Extra Pharmacopeia* (29th ed.) London: Pharmaceutical Press, 1989.

52. Rogers, L. Q., and Lutcher, C. L. Streptokinase therapy for deep vein thrombosis: A comprehensive review of the English literature. *Am. J. Med.* 88:389, 1990.

53. Rowbotham, B. J., et al. Plasma cross linked fibrin degradation products in pulmonary embolism. *Thorax* 45:684, 1990.

54. Salzman, E. W., et al. Management of heparin therapy. *N. Engl. J. Med.* 292:1046, 1975.

55. Sane, D. C., et al. Bleeding during thrombolytic therapy for acute myocardial infarction: Mechanisms and management. *Ann. Intern. Med.* 111(12):1010, 1989.

56. Sasahara, A. A. Therapy for pulmonary embolism. *JAMA* 229(13):1795, 1974.

57. Sharma, G. V. R. K., et al. Thrombolytic therapy. *N. Engl. J. Med.* 306(21):1268, 1982.

58. Singer, D., et al. Hemodynamic alterations following miliary pulmonary embolization in relation to the pathogenesis of the consequent diffuse edema. *Am. J. Physiol.* 191(3):437, 1957.

59. Sonnenblick, M., and Jacobsohn, W. Hyper-transaminasemia with heparin therapy. *Br. Med. J.* 3:77, 1975.

60. Spodick, D. H. Electrocardiographic responses to pulmonary embolism. *Am. J. Cardiol.* 30:695, 1972.

61. Spotnitz, H. M., et al. Pathophysiology and experimental treatment of acute pulmonary embolism. *Am. Heart J.* 82(4):511, 1971.

62. Stein, M., et al. Gas exchange after autologous pulmonary embolism in dogs. *J. Appl. Physiol.* 16(3):488, 1961.

63. Stewart, J. H., et al. Thrombolytic therapy. *Cleve. Clin. J. Med.* 56:189, 1989.

64. Talstad, I. Heparin therapy adjusted for body weight. *Am. J. Clin. Path.* 83(3):378, 1985.

65. Terrin, M., et al. Selection of patients with acute pulmonary embolism for thrombolytic therapy. *Chest* 95(5 Suppl.):279S, 1989.

66. Tillett, W. S., and Garner, R. L. The fibrinolytic activity of hemolytic streptococci. *J. Exp. Med.* 58:485, 1933.

67. Turpie, A. G. G., et al. Tissue plasminogen activator (rt-PA) vs heparin in deep vein thrombosis. *Chest* (4 Suppl.):173S, 1990.

68. USP DI. *Drug Information for the Health Care Professional* (11th ed.) United States Pharmacopeia Convention. Rockville, MD, 1991.

69. Verstraete, M., et al. Intravenous and intrapulmonary recombinant tissue-type plasminogen activator in the treatment of acute massive pulmonary embolism. *Circulation* 77(2):353, 1988.

7

Interstitial Lung Disease

Richard Carl Bernstein
Samuel V. Spagnolo

In view of the numerous causes (Table 7-1) of interstitial lung disease (ILD), we find it practical to divide ILD into categories based on the potential treatment options [12]. For example, lymphangitic spread of carcinoma will require antineoplastic treatment, and unusual interstitial lung infections (e.g., tuberculosis, blastomycosis) need the appropriate antimicrobial agents. Heart failure will be managed with diuretics, afterload reducers, and so forth. This leaves a group of disorders that are responsive to glucocorticoid and other antiinflammatory agents and a group with no drug treatment options other than support with supplemental oxygen [3,13]. This chapter will focus on the inflammatory disorders that involve the lung.

Most progressive antiinflammatory responsive ILD will cause abnormalities in lung architecture that leads to ventilation/perfusion mismatching causing hypoxemia. Initially this imbalance manifests only with exertion, but eventually it progresses to resting hypoxemia if the process is severe. Histologically these disorders start as inflammation in the pulmonary interstitium and development of irreversible fibrosis. This change in pulmonary architecture causes reduced lung volumes and decreased lung compliance, resulting in abnormal pulmonary mechanics. It is the abnormal lung mechanics and hypoxemia that cause the symptom of dyspnea [10,12].

Diagnosis

The diagnosis of the various ILDs is based on the specific type of disease process. A detailed history is important to determine if any

Table 7-1. Causes of interstitial lung disease

Sarcoidosis
Hypersensitivity pneumonitis
Idiopathic pulmonary fibrosis
Tuberculosis
Fungal infections
Pneumoconiosis
Congestive heart disease
Pulmonary vasculitis
Collagen vascular disease
Carcinoma (especially lymphangitic spread)
Eosinophilic diseases
Drug induced
Radiation pneumonitis
Atypical pneumonia
Lymphocytic infiltrative disorders

drug or occupational or recreational exposure is the cause. It is useful to identify other symptom complexes that could be consistent with collagen vascular diseases or other systemic diseases, thus enabling more specific treatment.

The physical examination in various ILDs may show a continuum ranging from no abnormalities to a severely dyspneic, cyanotic patient with diffuse crackles appreciated on auscultation of the chest. When a systemic disease is associated with ILD than other physical findings of these diseases, such as arthritis, subcutaneous nodules should be carefully searched for and documented [12].

The chest roentgenogram will frequently narrow the differential diagnosis based on specific radiographic patterns. Immunologic markers such as antinuclear antibody present in systemic lupus erythematosus and anti-SS antibodies associated with scleroderma are helpful in making a specific diagnosis [12].

Pulmonary function studies commonly reveal a decreased total lung capacity and decreased carbon monoxide diffusion capacity. The arterial blood gases may show a chronic respiratory alkalosis or hypoxemia associated with an increased alveolar-arterial oxygen tension gradient [1].

Radioactive lung scanning with gallium is frequently used to assess disease activity by demonstrating increased lung uptake if a major inflammatory component is present in the lung parenchyma [12]. Bronchoalveolar lavage with differential cell analysis reflects cellular inflammatory activity and may support a specific diagnosis (such as an increase in T-helper lymphocytes in sarcoidosis), but often the diagnosis must be confirmed by sampling of lung tissue. Lung tissue can be easily obtained by transbronchial lung biopsy, thoracoscopy with biopsy, or standard thoracotomy "open" lung biopsy [10,12]. The biopsy specimen is sent for appropriate cultures, special stains, general histologic evaluation, immunofluorescent staining, and possibly electron microscopy.

Treatment

The antiinflammatory agents most commonly used include the glucocorticoids, cyclophosphamide, and azathioprim. D-penicillamine causes high untoward effects in many cases [3,12], and we do not recommend its use in ILD at this time. Methotrexate is used extensively in rheumatoid arthritis and occasionally in other ILDs.

Glucocorticoid

Both prednisone (Deltasone) and methylprednisolone (Medrol) have similar characteristics, bioavailability, and side effects and can be discussed together. The comparative glucocorticoid potency of 5 mg of prednisone is equivalent to 4 mg of methylprednisolone, and both possess potent antiinflammatory properties. In ILD, the glucocorticoid will suppress neutrophil and lymphocyte function, decrease leukocyte migration, decrease immunoglobulin production, decrease secretion of proteolytic enzymes by the alveolar macrophage, and reduce the release of various chemotactic factors [5,12].

PHARMACOKINETICS

Prednisone and methylprednisolone are well tolerated after oral absorption. In the plasma, 90% or more of these agents are reversibly bound to two major proteins, corticosteroid-binding globulin and albumin. Glucocorticoids are metabolized by the reduction of the double bond in the 4,5 position, mainly in the liver, and are primarily excreted through the kidneys [5].

CLINICAL INDICATIONS

Glucocorticoids are indicated for ILD associated with systemic lupus erythematosus (SLE), rheumatoid arthritis, polymyositis and dermatomyositis, Sjögren's syndrome, Churg-Strauss syndrome, sarcoidosis, and eosinophilic pneumonia [3,10,12,13].

They are also frequently utilized for treatment of hypersensitivity pneumonitis and drug-induced ILD from such agents as amiodirone, methotrexate, and nitrofurantoin that are not responsive to drug withdrawal.

A glucocorticoid, in combination with cyclophosphamide is effective therapy for Wegener's granulomatosis and is frequently given as empiric therapy for idiopathic pulmonary fibrosis [2,4,6,7,9,11,15].

ADVERSE EFFECTS

Fluid and electrolyte disturbances occur, including sodium retention, fluid retention, and hypokalemic metabolic alkalosis. With chronic administration of a glucocorticoid, muscle weakness, osteoporosis, and compression fractures may develop. Peptic ulcer disease and pancreatitis are occasional GI complications. Impaired wound healing has been reported. Ocular complications include the development of cataracts and glaucoma. Chronic use may lead to the development of a Cushingoid appearance with a decreased glucose tolerance and secondary adrenocortical and pituitary unresponsiveness. The package insert should be reviewed prior to using this drug. **Patients on glucocorticoid therapy should not be vaccinated against smallpox. Other immunization procedures should not be done because of possible neurological complications and poor antibody response.**

DOSAGE AND ADMINISTRATION

Prednisone is available for oral use in 5-, 10-, and 20-mg tablets, and methylprednisolone is available for oral use in 4- and 8-mg tablets.

In ILD responsive to glucocorticoid treatment, the dosage of prednisone is started between 0.5 and 1.5 mg/kg/day up to 100 mg. The length of treatment and the rate of tapering is dependent on the specific condition. With all ILDs it is important that the lowest effective dosage be used for maintenance. Some diseases respond to alternate-day glucocorticoid therapy, which may decrease the adverse effects, including suppression of the hypothalamic-pituitary adrenal axis [12,13].

Cyclophosphamide

Cyclophosphamide (Cytoxan) is an alkylating agent chemically related to nitrogen mustard. It is biotransformed mainly in the liver to an active alkylating metabolite through a microsomal oxidase system. The metabolites interfere with growth of susceptible rapidly proliferating malignant cells. The antiinflammatory mechanisms of cyclophosphamide are not well understood.

PHARMACOKINETICS

Cyclophosphamide is well absorbed after oral administration, with greater than 75% bioavailability. Cyclophosphamide has a serum half-life of 3–12 hours, and approximately 75–95% is excreted as metabolites, with the remainder excreted unchanged in the urine. Plasma binding of the drug is low, but some metabolites are 60% protein bound [7,9].

CLINICAL INDICATIONS

Although not approved by the Food and Drug Administration (FDA), cyclophosphamide (usually given with prednisone) is effective therapy for Wegener's granulomatosis. Some efficacy has also been reported in idiopathic pulmonary fibrosis and lymphangiocentric granuloma [2,4,6,12]. Although cyclophosphamide has also been used in the treatment of general connective tissue diseases such as SLE, rheumatoid arthritis, Churg-Strauss, and polyarteritis nodosa [7], its use in these clinical situations remains controversial.

ADVERSE EFFECTS

The development of pulmonary interstitial fibrosis is a rare but serious complication. Cyclophosphamide also inhibits spermatogenesis in men and destroys follicular cells in women, causing infertility. Nausea and vomiting commonly occur, with diarrhea less frequent. Skin effects include rash and alopecia. Leukopenia is common and dose dependent, while thrombocytopenia occasionally occurs. Hemorrhagic cystitis may develop, which can lead to fibrosis. This can be prevented with increasing fluids to maintain good urine output.

DOSAGE AND ADMINISTRATION

Cyclophosphamide tablets are available in 25- and 50-mg tablets. Cyclophosphamide for parenteral use is available in 100-, 200-, 500-mg and 1- and 2-g vials.

For Wegener's granulomatosis, cyclophosphamide 1–2 mg/kg/day is given in addition to prednisone [4].

In idiopathic pulmonary fibrosis, parenteral cyclophosphamide 500–1800 mg given IV on a biweekly basis has recently been shown to be useful as a steroid-sparing agent [3]. If cyclophosphamide is given orally, low dosages — 1–2 mg/kg/day — are used. The package insert should be reviewed prior to using this drug.

Azathioprine

Azathioprine (Imuran) is an immunosuppressive antimetabolite derivative of 6-mercaptopurine. It has antiinflammatory actions, for which the mechanism is not known, but it has been shown to decrease delayed hypersensitivity and cellular toxicity to a greater extent than antibody response.

PHARMACOKINETICS

Azathioprine is well absorbed following oral administration and is approximately 30% bound to serum proteins. It is cleaved in vivo to mercaptopurine, with both the parent compound and metabolites oxidized or methylated in erythrocytes and the liver. It is also inactivated by conversion to 6-thiouric acid by xanthine oxidase. (If allopurinol, a xanthine oxidase inhibitor, is also given, the dosage of azathioprine must be decreased.)

CLINICAL INDICATIONS

Azathioprine is indicated in some conditions when steroids alone are insufficient for disease control or the steroid dosage cannot be successfully reduced without another antiinflammatory agent, such as in rheumatoid arthritis, idiopathic pulmonary fibrosis, and dermatopolymyositis [11,13,15]. Although not FDA approved, it is also used in conjunction with glucocorticoid and cyclophosphamide in Wegener's granulomatosis [12].

ADVERSE EFFECTS

Bone marrow suppression with leukopenia, thrombocytopenia, and macrocytic anemia may occur. There is an increased risk of opportunistic infections such as nocardia. Nausea and vomiting are common complications. Azathioprine can cause fetal harm and is teratogenic in laboratory animals. A skin rash is occasionally seen.

DRUG INTERACTIONS

Allopurinol-azathioprim dosage should be decreased to one-third or one-fourth the usual dosage in patients on allopurinol.

Caution: Angiotensin-converting enzyme inhibitors used with azothioprim may induce severe leukopenia.

DOSAGE AND ADMINISTRATION

The package insert should be reviewed prior to using this drug. Azathioprine is available in 50-mg tablets and 100-mg vials for injection. The usual dosage of azathioprine in most of the ILD-related conditions is 1–3 mg/kg/day [11,12,15].

Methotrexate

Methotrexate is a folic acid analogue that completely inhibits the enzyme dihydrofolate reductase, which is necessary for single carbon transfer in thymidylate synthesis. It is impairment of this enzyme that prevents DNA synthesis and results in its clinical effect.

PHARMACOKINETICS

Methotrexate is well absorbed from the GI tract and from IM injection. It is approximately 50% reversibly bound to plasma proteins. Methotrexate is cleared by glomerular filtration and active tubular secretion and is excreted mostly unchanged in the urine.

CLINICAL INDICATIONS

Methotrexate's main use in ILD is in the treatment of severe rheumatoid arthritis, polymyositis, and dermatomyositis, which does not respond to high-dosage corticosteroid [12].

ADVERSE EFFECTS

Methotrexate has been implicated as a cause of interstitial lung disease [12], although this is hard to differentiate from the underlying ILD in patients with rheumatoid arthritis and other connective tissue diseases of the lung. Lung injury may occur acutely at any time during therapy, even at dosages as low as 7.5 mg/week. This may require interruption of therapy.

Gastrointestinal toxicity occurs in two-thirds of the patients, with effects including bloating, nausea, diarrhea, and mouth ulcers, and requires interruption of therapy; otherwise, hemorrhagic enteritis and **death** from intestinal perforation may occur. Hyperenzymemia occurs, and hepatic toxicity as manifested on liver biopsy may occur in 20% of those receiving a cumulative dose greater than 1.5 g. Hepatic fibrosis and cirrhosis occur and may not be preceded by symptoms or abnormal liver function tests [8,14]. Alcohol is contraindicated in methotrexate recipients.

Methotrexate has been reported to cause fetal death or congenital anomalies and is not recommended for women of childbearing potential.

Methotrexate may produce marked bone marrow depression with resultant anemia, leukopenia, anemia, or thrombocytopenia.

Other side effects reported include dizziness, headaches, and vertigo, and the package insert should be reviewed prior to using this drug.

DOSAGE AND ADMINISTRATION

Periodic monitoring for toxicity, including CBC with differential and platelet counts, and liver and renal function tests are a mandatory part of methotrexate therapy. Periodic liver biopsies may be indicated in unusual situations.

Methotrexate is available in 20-mg, 50-mg, and 1-g vials for parenteral use and in 2.5-mg tablets (Rheumatrex Dose Pack). The dosage ranges from 5–15 mg given as a single oral or IM injection. Dosage should be reduced in renal failure, and extreme caution should be used in this situation.

DRUG INTERACTIONS

Severe and sometimes fatal marrow suppression and GI toxicity have been reported, with concomitant administration of methotrexate along with some nonsteroidal antiinflammatory drugs.

References

1. Bates, D. V. *Respiratory Function in Disease*. Philadelphia: W. B. Saunders, 1989.
2. Baughman, R. P., and Lower, E. E. Use of intermittent, intravenous cyclophosphamide for idiopathic pulmonary fibrosis. *Chest* 102:1090, 1992.
3. Costabel, U., and Matthys, H. Different therapies and factors influencing response to therapy in idiopathic diffuse fibrosing alveolitis. *Respiration* 42:141, 1981.
4. Fauci, A. S., et al. Wegener's granulomatosis: Prospective clinical and therapeutic experience with 85 patients for 21 years. *Ann. Intern. Med.* 98:76, 1983.
5. Goodman, L., and Gilman, A. *The Pharmacological Basis of Therapeutics* (8th ed.). New York: Macmillan, 1990.
6. Hoffman, G. S., and Leavitt, R. Y. Treatment of Wegener's granulomatosis with intermittent high-dose intravenous cyclophosphamide. *Am. J. Med.* 89:403, 1990.
7. Korvarsky, J. Clinical pharmacology and toxicology of cyclophosphamide: Emphasis on use in rheumatic diseases. *Semin. Arthritis Rheum.* 12:359, 1983.
8. Kreemer, J. M., and Joong, K. L. The safety and efficacy of the use of methotrexate in long-term therapy for rheumatoid arthritis. *Arthritis Rheum.* 29:822, 1986.
9. Moore, M. J. Clinical pharmacokinetics of cyclophosphamide. *Clin. Pharmacokin.* 20:194, 1991.
10. Murray, J. F., and Nadel, J. A. *Textbook of Respiratory Medicine*. Philadelphia: W. B. Saunders, 1988.
11. Raghu, G., et al. Azathioprine combined with prednisone in the treatment of idiopathic pulmonary fibrosis: A prospective double-blind, randomized, placebo-controlled clinical trial. *Am. Rev. Respir. Dis.* 144:291, 1991.
12. Schwartz, M. I., and King, T. E. *Interstitial Lung Disease*. Burlington, Ontario: BC Decker, 1988.

13. Turner-Warwick, M. Approaches to therapy (interstitial lung disease). *Semin. Respir. Med.* 6:92, 1984.

14. Whiting-O'Keefe, Q. E., et al. Methotrexate and histologic hepatic abnormalities: A meta analysis. *Am. J. Med.* 90:711, 1991.

15. Winterbauer, R. H., et al. Diffuse interstitial pneumonitis: Clinicopathologic correlations in 20 patients treated with prednisone/azathioprine. *Am. J. Med.* 65:661, 1978.

8

Lung Transplantation

James V. Palazzolo
Samuel V. Spagnolo

Organ transplantation has become the new frontier of medicine. With the success of renal transplantation, more clinical effort has been aggressively directed toward transplantation of other vital organs, such as the liver, pancreas, heart, and lung. Initial attempts at lung transplantation, however, met with dismal results. Difficulty in healing at the site of airway anastomosis was the major factor responsible for the failures. It was not until the mid-1960s that the first successful attempt at human lung transplantation was performed by Hardy and colleagues. The patient survived only 2 weeks, but the effort continued to spark attempts at lung transplantation.

Progress in renal, heart, and liver transplantation was due mainly to advances in immunosuppression. Side effects from immunosuppressive drugs, however, prevented similar progress in lung transplantation. Immunosuppressive treatment regimens consisted mainly of steroids, azathioprine, and antilymphocyte globulin. It was not until the discovery of cyclosporine and improvements in the surgical technique that the first successful single lung transplantation was completed by the Toronto Lung Transplant Group in 1983.

New developments in immunosuppressive therapy and operative techniques have continued to decrease morbidity and mortality significantly. During the past few years there has been a tremendous growth of lung transplant programs worldwide. By the end of 1991, over 1000 heart-lung and lung transplantations had been performed.

Initial lung transplantations were in the form of heart-lung combinations, due to the significant heart disease that candidates for lung transplantation possessed. Recently, attempts at double and single lung transplantation have proved that acquired heart disease can be partially reversed with lung transplants. Current indications for heart-lung transplants include individuals with septic pulmonary conditions, primary pulmonary disease (primary pulmonary hypertension and emphysema), irreversible cardiac dysfunction, congenital cardiac anomalies, or any combination of these. Double lung transplantation is also indicated in septic pulmonary disease (cystic fibrosis, bronchiolitis obliterans, and bronchiectasis), in addition to pulmonary fibrosis and severe emphysema. The indications for single lung transplantation have recently been expanded to include emphysema, pulmonary fibrosis, and primary pulmonary hypertension, as well as other end-stage lung diseases. It is the success thus far with single lung transplantation that has revealed the feasibility and potential benefit of such a procedure.

The goal of immunotherapy is to maintain a balance between immunosuppression and adequate host defenses. With the development of more effective and selective immune system modifiers, the incidence of postoperative graft rejection and infectious complications has decreased significantly. The ideal regimen for lung transplantation is currently being refined as investigations into additional selective immunosuppressive therapy continue.

Cyclosporine

Cyclosporine (Sandimmune) is a cyclic polypeptide composed of 11 amino acids and produced by the fungus *Tolypoclatium inflatum gams*. It is one of several antimicrobials produced by these fungi with the active metabolites cyclosporine A and C. Its immunosuppressive activity is through its inhibition of cell-mediated immune responses such as delayed hypersensitivity, allograft rejection, and graft-versus-host reactions.

MECHANISM OF ACTION

The exact mechanism of immunosuppression appears mainly to involve the inhibition of T helper cells, although some inhibition of T suppressor and cytotoxic cells also occurs. Cyclosporine inhibits the production and release of lymphokines such as interleukin 1 (lymphocyte activating factor) and interleukin 2 (T-cell growth factor) from T helper cells responsible for the activation of cytotoxic T cells. There appears to be no effect on the function of phagocytic cells, such as the macrophage, or significant inhibition of the beta-cell or humoral immune response.

The most important feature of cyclosporine immunosuppression is the absence of significant myelosuppression in therapeutic concentrations. In several studies using cyclosporine, bone marrow stem cell counts have been minimally affected or normal. This has greatly reduced the incidence of infectious complications posttransplantation.

INDICATIONS

Cyclosporine is used in combination with prednisone to maintain allograft lung and heart-lung transplants. Clinical studies indicate that cyclosporine may also be useful in the treatment of various autoimmune disorders, such as rheumatoid arthritis, inflammatory bowel disease, glomerulonephritis, and related diseases. In insulin-dependent diabetes mellitus, cyclosporine has been found to reverse the condition temporarily when given within 6 weeks of onset. Long-term therapy, however, has not been encouraging.

PHARMACOKINETICS

Cyclosporine pharmacokinetics are known to vary considerably among patients. Absorption from the GI tract is variable and incomplete. Peak serum concentrations of cyclosporine are reached in 3–4 hours. Approximately 60% of the drug is bound to erythrocytes, and 10–20% is bound to leukocytes. The remainder circulates in association with plasma lipoproteins. Plasma half-life approaches 6 hours.

Cyclosporine readily distributes in tissues with a large volume of distribution. Metabolism is primarily hepatic through the cytochrome P450 medicated oxidation of side chains. The majority of the drug and its metabolites are excreted in the biliary system, with less than 10% of a dose excreted in the urine. Cyclosporine is reported to cross the placenta and be excreted in breast milk.

DRUG INTERACTIONS

Low plasma levels resulting from increased clearance have been observed in patients receiving phenobarbital, phenytoin, isoniazid, rifampin, carbamazepine, and trimethoprim-sulfamethoxazole due to induction of the cytochrome system. Decreased clearance of cyclosporine, resulting in elevated blood levels, is associated with concomitant use of such drugs as erythromycin, ketoconazole, amphotericin B, cimetidine, diltiazem, metoclopramide, and imipenem. Increased immunosuppressive effects are noted with concurrent use of azathioprine, corticosteroids, cyclophosphamide, and verapamil. Close monitoring of cyclosporine blood levels is recommended.

CLINICAL TOXICITY

The most frequent and important adverse effect of cyclosporine is nephrotoxicity. Elevations of BUN and creatinine appear to be dosage related and decrease with discontinuing the drug. Mild nephrotoxicity can occur 2–3 months into therapy. BUN and creatinine elevations in mild nephrotoxicity can become stable in the range of 30–40 mg/dl and 2–2.5 mg/dl, respectively. The risk of severe cyclosporine-induced nephrotoxicity is increased when administered with other nephrotoxic agents. Clinically, cyclosporine nephrotoxicity may present with fluid retention, pedal edema, and a hyperchloremic, hyperkalemic metabolic acidosis. Gradual reduction in dosage with careful evaluation for several days to weeks is recommended. If patients are unresponsive to reductions in dosage, switching to therapy with azathioprine and prednisone may be considered. The use of steroids with cyclosporine has been shown to improve renal function.

Adverse cardiovascular effects of cyclosporine therapy include hypertension, which usually responds to antihypertensive therapy. Elevations in both systolic and diastolic values have been reported. Diastolic elevations may be more resistant to therapy.

Tremors, seizures, headaches, elevations in serum transaminases, serum bilirubin, and serum gamma glutamyl transferase have been reported with higher dosages early in treatment. These adverse effects usually respond to reductions in dosage.

Additional adverse effects include anorexia, abdominal discomfort, diarrhea, nausea, and vomiting. Hirsutism has been reported but appears not to be dosage dependent. Leukopenia, anemia, and thrombocytopenia can occur, although clinical studies in humans indicate that cyclosporine does not depress bone marrow function. Hypersensitivity reactions are exceedingly rare.

DOSAGE AND ADMINISTRATION

Cyclosporine is available in oral tablet and solution form. Both should be taken on a strict schedule in relation to meals and time of day. The addition of milk or juice to increase the palatability of the solution is encouraged. Care must be taken that a glass container is used; porous containers result in absorption of a portion of the drug, reducing the actual dosage. The container should also be rinsed with additional diluent and consumed to ensure complete dosing.

Dosage should be individualized routinely based on blood levels and serum creatinine. In lung transplantation, the usual initial oral dosage is 6 mg/kg as a single dose given 4–12 hours before surgery. This dosage is continued postoperatively as 3 mg/kg twice daily, adjusting for drug levels.

Intravenous dosing is reserved for those unable to tolerate oral dosing or if contraindicated. The IV infusion is one-third the oral dosage. Each ml of cyclosporine concentrate should be diluted in 20–100 ml of 0.9 normal saline or 5% dextrose solution and administered over 2–6 hours. Initial IV dose of 2–3 mg/kg is given 4–12 hours preoperatively. This dosage is continued daily postoperatively, adjusting to a serum trough level of 300–500 ng/ml, drawn within a half-hour before the fifth dose. The patient should be switched to oral dosing as soon as possible.

Azathioprine

MECHANISM OF ACTION

Azathioprine (Immuran) is a purine analogue. As an imidazole derivative of mercaptopurine, it functions as an antimetabolite, inhibiting both purine synthesis and its subsequent utilization in RNA and DNA synthesis. It was developed to function as a prodrug (precursor to mercaptopurine) to decrease the rate of metabolism of mercaptopurine. Reacting with sulfhydryl groups in compounds such as glutathione and cysteine, azathioprine allows the liberation of mercaptopurine locally at target sites. This is thought to enhance the antineoplastic effects of the drug locally.

In comparison with mercaptopurine, azathioprine generates less toxic immunosuppression. The exact mechanism for this is not entirely understood at present. It may be related to different pharmacokinetic properties and the metabolism of azathioprine at specific sites of the immune system.

PHARMACOKINETICS

Azathioprine reaches maximum serum levels 1–2 hours after oral administration. Approximately 30% of the drug is bond to plasma proteins. It is well absorbed from the GI tract and rapidly distributed in tissues throughout the body.

Due to the rapid removal of the drug from the circulation, serum levels are of limited use in monitoring therapy. Clinical effectiveness has been found to correlate best with tissue levels of thiopurine nucleotides.

Both azathioprine and mercaptopurine are extensively oxidized in the red blood cell and liver. Xanthine oxidase is the enzyme responsible for their conversion to inactive metabolites. With the inhibition of this enzyme by allopurinol, adjustment in dosing azathioprine is required whenever allopurinol is prescribed simultaneously.

CLINICAL TOXICITY

The most serious adverse effects of azathioprine are bone marrow suppression and GI disturbances. The severity of toxic effects depends on dosage and duration of therapy. Reduction of dosage or temporary withdrawal of the drug reverses these effects. Therapy should be maintained at the lowest effective therapy.

Infection is always a severe complication of bone marrow suppresion. With a direct relation to the extent of leukopenia, blood levels should be routinely monitored — weekly for the first several months of therapy, then biweekly, and eventually monthly. It is important to be aware of the potential delay in manifestations of infection. Anemia and thrombocytopenia have also been reported.

Azathioprine is mutagenic in animals and carries a risk of causing neoplasia in humans. Several studies have linked increased incidence of lymphomas and skin cancers with posttransplant immunosuppression. The combination of immunosuppressive agents may result in an even greater risk.

Nausea and vomiting usually occur within the first few weeks of therapy and quickly respond to dividing dosages or therapy after meals. Additional side effects include jaundice, steatorrhea, oral ulcerations, esophagitis, alopecia, fever, and arthralgia. Hepatotoxicity may occur at any time and is reversible when azathioprine is promptly discontinued. Periodic assessment of hepatic function is recommended.

DRUG INTERACTIONS

The use of allopurinol with azathioprine will lead to impaired metabolism of azathioprine, potentially increasing the extent of side effects. Simultaneous use may require a dosage reduction to one-quarter the normal dosage. Drugs known to induce leukopenia should be used with caution when administered with azathioprine. Azathioprine may reverse neuromuscular blockade.

DOSAGE AND ADMINISTRATION

Azathioprine may be given PO or IV. The oral route is preferred. The initial dosage is 1–2 mg/kg/day 1–3 days preoperatively. Following transplantation, the dosage is continued, adjusting for white blood cell count just below 5000/mm^3. Intravenous dosing may be carried out if patients are unable to tolerate oral administration at the same dosing level.

Azathioprine is distributed in 50-mg scored tablets and supplied in bottles of 100 tablets. The solution is supplied in 20-ml vials equivalent to 100 mg. It should be dissolved in 10 cc of sterile water and mixed gently to a clear solution prior to injection. It should be used within 24 hours of mixing. Additional dilution may be carried out with sterile dextrose or saline and can be infused in 5 minutes or over up to 8 hours (usual infusion time, 30–60 minutes). The vials should be protected from light and stored at 60–86°F.

Various regimens are currently under trial using azathioprine for maintenance of immunosuppression following transplantation. The combination of azathioprine and cyclosporine has a significant steroid-sparing effect. This has allowed favorable reduction in postoperative complications.

Antilymphocyte Globulin

MECHANISM OF ACTION

Antilymphocyte globulin (ATG) is an antibody preparation developed to stay acute episodes of rejection. It is one of several compounds from nonhuman sources found to result in the destruction of specific lymphoid cells active in the rejection process. Antithymocyte globulin can lower the number of thymus-derived antigen-reactive lymphocytes, as well as interfere with their normal function in rejection. Due to its equine origin, ATG possesses the ability to induce anti-idiotypic antibodies in persons with a hypersensitivity to horse protein. Rabbit antilymphocyte globulin (RATG) has been introduced more recently with the hopes of decreasing the incidence of the reaction.

INDICATIONS

The initial use of this product was for the reversal of acute graft-rejection episodes along with other immunosuppressive drugs. At present it is used most often prophylactically to avert the rejection process immediately after transplantation. In cases of overt graft rejection, however, it has been combined with both steroids and muromonab-CD_3 in an attempt to reverse the rejection process.

CLINICAL TOXICITIES

Serum sickness is the major concern. Severe anaphylaxis has been reported in only 1% of reactions. An intradermal skin test is recommended before the first dosing. A positive response of greater than 10 mm of erythema or swelling suggests increased risk for an anaphylactic reaction. Solutions more than 9–12 hours old should not be used.

Hematologic effects such as leukopenia, thrombocytopenia, and hemolysis have also been noted. Isolated cases of chest pain and pulmonary edema have been reported. Additional adverse effects are phlebitis, headache, seizure, nausea, vomiting, febrile episodes, hypotension, and rash. No adverse drug interactions have been reported.

DOSAGE AND ADMINISTRATION

Antithymocyte globulin is prepared from a 50-mg/ml solution for IV injection. There is no oral preparation available. Initial dosing may range from 2–4 mg/kg/day in normal saline. The preparation must be filtered during administration with pore sizes of 0.2–5 microns. The drug should be infused over at least 4 hours. Duration of treatment has been variable by regimen. It is usually administered for the first 3–10 days postoperatively and is replaced by low-dosage methylprednisolone, 0.1–0.8 mg/kg/day, with tapering. It may be repeated with increased dosage during acute rejection episodes. Undiluted solutions are unstable in acidic or dextrose solutions.

Muromonab-CD3

MECHANISM OF ACTION

Muromonab-CD3 (Orthoclone [OKT3]) is a monoclonal antibody to the CD3 antigen of T cells. It inhibits the recognition and transduction process of T cells responsible for graft rejection. The depletion of the CD3 antigen in lymphocytes occurs peripherally in the serum but not in the graft itself. It has not been found to interfere with other cell lines, thus providing a more selective form of immunosuppression.

INDICATIONS

Muromonab-CD3 has been indicated in patients with acute graft rejection in renal transplant patients. Only recently has it been employed in a few lung transplantation regimens for acute graft rejection. When given immediately postoperatively in renal transplants, it has allowed a reduction in the dosages of other immunosuppressants used. In addition, it has been found to be more effective in reversing acute rejections over conventional high-dosage glucocorticoid therapy or in steroid failures.

CLINICAL TOXICITIES

Muromonab-CD3 is a murine monoclonal antibody. The development of antiidiotypic antibodies to this preparation of a nonhuman source has been documented in individuals receiving the drug. The presence of these antibodies could decrease the effectiveness of further uses in certain individuals. Additional use should be done with caution. Some experts believe this drug should be used for only a single course of treatment.

One of the most important adverse effects of muromonab-CD3 in transplantation has been the production of pulmonary edema. This has occurred in less than 2% of patients following the first dose and was always associated with fluid overload. It is strongly recommended that patients not be in fluid overload when receiving this drug and remain under close medical observation for the initial 48–72 hours from initiation of therapy.

Approximately 6% of individuals develop an aseptic meningitis syndrome. Clinically, this appears as fever, chills, headache, and neck stiffness. It is more common in the initial few days of treatment, with a gradual subsiding of symptoms with continued treatment.

Additional adverse effects have been nausea, vomiting, diarrhea, wheezing, pruritus, pulmonary edema, chest pain, seizures, and tremors. As with all other immunosuppressants, complications with infection are reported with rates similar to those on corticosteroid therapy. Isolated cases of lymphoproliferative disorders have also been reported. These cases are more likely related to the total number of immunosuppressants used rather than a single drug.

DOSAGE AND ADMINISTRATION

Muromonab-CD3 is available only in a 1-mg/ml solution. It is supplied in packages of five ampules, with each ampule containing 5-ml solution. It should be stored in a refrigerator at 36–46°F. Shaking or freezing the solution should be avoided.

Inspection of the ampules for discoloration should be completed prior to use. The administered dosage should be filtered before use and is then injected directly IV, 2–5 mg daily, as an IV bolus over no more than 1 minute. It should not be administered concurrently with other drugs or by prolonged infusion. The administered dosage is continued for the 3–14-day course.

Most of the adverse reactions occur ½ to 6 hours after the first dose. To minimize acute reactions, a dose of methylprednisolone 1 mg/kg, as well as an antipyretic prior to the dosing and 100 mg of hydrocortisone 1 hour postdosing, are recommended.

Existing daily immunosuppressant therapy should be lowered during muromonab-CD3 therapy. Daily dosages of azathioprine should not exceed 25 mg. Prednisone therapy (or its equivalent) should be limited to 0.5 mg/kg/day. Cyclosporine therapy is recommended discontinued until 3 days prior to completion of muromonab-CD3 therapy. The maximum amount of this drug that can safely be given has not been established.

References

1. Borel, J. F., and Feurer, C. Biologic effects of cyclosporine A, a new antilymphocytic agent. *Agents Actions* 6:468–475, 1976.

2. Cooper, J. D., and Pearson, F. G. Technique of successful lung transplantation in humans. *Thorac. Cardiovasc. Surg.*, 93:173, 1987.

3. Elion, G. B., and Hitchings, G. H. Azathioprine. In A. C. Sartorelli and D. J. Johns (eds.). *Handbook of Experimental Pharmacology.* New York: Springer Verlag, 1975.

4. Ettinger, N. A., and Turlock, E. P. Pulmonary considerations in organ transplantation, Part 3. *Am. Rev. Respir. Dis.* 144:433–451, 1991.
5. Hardy, J., et al. Lung transplantation in man. *JAMA* 186:1065–1070, 1963.
6. Kriett, J. M., and Jamieson, S. W. Pulmonary transplantation. *Curr. Pulmonol.* 12:297–319, 1991.
7. McCarthy, P. M., and Starnes, V. A. Improved survival after heart-lung transplantation. *Thorac. Cardiovasc. Surg.* 99:54, 1990.
8. Modry, D. L., and Oyer, P. E. Cyclosporine in heart and heart-lung transplantation. *Can. J. Surg.* 28:274–280, 1985.
9. Patterson, G. A., and Cooper, J. D. Status of lung transplantation. *Surg. Clin. North Am.* 68:545, 1988.
10. Raju, A., and Mansel, J. K. Experience with single and double-lung transplantation. *Am. Rev. Respir. Dis.* 141(Suppl.):A410, 1990.
11. Reichart, B., and Reichenspurner, H. Heart-lung transplantation in 1990 — indications, surgical technique, postoperative complications and outcome. *Thorac. Cardiovasc. Surg.* 38:271–275, 1990.
12. Shennib, H., et al. Successful treatment of steroid-resistant double-lung allograft rejection with Orthoclone OKT3. *Am. Rev. Respir. Dis.* 144:224–226, 1991.
13. Trulock, E. P., and Egan, T. M. Single lung transplantation for severe obstructive pulmonary disease. Washington University Lung Transplantation Group. *Chest* 96:738, 1989.
14. Upjohn Company, Medical and Drug Information. Medical Library Services. Kalamazoo, MI.
15. Whitehead, B., and James, I. Intensive care management of children following heart and heart-lung transplantation. *Intensive Care Med.* 16:426–430, 1990.
16. Whitehead, B., and Helms, P. Heart-lung transplantation for cystic fibrosis. *Arch. Dis. Child.* 66:1022–1026, 1991.
17. Yacoub, M., and Khaghani, A. Single lung transplantation for obstructive airway disease. *Transplant. Proc.* 23:1213–1214, 1991.

9

Pulmonary Hypertension

Ann E. Medinger

Physiology

Pulmonary perfusion provides the transport medium for conveying respiratory gases between alveolar and systemic tissues: Pulmonary hypertension is high blood pressure in the pulmonary circulation, defined as mean pulmonary artery pressure (PAP) exceeding 25 mm Hg. The PAP is determined by four interrelated factors:

1. Flow generated by the right ventricle of the heart (Q).
2. Hydrostatic pressure in the pulmonary veins and in the left atrium of heart (Ppcw, Pla).
3. Alveolar pressure (PA).
4. Pulmonary vascular tone and patency (PVR).

The right ventricle of the heart is a low-pressure pump, generating an average flow of 5 liters/minute, a mean pressure of only 15 mm Hg to pump blood through the low-resistance pulmonary vascular circuit (normal pulmonary vascular resistance [PVR], 1.5–3 mm Hg/liter/minute). Features of the pulmonary vascular circuit that keep the work of the right heart low in contrast to left heart work include the following:

Proximity of the entire pulmonary vascular tree to the heart, requiring blood to be pumped only 15–20 cm against gravity.

Short length of the main pulmonary arterial trunk before branching. (Vascular resistance is directly proportional to vessel length and inversely proportional to collective diameter of parallel branches.)

Thin-walled compliant arterioles that dilate with increasing flow, keeping resistance low even with vigorous physical activity.

Presence of pulmonary vascular channels that are closed at rest and recruited when either pressure or flow increases across the lung.

Pulmonary hypertension occurs when rising pressure across the lung exceeds the pulmonary circulation's capacity for recruitment and dilation. It is caused by:

Increased pressure in the left atrium or pulmonary veins (left ventricular failure, mitral stenosis, venoocclusive disease).

Increased pulmonary vascular resistance (pulmonary vasoconstriction, vascular obstruction, pulmonic stenosis).

Increased blood flow through the lung (congenital heart disease).

Elevated alevolar pressure may also cause acute reversible pulmonary hypertension (e.g., positive pressure mechanical ventilation). Chronic pulmonary hypertension leads to right ventricular hypertrophy. Progressive pulmonary hypertension eventually causes right heart failure because the right ventricle is unable to meet the increasing workload imposed by the rising pulmonary vascular resistance.

Because of the built-in capacitance features of the pulmonary vascular tree (recruitment and dilation), mild to moderate pulmonary vascular restriction may occur without changing resting PAP. Hence, sedentary individuals may not become symptomatic from pulmonary hypertension until the disease is far advanced and the cardiac output has become low and fixed.

The most common cause of chronic pulmonary hypertension (Table 9-1) is pulmonary vasoconstriction secondary to alveolar hypoxia. Individuals with chronic lung disease who are unable to ventilate sufficiently to maintain alveolar oxygen tension above 70 mm Hg develop chronic diffuse pulmonary vasoconstriction; the smooth muscle of their pulmonary arterioles hypertrophies, giving the pulmonary vascular system enhanced vasoconstrictive properties.

Primary pulmonary hypertension (PPH) is occlusive pulmonary vascular disease of unknown origin. The World Health Organization has designated Etiologic and Morphologic classifications of PPH, responding to the fact that antemortem lung tissue is not obtained from most patients with PPH [4]. The Etiologic Classification requires an elevated PAP and exclusion of known causes of PPH, including thromboembolism and venoocclusive disease, as well as possible without an open lung biopsy. The Morphologic Classification has three histopathologic subsets: plexogenic pulmonary arteriopathy, pulmonary venoocclusive disease, and pulmonary thromboembolism. This apparent contradiction between the exclusion of thromboembolism and venoocclusive disease from the Etiologic Classification and its inclusion in the Morphologic

Table 9-1. Differential diagnosis of pulmonary hypertension

Primary causes	Secondary causes
Plexogenic arteriopathy	Alveolar hypoxic
Venoocclusive disease	Restrictive or obstructive lung disease
Pulmonary capillary hemangiomatosis	Chest wall deformity
	Hypoventilation-sleep apnea
	High altitude
	Pulmonary vascular obstruction
	Parasitic lung disease
	Pulmonary thromboembolism
	Pulmonary arteritis
	High pressure mechanical ventilation
	Sickle cell anemia
	Cardiogenic increased hydrostatic pressures
	Left ventricular failure
	Mitral stenosis
	Left atrial myxoma
	Pulmonic stenosis
	Congenital heart disease with left-to-right intracardiac shunt
	Partial anomalous pulmonary venous drainage

Classification reflects the fact that in spite of efforts to exclude these diseases antemortem, many postmortem autopsy studies of PPH find up to 55% incidence of thromboembolism among the histopathologic lung specimens. Some authors also include pulmonary capillary hemangiomatosis among the morphologic classes of PPH.

Diagnosis

Pulmonary hypertension is often asymptomatic until far advanced. When present, the symptoms include dyspnea, fatigue, syncope, and anginalike chest pain. Physical findings include an increase in the pulmonic component of the second heart sound (P2), palpable left parasternal thrust, a prominent presystolic "a" wave in the jugular veins, and an S_4 gallop rhythm heard best over the lower left sternal border. Patients may also have murmurs of tricuspid regurgitation and pulmonic insufficiency. When right heart failure occurs, additional signs appear: lower extremity edema, jugulovenous distention, hepatojugular reflux, and an S_3 gallop that varies with the respiratory cycle.

Although ECG, chest x ray, and echocardiographic findings may suggest pulmonary hypertension (Table 9-2), the definitive diagnosis requires measurement of the pulmonary artery pressure (normal mean PAP, 15 mm Hg; normal PVR, 1.5–3 mm Hg/liter/minute; normal Ppcw 5–10 mm Hg).

Once pulmonary hypertension is recognized, it is essential to search for underlying disease. Treatment prospects and prognosis are better for secondary pulmonary hypertension than for the primary condition. Testing to exclude underlying causes should include lung scan, pulmonary function tests, echocardiography, polysomnography, lower-extremity venography, or impedance plethysmography.

There is no general agreement about the need for pulmonary angiography and an open lung biopsy in the diagnosis of pulmonary

Table 9-2. Radiographic and cardiographic features of pulmonary hypertension

Chest x ray
- Prominant main pulmonary artery
- Enlarged hilar vessels
- Decreased peripheral vessels
- Prominant right ventricle in the retrosternal air space of the ECG
- Right axis deviation
- Right ventricular hypertrophy
- Right ventricular strain
- P Pulmonale

Echocardiogram
- Right ventricular enlargement
- Paradoxic septal motion
- Partial systolic closure of the pulmonic valve

hypertension. An angiogram is not needed if the lung scan is normal; one report of histologic specimens of PPH patients found a high correlation of patchy uptake on the lung scan with both venooclusive disease and chronic thromboembolism [12]. Open lung biopsy is the gold standard for excluding treatable causes of PPH and confirming the diagnosis; transbronchial biopsy does not provide enough tissue for accurate differentiation of PPH. Biopsy findings of plexogenic arteriopathy include medial hypertrophy, concentric intimal thickening, and plexiform lesions. Findings of venoocclusive disease are fibrous intimal proliferation with luminal occlusion of the septal veins, capillary congestion, and widening of alveolar septae with hemosiderin deposits in the interstitium and in alveolar macrophages. The findings of microthromboembolism include medial hypertrophy unevenly distributed, with predominant eccentric intimal thickening, bridging of the vascular lumen with fibrous bands, and the absence of plexiform lesions or involvement of pulmonary capillaries and veins.

Many authorities object to submitting individuals to the risk of open lung biopsy because medical science has such limited treatment offerings for PPH. However, a number of published autopsy and histopathology series have found a high incidence of chronic thromboembolism and other treatable conditions in patients with clinical PPH [3, 12, 19].

SECONDARY PULMONARY HYPERTENSION

Individuals with secondary pulmonary hypertension due to chronic thromboembolism and mitral stenosis may present primarily with the symptoms of pulmonary hypertension and have little evidence of their primary disease. However, individuals with secondary pulmonary hypertension due to chronic lung disease often have symptoms and physical findings typical of chronic lung disease predominating over the more subtle signs of pulmonary hypertension. These individuals become symptomatic at an earlier stage of their disease.

PRIMARY PULMONARY HYPERTENSION

Primary pulmonary hypertension is variable in its presentation. A national prospective study conducted by the National Institutes of Health to study PPH registered 187 patients between 1981 and 1985 [2, 13]. The study was based on the Etiologic Classification and did not require lung biopsy for confirmation of the diagnosis of PPH. The mean delay from onset of symptoms to diagnosis was found to be 2 years (up to 16 years delay). There was an overall female-to-male ratio of 1.7:1. Mean age was 36 years (range 1–81). The initial symptoms were dyspnea (60%), fatigue (19%), syncope and near syncope (13%), and chest pain (7%). Raynaud's phenomenon was present in 10% of patients; 6% of the cases were familial; and 29% of the registrants had mild symptoms and New York Heart Association (NYHA) functional classification of grade II. These individuals had a markedly better survival than those with grade IV. Women had a lower functional classification on entry into the registry and had a poorer prognosis.

Of the patients, 29% (69% of the women) had a positive antinuclear antibody test. Pulmonary function tests revealed mild restriction, a reduced carbon monoxide diffusing capacity, and mild hypoxemia with hypocapnia. Of the group, 58% had an abnormal lung scan, predominantly diffuse patchy patterns; 19% were receiving long-term drug therapy at the time of entry into the registry, primarily vasodilators; and 89% received long-term drug therapy over the course of their disease.

The mean survival was 2.8 years (34% had a 5-year survival); 26% of the deaths were from causes other than sudden death and right ventricular failure (readily attributable to PPH), including medication-related death.

Treatment

SECONDARY PULMONARY HYPERTENSION

The most effective treatment for pulmonary hypertension is reversal of the underlying primary cardiorespiratory condition causing hypertension: thrombolysis or anticoagulation for a thromboembolism, valve replacement of a stenotic mitral valve, weight loss for obesity hypoventilation syndrome, and so on (Table 9-3).

When the hypoxic lung disease causing pulmonary hypertension is irreversible, treatment with supplemental oxygen therapy to raise alveolar oxygen tension has been shown to reduce pulmonary hypertension and prolong life. Vasodilators are sometimes given as a last resort to treat refractory right heart failure in these patients; however, there is no evidence that vasodilator therapy prolongs life. In the chronic obstructive pulmonary disease (COPD) patient, vasodilator therapy can produce dangerous systemic hypotension, arrhythmias, and worsening of hypoxemia. Hence, it should be used only in those with reversible pulmonary hypertension in whom gas exchange does not deteriorate with therapy.

When chronic alveolar hypoxia and pulmonary hypertension are due to extrapulmonic factors, supplemental oxygen therapy may temporarily relieve pulmonary hypertension, but diagnosis and treatment of the underlying condition are key. Pulmonary hypertension due to obstructive sleep apnea syndrome resolves with tracheostomy; less drastic measures, including weight loss, pharmacologic therapy (protriptyline, progesterone), and nasal continuous positive airway pressure (CPAP) therapy may also give remarkable relief of apneas and pulmonary hypertension. Pulmonary hypertension due to progressive neuromuscular disease requires treatment with mechanical ventilation to correct hypoxemia and reverse pulmonary hypertension.

Patients with nonhypoxic pulmonary hypertension are not helped by supplemental oxygen therapy or mechanical ventilation. Table 9-3 outlines specific guidelines for diagnosis and treatment of common causes of secondary pulmonary hypertension.

Table 9-3. Diagnosis and treatment of secondary pulmonary hypertension

Condition	Diagnostic test	Treatment
Chronic lung disease	Chest X ray Pulmonary function tests	Bronchodilators Antiinflammatory agents Secretion management Continuous oxygen therapy
Pulmonary thromboembolism	Ventilation/perfusion lung scan Pulmonary angiogram	Anticoagulation Inferior vena cava interruption Embolectomy
Cardiogenic Left heart failure Mitral stenosis Left atrial myxoma Congenital shunt	Echocardiogram Cardiac catheterization with pressure, dye injection, and oxygen saturation measured	Diuretics, before and after load management Surgery
Pulmonary vasculitis Polyarteritis nodosa Lupus erthematosis Systemic sclerosis Wegener's granulomatosis	Serology, tissue biopsy	Corticosteroids Cytotoxic agents
Parasitic lung disease Schistosomasis	Parasite eggs in stool or urine	Praziquantel therapy
Sleep apnea syndromes	Polysomogram	Continuous positive airway pressure Tracheostomy Pharmacologic therapy
Neuromuscular diseases Postpolio syndrome Amyotrophic lateral sclerosis Progressive muscular dystrophy Myasthenia gravis	Pulmonary function tests	Mechanical ventilation
Sickle cell anemia	Peripheral smear Hemoglobin electrophoresis	Transfusion oxygen fluids
Cirrhosis of the liver	Liver function tests Liver biopsy Arterial blood gases on 100% oxygen	Lung transplant

PRIMARY PULMONARY HYPERTENSION

Endothelial dysfunction of the pulmonary vascular tree is recognized as an important component of pulmonary hypertension. The dysfunction may be caused by chemical, physical, or as-yet-undiscovered injury to the endothelium, but the net result is decreased production of the endogenous vasodilator prostacyclin and of endothelium relaxing factor, yielding vasoconstriction and promoting platelet adhesion and activation [5]. This understanding directs treatment efforts.

Primary pulmonary hypertension has been treated principally with anticoagulants and vasodilators; however, treatment is highly controversial because of its high risk compared to the wide variation in untreated survival reported for the disease. There are now a number of reports of long-term (up to 20 years) survival without treatment after diagnosis of PPH (34%, 5 years; 15%, 10 years). There are also reports of spontaneous improvement and regression [1]. PPH is no longer viewed as an inevitably rapidly fatal disease meriting high-risk treatment. There appears to be a bimodal distribution of patients: those with an accelerated course of death within months and those with a course slowly evolving over years [15]. Reports of treatment success with a variety of drugs have not been controlled studies and have failed to take into account this bimodal distribution of cases in their reports of long-term follow-up. No treatment has been prospectively proved to alter outcome of the disease.

Microthrombi are often found in the lungs of PPH patients at autopsy. The source of these thrombi is unknown; nearly all PPH patients have had none detected in a vigorous search for venous thrombosis antemortem. Although prospective trials of anticoagulation have failed to show clinical efficacy, at least one retrospective autopsy study of PPH patients, finding thromboemboli in 57% of the specimens, detected a significant difference in survival among the patients who had been treated with anticoagulant therapy [3]. Anticoagulant therapy may be helpful in prolonging life in PPH patients who have evidence of pulmonary thromboemboli, such as patchy uptake on the lung scan (Table 9-4).

Vasodilator therapy is based on the theory that PPH patients have hyperactive pulmonary vessels, which have a reversible vasoconstrictive component that eventually evolves into a fixed vascular obstruction. Vasodilator therapy is aimed at lowering pulmonary vascular resistance and right heart work. However, none of the vasodilators is selective for the pulmonary circulation; hypotension, gas exchange impairment, and sudden death are significant complications of this therapy in the dosage required to vasodilate the pulmonary vascular tree. Sudden death from vasodilator therapy for PPH can occur during titration of the medication with hemodynamic monitoring and during unmonitored, chronic, long-term use.

Vasodilator therapy may be helpful in prolonging the life of patients with PPH when given to individuals who have an accelerated course, with symptoms developing over months, or whose pulmonary vascular circulation can be shown to respond to vasodilators administered during central hemodynamic monitoring.

Table 9-4. World Health Organization Morphologic Classification of primary pulmonary hypertension: diagnosis and treatment

Condition	Diagnostic	Treatment
Plexogenic pulmonary arteriopathy	V/Q lung scan — normal lung biopsy	Vasodilators Anticoagulation?
Venoocclusive disease	V/Q lung scan — patchy hemodynamic: Ppcw increased with normal Pla, Plv Lung biopsy	Vasodilators? Anticoagulation?
Chronic pulmonary thromboembolism	V/Q lung scan — patchy pulmonary angiogram — lumenal filling defect	Anticoagulation Embolectomy
	Lung biopsy	Inferior vena cava interruption

V/Q = ratio of ventilation to perfusion; Ppcw = pulmonary capillary wedge pressure; Pla = left atrial pressure; Plv = left ventricular pressure

Because there is a high degree of spontaneous variability in PVR and PAP in PPH patients (up to 36% and 22%), hemodynamic response to vasodilation, measured in the cardiac catheterization laboratory must be high in order to be attributable to the tested vasodilator. The report of Reeves et al. [11] reviewing published reports of PPH patients indicates that patients tested in the cardiac catheterization laboratory and found to have greater than 30% reduction in PVR with pharmacologic therapy had a substantial chance (62%) of improvement when given chronic vasodilator treatment (by clinical or hemodynamic criteria). Those without this 30% response had little chance of improvement (6%) with chronic vasodilator therapy. The latter groups of individuals may have already progressed to fixed vascular obstruction. In this review, the initial measurements of PAP and PVR were not significant in discriminating responders from nonresponders. In the responders, long-term improvement was seen with a variety of vasodilating drugs. Reports indicate that 30–50% of PPH patients tested have a significant hemodynamic response to pulmonary vasodilation.

Although there is no general agreement about the need to perform pulmonary angiography and open lung biopsy in PPH patients to exclude all the other causes of pulmonary hypertension, experts agree that vasodilator therapy should not be undertaken without hemodynamic measurements demonstrating efficacy for the agent. Once treatment has begun with a drug proved hemodynamically useful in the individual, the patient should be carefully reevaluated at intervals. If there is no evidence of clinical improvement in activity level or quality of life, the treatment should be discontinued because the risk of sudden death is probably greater than the potential benefit to the individual.

Lung transplantation is the only treatment remaining for individuals with PPH for whom anticoagulant and vasodilator therapy are not helpful.

VASODILATOR THERAPY

The goal of vasodilator therapy in pulmonary hypertension is restoration of PAP to normal without diminishing cardiac output or systemic vascular resistance. Over 20 different vasodilating drugs have, at one time or another, been reported to be useful in treating primary pulmonary hypertension, but none of the currently available drugs is selective for the pulmonary circulation.

The categories that seem to have the longest or strongest record include direct-acting vasodilators and calcium channel blockers. Drugs that have been reported useful but are not detailed here are listed in Table 9-5.

The choice of vasodilator and dosage must be individualized. It is essential to base a trial of chronic therapy on the results of drug administration with hemodynamic monitoring. Individuals vary dramatically in their responses to the same drug; for all vasodilator medication categories, there are reports of success as well as failure, including death, in patients with PPH. Aggressive vasodilator therapy in PPH patients with fixed obstruction is likely to produce shock, heart failure, and cardiac arrest.

Prostacyclin is a useful initial screening agent to identify PPH patients whose pulmonary circulation will respond to vasodilator therapy [16]. Prostacyclin is especially well suited for hemodynamic testing of PPH patients:

It is a naturally occurring endogenous prostaglandin that acts on specific endothelial prostaglandin receptors, promoting vasodilation.
It is a potent vasodilator and predicts the hemodynamic positive and adverse effects of other vasodilators. Failure to respond to prostacyclin precludes response to other vasodilator drugs.
Adverse effects of vasodilation that may be lethal can be promptly terminated by stopping the infusion. It is short-lived; half-life is 1–2 minutes.

Prostacyclin is an investigational drug in the United States. Dosage is IV infusion of 1 ng/kg/minute for 15 minutes followed by increases of 1–2 ng/kg/minute q15min until the desired hemodynamic effect

Table 9-5. Vasodilators reported useful in treating primary pulmonary hypertension

Acetylcholine	Nitroglycerin
Captopril	Nitroprusside
Diazoxide	Minoxidil
Diltiazem	Phentolamine
Epoprostenal	Phenoxybenzamine
Flelodipine	Prazosin
Hydralazine	Prostacyclin
Isoproterenal	Terbutaline
Nifedipine	Tolazoline
Nitrendipine	Verapamil

is achieved, adverse effects occur, or a total of 12/ng/kg/minute has been given. Recent reports [8] suggest that acetylcholine may also be a useful short-acting agent for identifying responders in the catheterization laboratory. (Dosage is IV infusion rate of 1 mg/minute increased by 1–2 mg/minute q10min until the desired hemodynamic effects are seen, adverse reaction occurs, or a maximum of 10 mg/minute.)

Calcium Channel Blockers

Several calcium antagonists have been shown to lower pulmonary vascular resistance in primary pulmonary hypertension. They also inhibit platelet aggregation, which may be helpful in pulmonary hypertension. Sublingual nifedipine has been used as a rapidly acting vasodilator for testing pulmonary vascular responsiveness.

MECHANISM OF ACTION

Blockade of calcium channels inhibits vasoconstriction by decreasing the concentration of free intracellular calcium, required for the excitation contraction coupling of smooth muscle in arterial walls.

ADVERSE EFFECTS

Side effects of calcium channel blockers include dizziness, hypotension, headache, flushing, digital dysesthesia, hypothermia, nausea, dyspepsia, constipation, cough, wheezing, pulmonary edema, myocardial ischemia, bradycardia, palpitations, arterial-ventricular conduction disturbances, peripheral edema, polyuria, somnolence, insomnia, and rash.

DRUG INTERACTIONS

Use of calcium channel blockers with antihypertensive drugs can exacerbate sinus bradycardia by depressing the sinus node.

PHARMACOKINETICS

The effects of calcium channel blockers occur within 30–60 minutes of oral administration. Although first-pass hepatic metabolism may reduce bioavailability, repeated oral administration may increase bioavailability by saturating the hepatic enzymes. Elimination half-lives range from 1.3 to 5 hours; the agents are protein bound. Most agents have active metabolites with reduced vasodilating activity. Cirrhotic and geriatric patients require reduced dosage.

DOSAGE

Nifedipine (Procardia) is available in 10-and 20-mg capsules and 10-mg tablets (not available in the United States, however) [14]. Extended release tablets (Procardia XL), 30, 60, and 90 mg, are also available.

The **initial dosage** for adults is 20 mg PO every hour until a favorable hemodynamic response or adverse reaction occurs. The **subsequent daily dosage** is half the initial effective dosage q6–8hours.

Diltiazem (Cardizem) is available in tablets and capsules of 30, 60, 90, and 120 mg [14]. Extended-release capsules (Cardizem), 60, 90, and 120 mg, are also available.

The **initial dosage** for adults is 60 mg PO every hour until a favorable hemodynamic response or adverse reaction occurs. The **subsequent daily dosage** is half the initial effective dosage q6–8hours.

Direct-Acting Vasodilators

Organic Nitrates

Intravenous nitroglycerin has been found useful for diagnostic identification of PPH individuals with the potential for pulmonary vasodilation. Organic nitrates vasodilate the systemic and pulmonary arterial and venous circulation. Reduction in venous return to the right heart reduces pulmonary artery pressure independent of the drug's effect on the vascular tree.

MECHANISM AND SITE OF ACTION

Organic nitrates convert to the free radical nitric oxide (NO) in vivo, which activates guanylate cyclase to increase synthesis of guanosine monophosphate (GMP). A cyclic GMP-dependent kinase dephosphorylates the light chain of myosin, relaxing vascular smooth muscle's contractile state. Nitroglycerin has also been shown to induce the production of prostacyclin by human endothelial cells.

ADVERSE EFFECTS

Common side effects of organic nitrate administration include headache, dizziness, flushing, postural hypotension, blurred vision, and tachycardia. Rash, dry mouth, nervousness, twitching, and abdominal pain can also occur.

PHARMACOKINETICS

Organic nitrates are metabolized by reductive hydrolysis in the liver. Peak concentration of nitroglycerin occurs within 4 minutes of sublingual administration, and its half-life is 1–3 minutes. Metabolites are weak vasodilators and have a 40-minute half-life.

DOSAGE

Nitroglycerin is available in several forms and strengths:

Sublingual: 1/150 g.
Parenteral dextrose solution: 100 μg/ml, 200 μg/ml, 400 μg/ml; dilute in dextrose or normal saline.
Topical preparations: patch: 12.5, 25, 50, 75 mg; ointment: 2%.

For adults the dosage begins with an IV infusion, 10 μg/minute, increasing by 0.5 μg/kg q5min until pulmonary vasodilation is achieved or adverse effects develop. The maximum dosage is 120 μg/minute. Subsequent daily dosing begins with 2.5 mg transdermally over 24 hours, increasing every 3 days to achieve the target dosage. The dosage : area ratio must be kept constant.

Use of polyvinylchloride (PVC) tubing for infusion of nitroglycerin may increase the dosage required for an effect.

Hydralazine

MECHANISM AND SITE OF ACTION

Hydralazine's mechanism of directly relaxing arteriolar smooth muscle is unclear. It is suggested that it may be similar to the organic nitrates, releasing nitric oxide; other evidence suggests that hydralazine may interfere with the mobilization of calcium in smooth muscle. The vasodilation induced by hydralazine stimulates concomitant sympathetic discharge.

PHARMACOKINETICS

Although hydralazine is well absorbed from the GI tract, its bioavailability is low and is influenced by the individual's genetically determined rate of drug acetylation to its inactive form in bowel and liver. The half-life of hydralazine is 1 hour; peak concentration occurs 30–120 minutes after oral and 15–30 minutes after IV administration. The duration of its effect is 3–12 hours. Tachyphylaxis occurs.

ADVERSE EFFECTS

Principal adverse effects include headache, tachycardia, angina, palpitations, anorexia, nausea, vomiting, and diarrhea. Less frequently occurring side effects include rash, lupus erythematosis syndrome, hypotension, dyspnea, tremor, and peripheral neuritis.

DOSAGE

Tablets are available in strengths of 10, 25, 50, and 100 mg. The parenteral solution is 20 mg/ml.

For adults the **initial dosage** is 10 mg by IV infusion, repeated once after 10 minutes if pulmonary vasodilation or adverse effects have not occurred. The **subsequent daily dosage** is 25–50 mg PO q6h.

Anticoagulation (see Chapter 7)

References

1. Bourdillon, P.D.V., et al. Regression of primary pulmonary hypertension. *Br. Heart J.* 38:264–705, 1976.
2. D'Alonzo, G. E., et al. Survival in patients with primary pulmonary hypertension. *Ann Intern. Med* 115:343–349, 1991.
3. Fuster, V., et al. Primary pulmonary hypertension: Natural history and the importance of thrombosis. *Circulation* 70:580–587, 1984.
4. Hatano, S., et al. Primary Pulmonary Hypertension: report on a WHO meeting Geneva: World Health Organization, 1975.
5. Loscalzo, J. Endothelial dysfunction in pulmonary hypertension. *N. Engl. J. Med.* 327:117–119, 1992.
6. McManigle, J. E., et al. Treatment for primary pulmonary hypertension. *Chest* 96:900–905, 1989.
7. Packer, M. Vasodilator therapy for primary pulmonary hypertension. *Ann. Intern. Med* 103:258–270, 1985.
8. Palevsky, H. I., et al. Prostacyclin and acetylcholine as screening agents for acute pulmonary vasodilator responsiveness in primary pulmonary hypertension. *Circulation* 82:2018–2026, 1990.
9. Pearl, R. G., et al. Acute hemodynamic effects of nitroglycerine in primary pulmonary hypertension. *Ann. Intern. Med* 99:9–13, 1983.
10. Pepke-Zoba, J. et al. Inhaled nitric oxide as a cause of selective pulmonary vasodilation in pulmonary hypertension. *Lancet* 338:1173–1174, 1991.
11. Reeves, J. T., et al. The case for treatment of selected patients with primary pulmonary hypertension. *Am. Rev. Respir. Dis.* 134:342–346, 1986.
12. Rich, S., et al. Primary pulmonary hypertension: Radiographic and scintigraphic patterns of histologic subtypes. *Ann. Int. Med.* 105:499–502, 1986.
13. Rich, S., et al. Primary pulmonary hypertension: A national prospective study. *Ann. Int. Med.* 107:216–223, 1987.
14. Rich, S., et al. The effect of high doses of calcium-channel blockers on survival in primary pulmonary hypertension. *N. Engl. J. Med.* 327:76–81, 1992.
15. Robin, E. D. The kingdom of the near-dead; the shortened, unnatural life history of primary pulmonary hypertension. *Chest* 92:330–333, 1987.
16. Rozkovec, A. et al. Prediction of favorable responses to long-term vasodilator treatment of pulmonary hypertension by short-term

administration of Epoprostenol or Nifedepine. *Br. Heart J.* 59:696–705, 1988.

17. Rubin, L. J., et al. Oral hydralazine therapy for primary pulmonary hypertension. *N. Engl. J. Med.* 302:69–72, 1980.

18. Rubin, L. J., et al. Treatment of primary pulmonary hypertension with continuous intravenous prostacyclin. *Ann. Intern. Med* 112:485–491, 1990.

19. Wagenvoort, C. A. Primary pulmonary hypertension: A pathologic study of the lung vessels in 156 clinically diagnosed cases. *Circulation* 42:1163–1182, 1970.

10

Lung Cancer

Shakun Malik
Steven H. Krasnow

Lung cancer is the most common cancer in men (other than skin cancer) and the leading cause of cancer deaths in men and women. About 150,000 new cases occur yearly in the United States [2]. About 90% are attributable to tobacco abuse and thus are potentially preventable.

Lung cancer has four major histologic subtypes: squamous cell, large cell, adenocarcinoma, and small cell carcinoma. Small cell lung cancer is highly responsive to chemotherapy (drug therapy) and/or ratiotherapy, but it is rapid growing and usually metastatic at the time of diagnosis, making surgery infeasible in most cases. In contrast, the other histologic subtypes, despite differences in their biology and clinical characteristics, all exhibit slower growth and may be surgically curable; however, they respond poorly to radiotherapy and chemotherapy. Therefore, it is convenient to classify lung cancers as either small cell (SCLC) or nonsmall cell (NSCLC). Because chemotherapy has not prolonged survival in NSCLC, we shall consider chemotherapy agents used in SCLC unless otherwise specified.

Cancer is characterized by unregulated cell growth that becomes clinically evident when it compromises the function of vital organs. Cancer cells actually proliferate at a slower rate than corresponding normal cells in most instances. However, in normal tissues, cell production equals cell loss (except in growing or regenerating tissues); cell production exceeds cell loss in cancer because newly created cells fail to differentiate into nondividing cells and, in some cases, because the growth fraction (the percentage of actively dividing cells in a tissue) is greater.

Because chemotherapy usually targets dividing cells, an understanding of the cell division is useful in considering chemotherapy actions. The cell cycle (Fig. 10-1) describes the changes a cell undergoes during mitosis beginning from its resting state and ending with two daughter cells in their resting states. Nondividing cells that do not respond to stimuli to divide (the majority of cells in most tissues) are said to be in G_0 phase. Resting cells that can be stimulated to divide are said to be in G_1 phase. There is no way to distinguish these phases until a cell divides. The "S" defines the period of DNA synthesis wherein the diploid cell becomes tetraploid; in G_2, DNA synthesis is complete, and nuclear changes occur in preparation for M phase, or mitosis. This results in two diploid daughter cells in either G_0 or G_1 phase, completing the cell cycle. The cell cycle in normal cells is usually 24–48 hours in length; in malignant cells it is usually 72–120 hours.

Cell cycle kinetics describe important features of tumor cell production but do not predict the growth rate, which depends on the balance between cell production and cell loss. The growth fraction

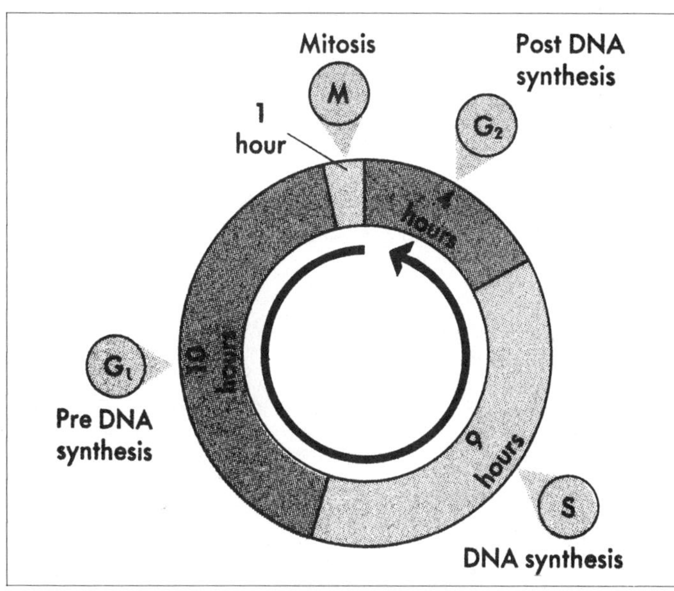

Fig. 10-1. The cell cycle. The process of cell division in a normal cell. Not shown are nondividing cells (said to be in G_0 phase) and cells that may leave the cell cycle by undergoing terminal differentiation. From: Watson, J. D. *Molecular Biology of the Gene* (3d ed.). Menlo Park, CA: W. A. Benjamin, 1976, p. 558. Reproduced with permission.

is an important determinant of overall cell production. Many factors contribute to cell loss, including genomic instability (a feature of most malignancies that results in lethal mutations), limitations in oxygen and blood supply that develop as a tumor grows, immune surveillance by the host, and effects of antitumor therapy. Overall tumor growth, ignoring the contributions of any particular factors, is usually measured as the clinical doubling time — the time it takes a tumor to double its volume. Tumors with very high cell production rates, assessed by tritiated thymidine uptake or mitotic index, may exhibit very long doubling times if cell loss is great. Conversely, a short doubling time can be seen in tumors with low cell production rates if cell loss is minimal.

When tumor cells are grown in culture media, they exhibit three phases of growth. After an initial lag phase during which the cells adapt to their environment, they grow exponentially until they exhaust their nutrient supply. The "Gompertzian" growth curve (Fig. 10-2) illustrates this growth pattern [37]. While the applicability of Gompertzian growth kinetics to human malignancy is somewhat controversial, it forms a framework for our understanding of tumor growth.

Using the average cell volume concept, it has been calculated that

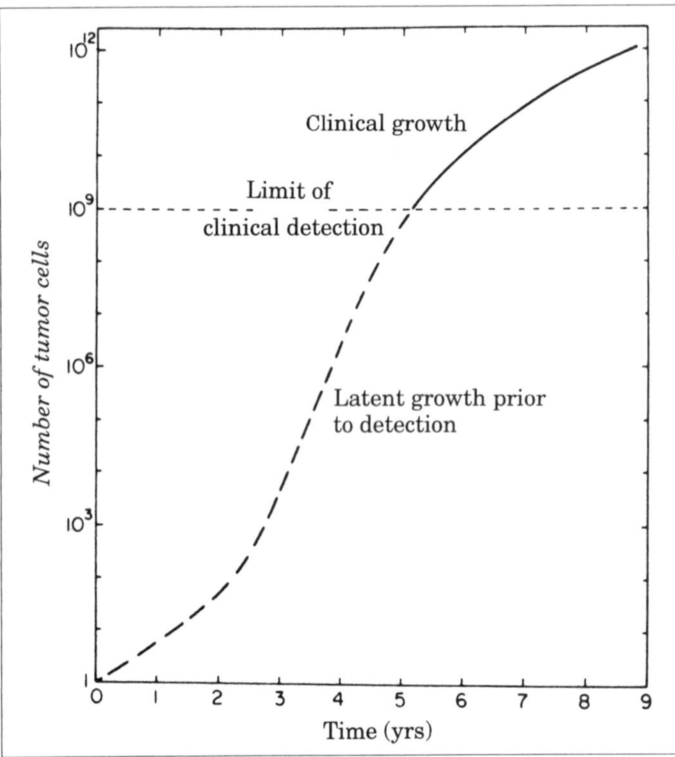

Fig. 10-2. The Gompertzian growth curve. The Gompertzian growth curve, indicating the approximate cell numbers believed to be applicable to human tumors during their growth. Note that clinical detection usually occurs late in the course of tumor growth. From: Tannock, I. F. Cell Proliferation. In I. F. Tannock and R. P. Hill (eds.), *The Basic Science of Oncology* (2d ed.). New York: McGraw-Hill, 1992, p. 156. Reproduced with permission of McGraw-Hill.

a tumor 1 cm in diameter (about the smallest clinically detectable tumor) contains about 10^9 cells. Assuming the tumor arose from one malignant cell, this represents 30 doublings. The average lethal tumor burden in humans is estimated at 10^{12} cells, which is 40 doublings. Average doubling times based on serial chest x-ray measurements of patients with untreated peripheral lung cancers are about 70 days for SCLC and about 87–134 days for NSCLC [48]. Thus, most cancers present late in their natural history, and their growth rate corresponds to the plateau phase of the Gompertzian curve. It is also apparent that most cancers arise years before they are first diagnosed. These considerations must be modified by many other variables. For example, the preclinical doubling time, which is probably much shorter, cannot be measured in most cases. Additionally, many of the cells in a tumor are not malignant cells but host-derived stromal cells and inflammatory cells. Finally, doubling times in individuals with similar tumors exhibit very wide variability.

Ideally, a chemotherapeutic agent should selectively destroy malignant cells, leaving normal cells unaffected. Unfortunately, malignant cells exhibit phenotypic properties that are usually qualitative or quantitative distortions of the corresponding normal cells from which they arose. Therefore, chemotherapy is usually nonspecific in its toxicity; its success relies largely on the ability of the host to recover more effectively than the tumor. Thus, chemotherapy is inherently toxic. As a corollary, chemotherapy's effectiveness is limited by toxicity to host tissues.

Since chemotherapeutic agents usually target proliferating cells, their toxicities are also greatest in normal tissues with the highest rates of cell turnover, such as bone marrow, mucosal epithelium, hair follicles, and germ cells. Thus, the major side effects of most chemotherapy agents are myelosuppression, GI toxicity such as mucositis and diarrhea, alopecia, and infertility. Nausea and vomiting are also frequent side effects of many agents; these are usually due to stimulation of the chemoreceptor trigger zone in the brainstem.

Because dosage-limiting toxicity renders chemotherapy agents marginally effective in most solid tumors, strategies have been developed to overcome this limitation. One method has been to use multiple chemotherapy drugs whose specific toxicities overlap, allowing maximal or near-maximal dosages of each agent. The efficacy of this approach was first demonstrated in the classic study of MOPP (mechlorethamine, Oncovin [vincristine], procarbazine, and prednisone) therapy in Hodgkin's disease [14]. The use of multiple agents has become the standard approach to most tumors in which chemotherapy is indicated.

Because it is generally accepted that there is a dose-response curve for chemotherapy, many methods of maximizing tolerable dosages have been implemented. The administration of chemotherapy by experienced personnel in settings where optimal supportive care modalities are available serves to minimize the perceived or actual need for dosage reductions or delays in treatment cycles. Methods to abrogate myelotoxicity with autologous or allogeneic bone marrow reconstitution [6,8], are effective in some hematologic malignancies but remain investigational in the treatment of solid tumors. Another approach to reduce toxicity is the use of cytokines, such as recombinant granulocyte colony stimulating factor (rG-CSF), to enhance marrow recovery following chemotherapy [21], and putative cytoprotective agents, such as WR2721, which is being investigated as an agent to selectively reduce toxicity from chemotherapy and radiotherapy in normal tissues [12].

Drug Resistance

A major factor limiting the effectiveness of chemotherapy is drug resistance; drug resistance may be present de novo or may emerge during treatment. Several mechanisms of drug resistance have been identified. Some common examples include gene amplification of a target enzyme or altered affinity of enzyme for drug, induction of

DNA repair mechanisms, decreased cellular uptake of drug, and increased drug metabolism. One of the most intensely studied mechanisms, referred to as multidrug resistance, confers resistance to vinca alkaloids, anthracycline antibiotics, and actinomycin D [22]. It was determined that these drugs were eliminated from cells by a membrane pump under the control of "P glycoprotein," the product of the mdr1 gene. The level of expression of this gene correlates well with resistance to these chemotherapy agents, and high levels were detectable in previously untreated resistant tumors and in some tumors at relapse after treatment. Attempts at blocking P glycoprotein with calcium channel blockers (through an unknown mechanism independent of their effects on calcium homeostasis) are effective in vitro [27] but have met with limited success in clinical trials.

Chemotherapy effectiveness may be limited by factors other than cellular mechanisms of resistance. The drugs must also reach tumor cells in adequate concentrations. Tumors exhibit high interstitial pressures that reduce blood flow [30]. In addition, abnormalities of red blood cell deformability, a major determinant of blood flow at the capillary level, have been described in cancer patients [9]. Finally, some tumors or their metastases are located in sanctuary sites, such as the brain and the testes, that provide pharmacologic barriers to many drugs delivered through the bloodstream.

Response to Treatment

The effectiveness of any cancer treatment depends on several prognostic factors, most of which relate to the status of the host. Perhaps the best predictor of response to chemotherapy, and of survival duration, is referred to as performance status, an assessment of functional impairment caused by cancer that is easily done by any clinician. The Karnofsky scale [32] and the Zubrod scale [51] are both widely used, but the latter (Table 10-1) is briefer and easier to remember. In this five point scale (0–4) performance is rated from asymptomatic (PS-0) to bedridden (PS-4), with intermediate scores determined by time spent in bed during waking hours. Patients with performance status 0 or 1 tolerate chemotherapy much better than those with lower scores. Chemotherapy is rarely, if ever, indicated for PS-4 patients. Performance status correlates well with other prognostic factors but is also predictive independently of them.

Other important prognostic factors (Table 10-2) for treatment re-

Table 10-1. The ZUBROD (ECOG) performance status scale

Score	Definition
0	Asymptomatic
1	Symptomatic, fully ambulatory
2	In bed <50% of waking day
3	In bed >50% of waking day
4	Bedridden

Table 10-2. Prognostic factors for survival in lung cancer patients

1. Tumor stage
2. Performance status
3. Weight loss
4. Prior chemotherapy or radiotherapy

sponse and survival are stage of the cancer, weight loss [15], and prior treatment. The last is clear from virtually all studies in which chemotherapy is administered to previously treated and untreated patients. The reasons may include the possibility that unresponsive or relapsed patients are further along in the natural history of their disease when the subsequent treatment is instituted. There may also be cross-resistance between the prior and subsequent treatment [18]. Finally, several routine laboratory measurements, such as hematocrit and serum lactic dehydrogenase (LDH), levels may be useful prognostic indicators in cancer patients [11].

The extent of cancer, or its stage, is a critical prognostic factor by definition because tumor staging is designed to create groups of patients according to prognosis. Most cancers, including lung cancer, are staged according to a TNM classification (T refers to the size of the primary tumor; N refers to the location and extent of regional nodal metastases; M refers to the presence of distant metastases) established and periodically revised by authoritative bodies such as the American Joint Committee on Cancer (AJCC). Lung cancer is assigned a stage from I to IV based on these criteria [1] (Table 10-3). Most patients with NSCLC are unresectable at presentation (stage IIIb-IV) and have a median survival of around 6 months.

Because most SCLC patients are presumed to be metastatic at diagnosis, they are operationally staged as limited or extensive. In limited-stage disease, detectable tumor is confined to the chest such that it can be encompassed in a single radiation port (this may include contralateral supraclavicular nodes or chest wall extension but not contralateral pulmonary tumor or malignant pleural effusions). Extensive-stage disease refers to more advanced tumor. Approximately one-third of SCLC patients present with limited-stage disease; their median survival is about 15 months compared with about 8 months for patients with extensive disease. However, it is not this difference in median survival that is significant between the two stages; rather it is the 10–20% of limited-stage patients who achieve long-term survival compared with virtually no patients presenting with extensive-stage disease.

The results of chemotherapy in SCLC depend on the stage. For limited-stage patients (most of whom have good performance status), overall response rates exceeding 70–90% can be expected with about 50% complete responses (disappearance of all detectable tumor for more than 1 month). As noted, 10%–20% will live beyond 5 years. For extensive-stage patients with good performance status, response rates of about 50% are seen, with around 20–30% complete responses but only rare long-term responders. Prognosis in these

Table 10-3. TNM staging schema for lung cancer

T lesion

TX: primary tumor cannot be assessed or diagnosis by sputum cytology or bronchial washings without visualized lesion

T0: No evidence of primary tumor

Tis: Carcinoma in situ

T1: Tumor <3 cm in diameter surrounded by lung or visceral pleura with no tumor in a main bronchus

T2: Tumor with any of the following:
- Greater >3 cm in diameter
- Involving a main bronchus but >2 cm from main carina
- Invading visceral pleura
- Lobar atelectasis or obstructive pneumonitis not involving whole lung.

T3: any size tumor with any of the following features:
- Invasion of chest wall, diaphragm, mediastinal pleura, or pericardium
- Tumor <2 cm from main carina but not involving it
- Whole lung atelectasis or postobstructive pneumonitis

T4: Tumor of any size with any of the following features:
- Invasion of mediastinum, heart, great vessels, trachea, esophagus, vertebral bodies, main carina
- Malignant pleural effusion

N lesion

NX: regional nodes cannot be assessed

N0: No regional lymph nodes involved

N1: Involvement of ipsilateral peribronchial or hilar nodes

N2: Involvement of ipsilateral mediastinal or subcarinal nodes

N3: Involvement of contralateral nodes, ipsilateral or contralateral scalene or supraclavicular nodes

M lesion

MX: Distant metastases cannot be assessed

M0: No distant metastases

M1: Distant metastases

Stage groupings			
Occult	TX	N0	M0
Stage 0	Tis	N0	M0
Stage I	T1-2	N0	M0
Stage II	T1-2	N1	M0
Stage IIIA	T1-2	N2	M0
	T3	N0-2	M0
Stage IIIB	Any T	N3	M0
Stage IV	Any T	Any N	M1

patients varies with the number of metastatic sites and with performance status.

In oncology, an objective response is usually understood to mean at least a 50% reduction in the size of all evaluable lesions without the appearance of new lesions for at least 1 month. For measurable lesions, the product of the longest perpendicular diameters of a lesion is used to determine this. A complete response refers to disappearance of all clinical evidence of tumor with return of laboratory tests and performance status to baseline for at least 1 month. A partial response is an objective response less than a complete response. While some investigators use terms such as *minor* or *minimal* response to signify lesser degrees of response or subjective improvement, these have no clinical significance. It is also important to realize that longer survival in responders compared to nonresponders in a single-arm study does not necessarily imply causation by the treatment under study because responses occur more often in patients with better prognostic factors. Any published study should provide definitions of the response criteria used to allow meaningful evaluation of the results.

New drugs with antitumor potential are selected for clinical trials based on several factors, including their anticipated actions based on molecular structure, antitumor profile in preclinical studies, both in vitro and in animal, and expected toxicity profile. Initial clinical trials (phase I trials) establish an appropriate dosage and schedule of administration. They are usually conducted in patients with advanced cancer unresponsive to available treatments. Since the major end point of a phase I trial is a recommended dosage rather than a response rate (although responses do occur in these trials), the presence of evaluable tumor is not essential; however, end organ function (e.g., liver and kidneys) should be relatively normal. In phase II trials, the activity of a drug or regimen, in dosages defined in phase I studies, is tested in specific tumor types. Here, it is essential to select patients with evaluable tumors and to define carefully the prognostic factors that may influence outcome. If a regimen is active in phase II trials, it may be tested in phase III trials in which patients are randomly allocated to receive the best standard therapy or the investigational therapy. All investigational clinical trials require that appropriate informed consent be obtained from participants. The principles of clinical trial design, including stratification for prognostic factors and appropriate response criteria, have developed largely over the past two decades. Accurate data on drugs developed prior to that time are often lacking.

Although this chapter focuses on pharmacologic therapy of lung cancer, it must be stressed that modern cancer treatment, including that for lung cancer, involves multimodality approaches. The treatment with the greatest impact on NSCLC is surgery, with radiotherapy contributing effective symptom palliation in advanced disease. The role of radiotherapy in SCLC is discussed below.

Chemotherapy Drugs in Lung Cancer

Any physician prescribing or administering chemotherapeutic agents must have a thorough knowledge of drug metabolism and side effects and should have access to good supportive care modalities. Chemotherapy toxicities often require skilled fluid and electrolyte management, nutritional support, and management of sepsis. Aggressive use of modern antiemetics regimens is essential with many chemotherapy regimens. Psychological support and the need to help patients deal with their disease is best achieved with a multidisciplinary effort by physicians, nurses, social workers, support groups, and other ancillary staff.

Chemotherapy dosages are usually calculated according to patient body surface area, which is derived from height and weight. While charts are usually consulted to derive the surface area, a simplified formula has been shown to be accurate in most circumstances [43]:

$$BSA(m^2) = \sqrt{Ht(cm) \times Wt(kg)/3600}$$

Drug dosages may also need to be modified for abnormal renal or hepatic function (depending on the drugs used), severity of toxicity with previous cycles, or performance status. The commonly used chemotherapeutic agents are classified by their presumed mode of action, origin, or structure, although some drugs do not fit clearly into any single group. Only drugs currently useful in lung cancer treatment will be described in detail. Important toxicities of each agent will be described; rare and minor toxicities or side effects may be omitted.

Alkylating Agents

Alkylating agents fall into the following categories:

Nitrogen mustards
- Cyclophosphamide
- Iphosphamide
- Mechlorethamine (HN2)
- Chlorambucil
- Melphalan

Alkyl sulfonates
- Busulfan

Nitrosoureas
- Carmustine (BCNU)
- Lomustine (CCNU)
- Semustine (methyl-CCNU)
- Streptozocin

Triazenes
- Dacarbazine

Platinum coordinate compounds
- cis-platinum (Platinol)
- Carboplatin (Paraplatin)

MECHANISMS OF ACTION

Alkylating agents are usually inactive until they are metabolized into electrophilic intermediates. These reactive intermediates form covalent bonds with macromolecules, including nucleic acids, most commonly by alkylation of guanine moieties. Some have two reaction sites (bifunctional alkylating agents), which enable them to cross-link DNA either within one strand or across both strands, or to link it to another macromolecule such as a protein. Agents in this group are both cytotoxic and carcinogenic. Alkylating agents are not cell cycle specific; that is, they are effective even in resting cells; however, their cytotoxic action is not expressed until the cell attempts to progress through the cell cycle. Since DNA replication is impaired, cells cannot progress through S phase to G2 phase. Alkylating agents react with macromolecules of all tissues but are most toxic where rapid cell division occurs (e.g., bone marrow, mucosal epithelium, and gonads). Normal DNA repair mechanisms have more time to reverse the damage done by alkylating agents in slowly dividing cells.

MECHANISMS OF RESISTANCE

Acquired resistance is common with alkylating agents but incompletely understood. Multiple processes appear to contribute to resistance, including decreased cellular uptake of drug, accelerated metabolism of active intermediates, and induction of DNA repair mechanisms. Cross-resistance with other alkylating agents is common.

Cyclophosphamide

The development of cyclophosphamide (Cytoxan) was undertaken in an attempt to create a mechlorethamine (nitrogen mustard) analogue with greater selective toxicity for tumor cells. While this was not fully successful, a more favorable toxicity spectrum and greater stability has made this the most commonly used alkylating agent. It is active in lymphomas, myeloma, pediatric malignancies, ovarian carcinoma, sarcomas, and breast cancer. Cyclophosphamide was moderately active as a single agent in SCLC [17,38].

PHARMACOLOGY

Cyclophosphamide must be biotransformed in the liver by mixed function oxidases (p450 enzymes) to active alkylating metabolites. Several intermediates are formed; it is not clear which ones are critical in its therapeutic actions. Subsequent metabolism of these intermediates to inactive forms then occurs, with rapid renal clearance. The parent drug is eliminated slowly and has a plasma half-life of about 7 hours. Because the interaction of activated drug metabolites with DNA is an all-or-none phenomenon and because of the persistence of the parent drug in the circulation, induction of p450 enzymes by drugs such as phenobarbital has little effect on drug action. Instead, final drug detoxification and clearance play larger roles in pharmacokinetics.

ADVERSE REACTIONS

Hematologic

Neutropenia is common, with nadir counts occurring 7–10 days after administration and recovery after about 2–3 weeks. Thrombocytopenia occurs in the same time frame but is usually less severe. Anemia occurs occasionally.

Gastrointestinal

Nausea and vomiting are common, particularly with high dosages. Anorexia, diarrhea, and oral mucositis may occur.

Dermatologic

Alopecia is common but reversible after drug discontinuation.

Lung

Interstitial pulmonary fibrosis is a well-described but uncommon idiosyncratic reaction to this drug. It is more common with busulfan, in which it occurs after prolonged administration.

Genitourinary

Hemorrhagic cystitis can develop with high dosages, but is most common with prolonged oral administration and with the cyclophosphamide analogue iphosphamide. Rarely, it may be severe or even fatal. It is thought to be due to bladder irritation caused by high urinary concentrations of the metabolite acrolein. It can be decreased by maintaining good hydration, advising frequent urination, and administering morning dosage to minimize bladder contact. Patients should not have any genitourinary tract obstruction or should be catheterized for free urinary flow. Administration of sulphydryl containing compounds such as *N*-acetylcysteine or mesna (2-mercaptoethanesulfonate), which react readily with acrolein, may reduce the incidence of this toxicity.

Local

Cyclophosphamide is not a vesicant.

Secondary malignancies

Most alkylating agents, including cyclophosphamide, are mutagenic as well as cytotoxic and may result in posttherapeutic malignancies in long-term survivors of SCLC. These are usually leukemias, but an increased frequency of other solid tumors occurs as well. The most common solid tumor in lung cancer survivors is NSCLC, but this is probably related to field carcinogenesis — the concept that the entire bronchial mucosa is at risk of carcinogenesis, usually from tobacco use.

DOSAGES

Cyclophosphamide is available in 25-mg and 50-mg tablets for oral administration. Vials are available containing 100-mg, 200-mg, 500-mg, 1-g, and 2-g powder for IV administration after reconstitution with sterile water.

The dosage range is highly variable. In the treatment of lung cancer, it is rarely used as a single agent, and IV administration is the rule. Common dosages are 400–1500 mg/m^2 every 3 weeks in the absence of undue toxicity.

Lomustine

Lomustine (CCNU, CeeNU), a bifunctional alkylating agent, is a nitrosourea, one of a group of compounds developed because they are highly effective in many animal models and because their high lipid solubility renders them capable of crossing the blood-brain barrier, suggesting utility in CNS malignancies. Unfortunately, their promise in preclinical studies did not hold up in clinical trials, and they remain of limited usefulness in a few malignancies, including brain tumors and melanoma. Because most chemotherapy drugs do not cross the blood-brain barrier and because brain metastases occur frequently in SCLC, lomustine was incorporated into some regimens in the hope that it would decrease the incidence of brain metastases developing in patients otherwise in complete remission. This hope was not realized; nevertheless, lomustine has shown modest activity in SCLC [17].

PHARMACOLOGY

Lomustine is well absorbed after oral administration. In contrast to the nitrogen mustards, spontaneous nonenzymatic degradation to electrophilic intermediates occurs as well as enzymatic metabolism. The active metabolites exhibit plasma half-lives up to 48 hours. Most of the drug and its metabolites are excreted renally. Accumulation of active metabolites in the cerebrospinal fluid occurs rapidly.

TOXICITY

Hematologic

The nitrosoureas cause delayed myelosuppression compared with most other chemotherapeutic agents. White count and platelet nadirs occur about 4 weeks after treatment, and recovery is by 6 weeks. Therefore, in combination regimens, these drugs are usually administered with every other cycle. Bone marrow toxicity is also cumulative. While this does not usually limit initial therapy of SCLC, it may reduce tolerance to subsequent chemotherapy if it is needed.

Gastrointestinal

Moderate nausea and vomiting are common after administration of lomustine.

Diarrhea and mucositis

Both are common.

Lung

Interstitial fibrosis has occasionally been reported.

Local

Lomustine is not a vesicant.

Secondary malignancies

As with other alkylating agents, posttherapeutic malignancies may occur.

DOSAGES

Lomustine is available in 10-mg, 40-mg, and 100-mg tablets. The usual dosage is 130 mg/m^2 as a single agent and 100 mg/m^2 when used in combination chemotherapy.

Cis-platinum

Cis-platinum's (Platinol) clinical potential was discovered serendipitously when bacterial growth inhibition in electromagnetic fields was found to be caused by platinum coordinate compounds arising from platinum electrodes. It is currently one of the most widely used chemotherapy agents because of its broad antitumor spectrum of activity. It is, unfortunately, also highly toxic, and newer analogues are being sought with more favorable toxicity profiles. It is a drug of choice in regimens for germ cell tumors, head and neck cancer, and ovarian carcinoma and is active in esophagus cancer, bladder cancer, sarcomas, and lymphomas. In SCLC, few good phase II studies in previously untreated patients were performed; the modest results demonstrated in previously treated patients [23] underestimate its potential, which was subsequently realized in combination regimens in previously untreated patients.

PHARMACOLOGY

Cis-platinum consists of a central platinum atom bound to two chlorine and two ammonia groups. The cis configuration is necessary for cytotoxic activity, the trans isomer being inactive. Activation occurs intracellularly where the low chloride concentrations result in replacement of the chloride moieties with water molecules, resulting in a positively charged complex (see Fig. 10-3). These react with electrophilic sites on the DNA molecule, most commonly at the N7 position on guanine or the C3 position on cytosine. Intrastrand links appear to be critical to its action. Following an IV dose, cis-platinum concentrates in liver, kidneys, and intestines. The terminal plasma half-life of the parent drug is about 30 minutes, but extensive covalent binding to plasma proteins and erythrocytes occurs. Cisplatinum penetrates CNS poorly. The drug is primarily excreted by the kidneys, with 20–75% excreted within 24 hours. The remainder is probably tissue bound.

ADVERSE REACTIONS

Hematologic

Marrow suppression is usually mild. A chronic normochromic, normocytic anemia may be seen. Occasionally, hemolytic reactions occur.

Gastrointestinal

Severe vomiting, sometimes without nausea, typically follows administration by about 4 hours and is felt to be mediated by stimulation of the chemoreceptor trigger zone in the brainstem. It may be dose limiting and is best prevented with very aggressive antiemetic therapy employing a selective 5-hydroxytryptamine antagonist such as ondansetron (Zofran) in combination with dexamethasone 10–20 mg IV and a sedative or antihistamine. Delayed emesis and profound anorexia may develop a few days after resolution of acute emesis. It is refractory to available treatments and may require IV fluid support. Mucositis occurs uncommonly. Diarrhea occurs often and may be severe, requiring fluid and electrolyte replacement.

Dermatologic

Reversible alopecia may occur.

Renal

This is frequently a dosage-limiting toxicity of cis-platinum therapy and has been the subject of intense investigation. It may be seen after a single dose and is manifest as a rising BUN, creatinine levels, and uric acid levels, usually during the second week after therapy. The drug is especially toxic to the distal renal tubule and collecting system, but reduced glomerular filtration, proteinuria, and magnesium wasting also occur. The underlying basis for cis-platinum nephrotoxicity is still unclear. Nephrotoxicity can be minimized by pretreatment IV hydration (at least 1 liter over 4–6 hours) and by administration of IV mannitol 25–50 g before and after cis-platinum administration. Nephrotoxicity is enhanced by concomitant therapy with aminoglycoside antimicrobials, nonsteroidal antiinflammatory drugs (NSAIDs), and other nephrotoxic drugs, which should all be used with the greatest caution, if at all, in patients receiving cis-platinum. While serum BUN and creatinine usually return to normal within a few weeks, persistent decreases in creatinine clearance are usually measurable. Cis-platinum should not be administered to patients with creatinine clearances under 55 cc/minute.

Metabolic

Severe and life-threatening electrolyte disturbances associated with nephrotoxicity may occur and require extreme vigilance. Severe renal magnesium wasting has been demonstrated and may result in secondary hypocalcemia, occasionally with tetany. Refractory hypokalemia with daily losses exceeding 200 mEq may occur. Hypophosphatemia also occurs. These problems may be exacerbated by vomiting, prolonged periods of anorexia, or both. Electrolytes should be normal prior to treatment and monitored frequently; aggressive replacement of potassium and magnesium is indicated if serum levels drop. Electrolyte imbalances may be exacerbated by nephrotoxic antimicrobials such as aminoglycosides and by extended spectrum penicillins.

Neurologic

Peripheral neuropathy is cumulative, usually appears after more than six cycles of treatment, and may be severe and dosage limiting. It is usually manifest clinically as sensory paresthesias in a stocking and glove distribution. Decreased proprioception and vibratory sensation may occur, and nerve conduction velocity is impaired. Segmental demyelination has been seen histologically. Motor dysfunction occurs in severe cases.

Ototoxicity

High-frequency hearing loss, occasionally with tinnitus, occurs commonly, especially in elderly patients, and is associated with damage to the organ of Corti. It may occur after the first treatment and is cumulative. Audiograms are recommended prior to starting of cis-platinum and before each cycle.

Allergic

Hypersensitivity reactions sometimes occur, manifest as facial flushing, angioneurotic edema, or urticaria; anaphylaxis occurs rarely. Management is with antihistamines and corticosteroids; epinephrine is rarely needed.

Vascular

Several reports link cis-platinum administration to acute and delayed arterial vascular events, including myocardial infarction and stroke, but a definite association is difficult to establish because of the frequency of these events in the adult population receiving chemotherapy. Raynaud's phenomenon has been definitely linked to cis-platinum in combination with bleomycins and vinblastine in patients with germ cell tumors.

Local

Cis-platinum is not a vesicant.

Secondary Malignancies

There are few reports establishing posttherapeutic malignancies, but these might be expected because cis-platinum is genotoxic and mutagenic.

DOSAGES

Vials containing 10-mg or 50-mg powder are available for IV administration. **Note:** Administration equipment containing aluminum parts must be avoided. They react with cis-platinum, inactivating it. The usual dosage is 50–100 mg/m^2 IV every 3–4 weeks. Equivalent dosages divided into 5 daily doses or as continuous infusions are also used.

Carboplatin

Carboplatin (Paraplatin) is a second-generation platinum coordinate compound developed in the hope that its toxicity profile would be improved over cis-platinum while retaining its broad spectrum of antitumor activity. Carboplatin does exhibit far less nephrotoxicity, ototoxicity, and neurotoxicity and is less emetogenic but at the expense of dosage-limiting hematologic toxicity. Its full spectrum of activity is still under investigation but appears promising.

In SCLC, phase II studies yielded response rates in previously untreated patients to be around 50%, with about 10% complete responders [3].

PHARMACOLOGY

A bidentate carboxycyclobutane moiety replaces the two chlorine atoms of cis-platinum, resulting in a more stable compound that is more slowly aquated and is only 10–20% protein bound in plasma. The terminal half life is 7.5–20 hours. The kidneys eliminate most of the drug, with 50–70% eliminated within 24 hours. Carboplatin dosages must be adjusted for decreased renal function; this may be done empirically, but several formulas exist for greater accuracy [5,52].

TOXICITY

Hematologic

Marrow suppression is dosage limiting, with thrombocytopenia often greater than neutropenia. Nadir counts occur in 7–10 days, and recovery is usually by 4 weeks.

Gastrointestinal

Nausea and vomiting are very common, but in contrast to cisplatinum, they are usually easily controlled with standard antiemetics.

Dermatologic

Mild reversible alopecia occurs rarely. Hypersensitivity rashes may also occur occasionally.

Nephrotoxicity

Subclinical decreases in renal function have been measured, but clinically significant renal impairment is rare except at very high dosages and after cis-platinum therapy. Unlike cis-platinum, renal tubular excretion of carboplatin does not occur.

Neurotoxicity

Mild peripheral neuropathies have occasionally been reported.

Local

Carboplatin is not a vesicant.

Secondary Malignancies

There are no adequate data, but the potential must be presumed from the mechanism of action.

DOSAGES

Vials are available containing 50-mg, 150-mg, or 450-mg powder for reconstitution, respectively, with 5-ml, 15-ml, or 45-ml sterile water or saline or 5% dextrose. The usual dosage is 200–400 mg/m^2 IV every 3–4 weeks.

Antimetabolites

Examples are the folic acid analogues methotrexate and trimetrexate; the pyrimidine analogues 5-flurouracil and cytarabine (cytosine arabinoside); and the purine analogues 6-mercaptopurine and 6-thioguanine.

MECHANISMS OF ACTION

Antimetabolites are structurally similar to normal metabolic substrates required for synthesis of purines, pyrimidines, and nucleic acids. They impair cellular functions by substituting for normal precursors in vital physiologic reactions or by blocking these reactions, leading to strand breaks and premature chain terminations. They must be present at cytotoxic concentration during DNA synthesis (S phase) to be effective and thus tend to be cell cycle specific. For this reason and because of their short plasma half-life, they are often more effective when administered by prolonged IV infusion. Secondary malignancies are usually not attributable to antimetabolites. The specific mechanisms of actions and other pharmacologic features of the antimetabolites vary widely among different preparations. The most commonly used antimetabolite in lung cancer is methotrexate, and further discussion will be limited to this drug.

Methotrexate, an analogue of folic acid (pteroylglutamic acid) (Fig. 10-3), acts as an inhibitor of the enzyme dihydrofolate reductase (DHFR). Folates are essential nutrients that, when reduced to tetrahydrofolate (FH_4) by DHFR, serve as a coenzymes in reactions in which one carbon transfers occur. The one-carbon moieties are attached to positions 5 or 10 of the pteridine ring (or bridge them) and are transferred in a number of reactions. One of these is the conversion of 2-deoxyuridine monophosphate (dUMP) to thymidylate by the enzyme thymidylate synthetase, the rate-limiting step in DNA synthesis.

When reduced folate transfers a methyl group to dUMP to form thymidylate, the FH_4 is oxidized to dihydrofolate (FH_2). Before it can serve as an acceptor of another methyl group, it must be converted back to FH_4 by DHFR. Inhibition of DHFR by methotrexate traps folate in its oxidized state, disrupting DNA synthesis. There are two methods to bypass this block pharmacologically: (1) supply enough thymidine, which can be converted to thymidylate by the enzyme thymidine kinase, or (2) supply leucovorin (citrovorum factor), which is reduced and metabolically active without the need for reduction by DHFR. The latter is useful clinically because it can ameliorate the toxicities of methotrexate, which result, in part, from its inhibition of multiple reactions involving one-carbon transfers.

MECHANISMS OF RESISTANCE

At least three mechanisms of acquired resistance to antifols have been clearly demonstrated: (1) decreased cellular uptake of meth-

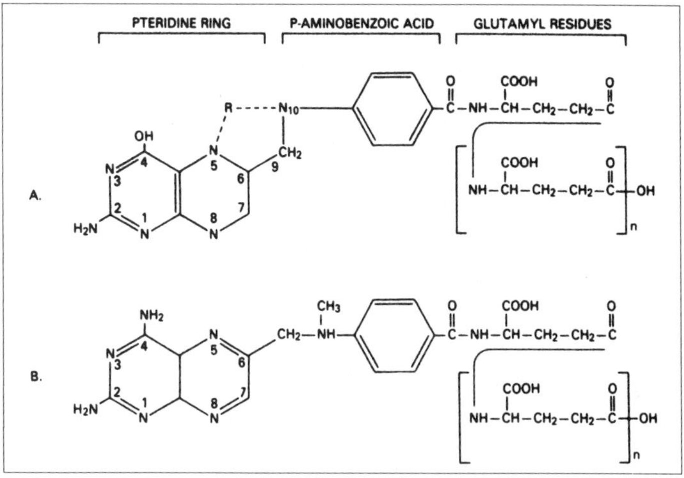

Fig. 10-3. Structures of tetrahydrofolate and methotrexate. The R group in the tetrahydrofolate molecule represents one-carbon moieties; these are carried on the nitrogen atom at position 5 or 10 or form a bridge between the two. Reduction of folates to the tetra-hydro form requires the enzyme dihydrofolate reductase. Methotrexate is also a substrate for this enzyme. From Jolivet, J., et al. The pharmacology and clinical use of methotrexate. *N. Engl. J. Med.* 309:1104, 1983. Reproduced with permission from *The New England Journal of Medicine.*

otrexate, (2) production of DHFR isoenzymes with decreased affinity for methotrexate, and (3) DHFR gene amplification. The last may result in DHFR concentrations hundreds of times higher than those prior to treatment.

Methotrexate

Methotrexate (Methotrexate) is one of the oldest chemotherapy agents in use. It was the first agent shown to be curative as a single agent when it was used in gestational choriocarcinoma. It can also be curative in regimens used for pediatric leukemias. It is active in osteogenic sarcoma and in adult lymphomas. Although no good single-agent trials in SCLC have been performed, activity has been suggested [54]. A comparison of high-dosage versus low-dosage methotrexate in a combination regimen, in the hope that high-dosage methotrexate would cross the blood-brain barrier and prevent CNS metastases, showed no difference in systemic response rates or in the incidence of brain metastases [25].

PHARMACOLOGY

Oral absorption appears to be saturable and thus dose dependent. Peak serum levels are reached within 1–2 hours. Methotrexate is well absorbed from the IM route. The drug does not penetrate the cerebrospinal fluid (CSF) in therapeutic amounts but is one of the few chemotherapeutic agents that can be safely administered by the intrathecal route (others are cytosine arabinoside and 6-mercaptopurine) for management of carcinomatous meningitis. Methotrexate competes with reduced folates for active transport across cell membranes by means of a single carrier–mediated active transport process. At serum concentration of more than 100 micromoles, passive diffusion becomes a major pathway by which effective intracellular concentration can be achieved. Methotrexate, like physiologic folates, undergoes intracellular polyglutamation; the decreased membrane permeability of these forms may serve to retain the drug intracellularly. Methotrexate is 50% protein bound in plasma and can be displaced by various drugs (e.g., sulfonamides, salicylates, tetracyclines, and phenytoin), thus increasing its toxicity. Severe and sometimes fatal bone marrow suppression and GI toxicity have been reported with concomitant salicylate use. Other antineoplastic agents such as vincristine and etoposide may block methotrexate efflux from cells, enhancing toxicity. The terminal elimination half-life is about 7 hours. Prolongation of the latter can result in severe toxicity. Methotrexate diffuses freely into pleural effusions and other "third spaces" from which slow efflux can greatly extend its half-life. It is important that such third spaces be drained prior to methotrexate administration. Renal excretion is the primary route of elimination, occurring by glomerular filtration and active tubular secretion. Methotrexate clearance rates vary widely and are generally decreased at higher dosages. The potential for toxocity from high-dosage regimens can be reduced by hydration, alkalinization of urine, and administration of leucovorin.

TOXICITY

Hematologic

Leukopenia and thrombocytopenia are common and may be dosage limiting. Nadir counts occur in about 7–10 days with recovery by 3 weeks. Bone marrow suppression is often less severe with high-dosage methotrexate followed by leucovorin.

Gastrointestinal

Nausea and vomiting are mild with low dosages but may be more severe at high dosages. Stomatitis can be severe and dosage limiting.

Dermatologic

Rash, pruritus, and alopecia are common.

Hepatic

Transient serum enzyme elevations are common. Hepatotoxicity and cirrhosis may be seen with prolonged oral use, a regimen used only in rheumatologic (nonmalignant) conditions.

Lung

Methotrexate-induced interstitial lung disease is uncommon and idiosyncratic but can be severe and irreversible.

Renal

Nephrotoxicity leading to acute renal failure can be seen when high dosages (over 1 g) are used. Renal toxicity is primarily due to the precipitation of methotrexate and 7-hydroxymethotrexate in the renal tubules. Alkalinization of the urine and vigorous hydration minimize this risk.

Neurologic

Following intrathecal use, acute chemical arachnoiditis, motor dysfunction seizures, and coma uncommonly occur. Delayed clearance from the CNS increases the risk of complications, and monitoring of CSF levels may be helpful in deciding on leucovorin administration and subsequent dosing.

Local

Methotrexate is not a vesicant.

Secondary Malignancies

These have not been reported with methotrexate.

DOSAGES

Methotrexate is available as 2.5-mg tablets for oral use. Vials containing up to 250-mg powder are available for IM or IV administration. "Low-dosage" treatment usually consists of 30–40 mg/m^2 weekly. "Intermediate-dosage" regimens in the range of 100–200 mg/m^2 are common. Dosages higher than 50 mg/m^2 require leucovorin administration 24 hours later. "High-dosage" treatment, sometimes in the range of 10–20 g/m^2, requires vigorous hydration, urine alkalinization and other special supportive care. For intrathecal administration, 12 mg/m^2 in preservative-free saline is instilled every few days until spinal fluid is free of malignant cells, and then less frequently.

Antimicrobials

Examples of anthracycline antimicrobials are doxorubicin (Adriamycin), daunorubicin (Daunomycin), and mitoxantrone (Novantrone). Other antimicrobials are bleomycin (Blenoxane), dactinomycin (cosmegen), and mitomycin C (Mutamycin).

MECHANISM OF ACTION

Antimicrobials are biologic products of bacteria or fungi. They form a diverse group of compounds with no common mechanism of action. The activities of the anthracyclines, the most widely used representatives of this group, are especially enigmatic. They intercalate nucleic acids, interfering with DNA and RNA synthesis; inhibition of topoisomerase II activity by stabilizing enzyme-DNA complexes appears to be critical to their action. They are also metabolized by cytochrome p450 enzymes to produce free radical intermediates with potentially damaging effects on DNA. However, interaction with the plasma membrane appears to be critical for their activity. Anthracycline loaded cells are viable when efflux is prevented by cold temperatures or, upon warming of these cells, when extruded drug is absorbed by a calf thymus DNA [53]. Despite these unexplained factors, the interactions with DNA render the anthracyclines mutagenic and carcinogenic.

MECHANISM OF RESISTANCE

Anthracyclines, as well as vinca alkaloids and dactinomycin, are subject to pleiotropic resistance. Decreased availability or affinity of topoisomerase II for the drug may also occur.

Doxorubicin

Doxorubicin (Adriamycin) is the most widely used anthracycline antimicrobial. It is active in Hodgkin's disease (part of the ABVD regimen), non-Hodgkin lymphomas (part of the CHOP regimen and others), breast cancer and sarcomas, and pediatric malignancies. Moderate activity was demonstrated in small, single-agent trials in SCLC [23]. It forms a deep-red pigment in solution. It varies in structure from daunorubicin by a single hydroxyl group, although use of the latter analogue is restricted to acute leukemias.

PHARMACOLOGY

Intravenously administered doxorubicin is rapidly cleared from the plasma and undergoes significant tissue binding. The terminal elimination half-life is 24–48 hours. Both unchanged drug and several metabolites are excreted. Hepatic metabolism and biliary excretion accounts for most of its disposition; 5–10% is excreted by the kidney, mostly in the first 6 hours, during which time the urine may appear red. It does not cross blood-brain barrier. Doasges must be adjusted in the face of impaired liver function.

TOXICITY

Hematologic

Leukopenia is very common, with nadir counts occurring at 10–14 days and recovery by about 3 weeks. It may be dosage limiting. Thrombocytopenia is less common than leukopenia.

Gastrointestinal

Nausea and vomiting occur frequently and are usually moderate in severity. Mucositis occurs commonly.

Dermatologic

Alopecia is common but reversible. Erythematous streaking along the infusion site is a common, transient idiosyncratic reaction that must be distinguished from extravasation.

Cardiac

Cumulative cardiac toxicity manifest as congestive cardiomyopathy occurs regularly; the incidence begins to rise steeply at cumulative dosages exceeding 500 mg/m^2, and higher dosages usually should not be administered. Newer anthracyclines such as mitoxantrone may exhibit less cardiotoxicity, but adequate experience with it in lung cancer is lacking. There is evidence that a weekly dosing schedule increases the cardiac tolerance to doxorubicin. Lower thresholds for cardiac toxicity are seen in the elderly, patients with preexisting heart disease, or those with prior mediastinal irradiation. A decline in cardiac ejection fraction is an early indicator of doxorubicin cardiotoxicity; echocardiography and radionuclide angiography are indicated at baseline and periodically throughout treatment. Endomyocardial biopsy is the most sensitive indicator, and serial biopsies have been used to monitor toxicity; however, this is not widely practiced. Acutely, doxorubicin can cause atrial and ventricular arrhythmias, ST-T changes on electrocardiogram, or both in a small percentage of patients. These are usually of no clinical significance.

Local

Anthracyclines are potent vesicants, and extreme care must be used to prevent extravasation of drug around the infusion site. Extravasation frequently results in extensive necrosis of skin, soft tissues, and muscle, requiring plastic surgery and skin grafting. There is no agreed-on management of suspected extravasation because no measures have been proved to ameliorate this toxicity. Preventive measures include selection of large veins away from the hand or elbow joints, avoiding any undue trauma during venipuncture, ensuring good inflow and backflow through the line, and leaving the needle entry site untaped for monitoring. If a site near a joint must be used, an arm board to stabilize the joint is desirable. Infusions should be into the side arm of a freely running IV infusion of saline or dextrose/saline. Infusions must be constantly monitored. Most of these measures can be obviated if a long-term indwelling catheter (e.g., Hickman or Groshong catheter) or subcutaneous port is employed.

Potentiation of Other Agents

Doxorubicin may potentiate the toxicity of other anticancer therapies. Exacerbations of cyclophosphamide-induced hemorrhagic cystitis, 6-mercaptopurine–induced hepatotoxicity, and radiation toxicity have been reported to be increased with concomitant use. A radiation "recall" phenomenon has been described in which local toxicity within a prior radiation field is exacerbated by doxorubicin administration.

Secondary Malignancies

Doxorubicin is mutagenic and presumed to be carcinogenic.

DOSAGES

Vials containing 10 mg or 50 mg are available for IV administration after reconstitution with sterile saline. The usual dosage is 50–75 mg/m^2 IV every 3 weeks.

Mitomycin C

Mitomycin C (Mutamycin) is a naturally occurring antimicrobial that acts as a bifunctional alkylating agent after intracellular metabolism. It forms a deep blue solution upon reconstitution. It has modest activity in a GI malignancy, breast cancer, head and neck cancers, and lymphomas. It is moderately active in NSCLC, but its toxicity limits its use [47]. It is useful intravesically in the management of superficial bladder cancer.

PHARMACOLOGY

Mitomycin C is poorly absorbed after oral administration. After IV administration, it exhibits a plasma half-life of 35 minutes. It is metabolized in the liver, and dosages should be adjusted for hepatic dysfunction, although specific guidelines are lacking. Minimal amounts are excreted in either urine or bile. Its metabolites are unknown.

TOXICITY

Hematologic

Delayed and cumulative myelosuppression is often dosage limiting, with nadir counts at 4 weeks and recovery by 6 weeks. Both neutropenia and thrombocytopenia may be severe. Mitomycin C can occasionally induce a characteristic microangiopathic hemolytic anemia associated with renal failure (hemolytic uremic syndrome). This may occur long after discontinuation of the drug, and its pathogenesis is unknown.

Gastrointestinal

Nausea and vomiting are usually moderate. Stomatitis and diarrhea may occur.

Dermatologic

Reversible alopecia and allergic dermatitis may occur.

Pulmonary

Irreversible interstitial pneumonitis similar to that seen with busulfan and, less commonly, with other alkylating agents may occur and may be fatal. It is probably mediated by oxygen-free radicals resulting in lipid peroxidation. It is not dosage related. Cough, dyspnea, and fever associated with interstitial infiltrates are characteristic. The syndrome may respond dramatically to corticosteroids.

Cardiac

Mitomycin C may potentiate the cardiotoxicity of doxorubicin.

Local

Mitomycin C is a vesicant and great care must be taken in administration through a peripheral line.

Secondary Malignancies

Mitomycin C is mutagenic and presumed to be carcinogenic.

DOSAGES

Vials containing 5-mg and 20-mg powder are available for reconstitution with saline or sterile water. The usual dosage is 10–20 mg/m^2 IV every 6 weeks.

Plant Alkaloids

Alkaloids are complex organic bases that are formed in plants. Vinca alkaloids represent natural or semisynthetic drugs derived from the periwinkle plant, *Vinca rosea*. Epipodophyllotoxins are semisynthetic derivatives of podophyllotoxin, extracted from the mandrake root, *Podophyllum peltatum*. Examples of the vinca alkaloids are vincristine (Oncovin), vinblastine (Velban), and vindesine (Eldisine). Examples of epipodophyllotoxins are Etoposide (VP-16-213; VePesid) and teniposide (VM-26).

MECHANISMS OF ACTION

Vinca alkaloids bind to the cytoplasmic structural protein tubulin, an essential component of microtubules, which comprise the mitotic spindle apparatus and are involved in other cellular functions such as axonal transport in neurons. Binding of vinca alkaloids to tubulin results in the disruption of microtubule assembly, causing cycling cells to arrest in metaphase. Thus, these agents are cell cycle specific. Neuropathy, seen as the primary toxicity of these drugs, probably results from their action on microtubules in the long axon of nerves.

The epipodophyllotoxins also bind to tubulin but at a different site from that of the vinca alkaloids; however, they do not disrupt mitotic spindle assembly and, in contrast to the vinca alkaloids, cause cell cycle arrest at the S-G2 interface. The presence of single-strand DNA breaks led to the discovery that these agents inhibit topoisomerase II, an enzyme needed to effect DNA conformational changes during replication.

MECHANISM OF RESISTANCE

Mutations in tubulin resulting in decreased affinity for vinca alkaloids has been described. Vinca alkaloid efflux is also under the control of the P-170 glycoprotein and is subject to pleiotropic resistance, as are the epipodophyllotoxins. Resistance in the latter also may result from decreased topoisomerase II levels in the cell, decreased affinity of topoisomerase II for the drugs, or accelerated DNA repair mechanisms. Cells resistant to etoposide show complete cross-resistance to teniposide. However, vincristine and vinblastine, despite remarkable similarities in structure, do not exhibit cross-resistance.

Vincristine

Vincristine (Oncovin) is active primarily in hematologic malignancies. Its congener vinblastine has been used extensively in germ cell tumors but is being replaced by etoposide. Vindesine is a newer analogue whose role is being defined in clinical trials. Vincristine has shown significant activity in SCLC [16].

PHARMACOLOGY

About half an administered dosage of vincristine is plasma protein bound; the drug also has great affinity for blood elements, especially platelets. The plasma terminal half-life is about 150 minutes. Vincristine does not cross the blood-brain barrier. It is metabolized principally by the liver, and dosage adjustments are needed for hepatic dysfunction. Metabolic products appear rapidly in bile. About 70% is excreted in stool and only about 12% by the kidneys. Vincristine may decrease plasma phenytoin levels, which must be monitored in patients receiving it.

TOXICITY

Hematologic

Marrow suppression is mild in the usual dosing scheme. Platelet counts may actually rise (vinblastine has been explored, with little success, as a treatment for idiopathic thrombocytopenic purpura. Neutropenia was dosage limiting on a continuous IV infusion schedule of vincristine.

Gastrointestinal

Acute nausea and vomiting are unusual or mild. Constipation leading to obstipation, abdominal pain, and ileus leading to intestinal perforation may occur due to autonomic neuropathy. Anorexia is common. Aggressive laxative use and close monitoring are necessary. Mucositis may occur.

Dermatologic

Alopecia is usually reversible, with some hair growth even while patient is still on therapy.

Neurologic

Peripheral and autonomic neuropathy are cumulative and frequently dosage limiting. Risk factors include advanced age, preexisting neuromuscular disease, or use of concomitant neurotoxic drugs. Sensory paresthesias are the earliest symptoms, and loss of deep tendon reflexes the earliest sign. Progression to foot drop, wrist drop, ataxia, and paralysis may occur with continued treatment.

Severe cases can also be accompanied by cranial nerve palsies or seizures. While mild paresthesias or loss of deep tendon reflexes may not require drug discontinuation, more severe symptoms or progressive neuropathy, including autonomic neuropathies, require dosage reduction or discontinuation. In a recent study, coadministration of glutamic acid decreased vincristine toxicity [29].

Genitourinary

Bladder atony, incontinence, and urinary retention may occur as features of autonomic neuropathy.

Endocrine

The syndrome of inappropriate antidiuretic hormone (SIADH) with severe hyponatremia and seizures may occur uncommonly.

Local

These drugs are potent vesicants, and extreme caution is needed when peripheral IV lines are used.

Secondary Malignancies

Vincristine is mutagenic and presumed to be carcinogenic.

DOSAGES

Vials containing solutions of 1 mg, 2 mg, or 5 mg for reconstitution with sterile water or saline are available. The usual dosage is 1.4 mg/m^2 (maximum 2 mg) IV every 3 weeks.

Etoposide

Etoposide (VP-16-213, Vepesid) represents an important advance because of its relatively low toxicity. It is highly active in lymphomas and in germ cell tumors (where it is now a drug of choice). Numerous studies using a wide variety of dosages and schedules demonstrate it to be one of the most active agents in SCLC [23]. Equivalent oral dosages are twice those of IV dosages because of limited absorption. Daily oral dosages of 50 mg/m^2 in 14–21-day cycles are being used in SCLC for poor-risk patients.

PHARMACOLOGY

Rapid IV infusion or infusion of undiluted drug can result in acute hypotension and bronchospasm. Current recommendations call for infusion over at least 30 minutes. Furthermore, the drug is not fully miscible with aqueous solutions and must be agitated prior to infusion. After IV administration, etoposide exhibits a terminal half life of 4–11 hours. It crosses the blood-brain barrier poorly. It is highly protein bound in plasma, and decreased serum albumin causes increased renal clearance. Urine is the main source of excretion, with a minor fraction eliminated in stool. Dosages must be reduced in the presence of renal impairment. Only about 50% of an oral dosage is absorbed so the oral dosage must be doubled for equal bioavailability. The metabolism and excretion of orally and intravenously administered etoposide are otherwise similar.

TOXICITY

Hematologic

Marrow suppression is only mild to moderate but may constitute the dosage-limiting toxicity. It is not cumulative. Nadir neutrophil and platelet counts occur between 7 and 14 days and normalize within about 3 weeks.

Gastrointestinal

Nausea and vomiting are usually mild. Mucositis is uncommon.

Dermatologic

Reversible alopecia occurs frequently.

Cardiovascular

Hypotension may occur with rapid IV administration with no ECG changes or cardiac toxicity. If it occurs, infusion should be stopped immediately and the patient placed in the Trendelenburg position and given rapid IV fluid administration. The problem can be avoided by proper dilution and mixing of the drug and administration over at least 30 minutes.

Allergic

Allergic reactions characterized by fever, chills, tachycardia, and dyspnea occur in some patients within minutes of starting an infusion. It is usually reversible with IV diphenhydramine (Benadryl), after which resumption is usually uneventful. For severe reactions, discontinuation should be considered.

Neurologic

A mild peripheral neuropathy occurs in some patients; however, synergistic neurotoxicity may exist in the vinca alkaloids, and great caution should be exercised in patients treated previously with a vinca alkaloid.

Local

Etoposide is not a vesicant.

Secondary Malignancies

Despite few clinical data, etoposide is mutagenic and presumed to be carcinogenic.

DOSAGES

Liquid-filled capsules of 50 mg for oral administration, and vials of 100 mg/5 ml for IV administration are available. Dilution with 5% dextrose or saline to concentrations under 0.4 mg/ml is necessary to prevent precipitation. Intravenous doses are usually 100 mg/m^2

daily for 3 consecutive days or every other day for 3 days. Cycles are repeated every 3 weeks.

Investigational Agents

Some newer drugs under investigation appear to be active in lung cancer and will probably play roles in future management. One of these is edatrexate (10-ethyl-10-deaza-aminopterin), an antifol that is more greatly polyglutamated intracellularly than methotrexate and appears to enhance the activity of other chemotherapeutic agents in NSCLC [36]. Another drug of interest is camptothecan-11, a semisynthetic derivative of the plant alkaloid camptothecan, which had failed previous clinical trials. Camptothecans are potent inhibitors of topoisomerase I. It has exhibited significant activity in a phase II trial in NSCLC patients [20]. The novel antineoplastic drug taxol (Paclitaxel), derived from the bark of the western yew tree (*Taxus brevifolia*), has recently been marketed for treatment of ovarian cancer. Its activity is being explored in many other tumors, and preliminary data indicate significant activity in metastatic NSCLC [7]. Finally, retinoids such as 13-cis-retinoic acid and all-trans-retinoic acid, vitamin A analogues that induce terminal squamous differentiation in epithelial cells, are undergoing clinical trials in both SCLC and NSCLC. 13-cis-retinoic acid has been shown to prevent second primary squamous cell head and neck cancers in high-risk individuals [26].

Combination Chemotherapy Regimens in Lung Cancer

SMALL CELL LUNG CANCER

The superiority of multidrug compared to single-agent chemotherapy in SCLC has been clearly demonstrated [39]. Evidence for dosage intensification of individual drugs was also provided [10], although a more recent study failed to confirm this [31]. Several regimens are highly active in SCLC. Unfortunately, despite innumerable combinations and permutations of chemotherapy drugs, few significant improvements in outcome have occurred since the 1970s. Reported differences among studies are usually attributable to variability of patient prognostic factors rather than to the regimens themselves. Alternating regimens designed to be "non-cross resistant" have been tried; despite some conflicting results, survival does not appear to be improved by this approach [28]. Dosage intensification with cytokines such as granulocyte colony stimulating factor (GCSF) to maintain neutrophil counts have also failed to improve survival [13]. While higher response rates and lower toxicity (using neutropenia as the index of toxicity) have been claimed for cisplatinum-based regimens, no survival advantage has accrued [45].

One important recent finding is that prolonged courses of chemotherapy after maximum tumor response produces minimal survival prolongation in SCLC, especially considering the additional toxicity [50]. Since maximal tumor regression usually has occurred within the first 12 weeks after chemotherapy is instituted, treatment beyond 4–6 months is inadvisable.

Another recent finding of clinical relevance is that single-agent, oral etoposide is reasonably active and well tolerated in elderly or otherwise poor risk SCLC patients, including those refractory after prior treatment [24]. However, any survival advantage for this approach is modest at best. The role of this route and schedule in combination with other drugs has yet to be determined.

Small cell lung cancer is moderately sensitive to radiotherapy. Sequential chemotherapy and radiotherapy in patients with limited-stage disease results in good local control but no improvement in survival, with most patients relapsing outside the chest [33]. Concurrent chemotherapy and radiotherapy in patients with limited-stage disease appears to improve response rates and survival but at the cost of increased toxicity [4]. In a recent study, chemotherapy consisting of cis-platinum and etoposide with concurrent radiotherapy was better tolerated and produced more long-term survivors than previous regimens [41]. These findings require confirmation.

The other major role for radiotherapy in limited-stage SCLC is in prophylactic cranial irradiation (PCI) to prevent the emergence of brain metastases [44]. Since most chemotherapy drugs penetrate the blood-brain barrier poorly, the brain remains a sanctuary site for metastatic tumor. Only complete responders with a prospect for long-term survival should receive PCI because other patients will probably die of systemic disease rather than brain metastases. Significant toxicity may be associated with PCI, and not all investigators advocate its use [19].

A reasonable chemotherapy regimen for patients with SCLC might consist of etoposide 100mg/m^2 IV for 3 consecutive days, with cis-platinum 100 mg/m^2 IV on the first day. In the case of limited-stage disease, concurrent chest radiotherapy should be considered. At least four monthly cycles would be given in the absence of disease progression or undue toxicity. If a complete response were achieved, two additional cycles would be given as well as PCI. For patients with renal compromise or other contraindications to cis-platinum, carboplatin might be substituted at a dosage of 300 mg/m^2 IV on the first day of each cycle (but additional reductions would be needed for renal compromise, as discussed above). Regimens not containing a platinum coordinate compound include combinations of cyclophosphamide, doxorubicin, and etoposide (previously, vincristine would be used instead of etoposide) or cyclophosphamide, methotrexate, and lomustine.

NONSMALL CELL LUNG CANCER

The treatment of choice for NSCLC is surgery. Unfortunately, the majority of patients diagnosed with this disease are either inoperable or unresectable, and the relapse rate following curative resections is high. Radiotherapy may provide good palliation of symptoms caused by lung cancer, but it has not been demonstrated to extend survival.

Chemotherapy of unresectable NSCLC is unsatisfactory. Virtually all single agents considered active produce partial response rates in the range of 10–20%, with virtually no complete responses. Cis-platinum-based regimens have generally produced higher response rates than regimens not containing this drug [13]. Although numerous small trials in single institutions have reported high response rates for various regimens, larger trials suggest that the most active regimens produce overall response rates of around 30%, with under 5% complete responses and virtually no long-term survivors.

A randomized trial [46] compared four regimens considered most active in NSCLC: (1) cyclophosphamide, doxorubicin, methotrexate and procarbazine (CAMP); (2) mitomycin, vinblastine, and cis-platinum (MVP); (3) etoposide and cis-platinum (VP-P); and (4) vindesine and cis-platinum (VDA-P). Overall response rates were: CAMP, 17%; MVP, 31%; VP, 20%; and VDA-P, 25%. Only 15 complete responses were seen in the 486 patients entered, and the median survival of 24.5 weeks did not differ significantly among the four groups. An excess of treatment-related deaths was seen among patients who were performance status 2, suggesting that only fully ambulatory patients are suitable for treatment. This study illustrates the limitations of currently available chemotherapy in NSCLC.

Several randomized studies have looked at chemotherapy versus supportive care only in NSCLC [55]. These trials have demonstrated a small survival advantage (not statistically significant in all studies) for patients in the chemotherapy arm. However, none of the studies has performed adequate quality-of-life assessments to determine if these small differences warrant the toxicity, time, and expense of chemotherapy.

Radiotherapy clearly provides a palliative role in advanced NSCLC. Used as adjuvant treatment of locally advanced disease after complete resection, it may improve local control but does not prolong survival [40]. Several trials have explored the use of cis-platinum-based chemotherapy regimens with or without radiotherapy as adjuvant therapy for resected locally advanced tumors (those at high risk of recurrence). Some of these studies did demonstrate a survival advantage for the combined modality arm [34,49]. However, the survival curves at the times of publication of these studies suggest no clinically important increase in long-term survivors, and none of the studies provided adequate quality-of-life assessments to recommend this approach. Other studies have suggested no benefit from this approach [35,42].

Conclusions

Despite the responsiveness of SCLC to chemotherapy and radiotherapy, the ultimate outlook is dismal for the vast majority of patients. Newer drugs and approaches are needed. This is even more true for NSCLC. Chemotherapy should not routinely be recommended for patients with NSCLC outside the context of an investigational clinical trial. Emphasis on prevention is also more sensible than attempting to cure advanced disease; however, appropriate drugs and technology must be available. Obviously, the most effective step would be to convince smokers to quit their habit, but smoking-cessation strategies have thus far met with limited long-term success.

References

1. American Joint Committee on Cancer. *Manual for Staging of Cancer* (4th ed.). Philadelphia: J. B. Lippincott, 1992.
2. Boring, C. C., et al. Cancer statistics, 1991. *CA* 41:19–36, 1991.
3. Bunn, P. A., Jr. Review of therapeutic trials of carboplatin in lung cancer. *Semin. Oncol.* 16 (Suppl. 5):27–33, 1989.
4. Bunn, Jr., P. A., et al. Chemotherapy alone or chemotherapy with chest radiation therapy in limited stage small cell lung cancer. *Ann. Intern. Med.* 106:655–662, 1987.
5. Calvert, A. H., et al. Carboplatin dosage: Prospective evaluation of a simple formula based on renal function. *J. Clin. Oncol.* 7:1748–1856, 1989.
6. Champlin, R. E., and Gale, R. P. Role of bone marrow transplantation in the treatment of hematologic malignancies and solid tumors: Critical review of syngeneic, autologous and allogeneic transplants. *Cancer Treat. Rep.* 68:145–161, 1984.
7. Chang, A., et al. Phase II study of taxol in patients with stage IV non-small cell lung cancer (NSCLC): The Eastern Cooperative Oncology Group (ECOG) results. *Proc. Am. Soc. Clin. Oncol.* 11:293, 1992.
8. Cheson, B. D., et al. Autologous bone marrow transplantation. *Ann. Intern. Med.* 110:51–65, 1989.
9. Cohen, M. H. Influence of tumor burden on red blood cell deformability in small cell lung cancer patients. *Ann. Clin. Res.* 13:387–391, 1981.
10. Cohen, M. H., et al. Intensive chemotherapy of small cell bronchogenic carcinoma. *Cancer Treat. Rev.* 61:349–354, 1977.
11. Cohen, M. H., et al. Laboratory parameters as an alternative to performance status in prognostic stratification of patients with small cell lung cancer. *Cancer Treat. Rep.* 65:187–195, 1981.
12. Constine, L. S., et al. Protection by WR-2721 of human bone marrow function following irradiation. *J. Radiat. Biol. Oncol. Phys.* 12:1505–1508, 1986.
13. Crawford, J., et al. Reduction by granulocyte colony-stimulating factor of fever and neutropenia induced by chemotherapy in patients small-cell lung cancer. *N. Engl. J. Med.* 325:164–170, 1991.
14. DeVita, V. T., et al. Carbone PP: Combination chemotherapy in the treatment of advanced Hodgkin's disease. *Ann. Intern. Med.* 73:891–895, 1970.

15. Dewys, W. D., et al. Prognostic effect of weight loss prior to chemotherapy in cancer patients. *Am. J. Med.* 69:491–497, 1980.

16. Dombernowsky, P., et al. Vincristine (NSC-67574) in the treatment of small-cell anaplastic carcinoma of the lung. *Cancer Treat. Rep.* 60:239–240, 1976.

17. Edmonson, J. H., et al. Cyclophosphamide and CCNU in the treatment of inoperable small cell carcinoma of the lung. *Cancer Treat. Rep.* 60:925–932, 1976.

18. Ensley, J. F., et al. Correlation between response to cisplatinum-combination chemotherapy and subsequent radiotherapy in previously untreated patients with advanced squamous cell cancers of the head and neck. *Cancer* 54:811–814, 1984.

19. Fleck, J. F., et al. Is prophylactic cranial irradiation indicated in small-cell lung cancer? *J. Clin. Oncol.* 8:209–214, 1990.

20. Fukuoka, M., et al. A Phase II study of CPT-11, a new derivative of camptothecin, for previously untreated non-small-cell lung cancer. *J. Clin. Oncol.* 10:16–20, 1992.

21. Glaspy, J. A., and Golde, D. W. The colony-stimulating factors: Biology and clinical use. *Oncology* 4:25–32, 1990.

22. Goldstein, L. J., et al. Expression of a multidrug resistance gene in human cancers. *J. Natl. Cancer Inst.* 81:116–124, 1989.

23. Grant, S. C., et al. Single-agent chemotherapy trials in small-cell lung cancer, 1970 to 1990: The case for studies in previously treated patients. *J. Clin. Oncol.* 10:484–498, 1992.

24. Greco, F. A., et al. Chronic daily administration of oral etoposide. *Semin. Oncol.* 17 (Suppl. 12):71–74, 1990.

25. Hande, K. R., et al. Randomized study of high-dose versus low-dose methotrexate in the treatment of extensive small cell lung cancer. *Am. J, Med* 73:413–419, 1982.

26. Hong, W. K., et al. Prevention of second primary tumors with isotretinoin in squamous-cell carcinoma of the head and neck. *N. Engl. J. Med.* 323:795–800, 1992.

27. Huet, S., and Robert, J. The reversal of doxorubicin resistance by verapamil is not due to an effect on calcium channels. *Int. J. Cancer* 41:283–286, 1988.

28. Ihde, D. C. Drug therapy: Chemotherapy of lung cancer. *N. Engl. J. Med.* 327:1434–1441, 1992.

29. Jackson, D. V., et al. Amelioration of vincristine neurotoxicity by glutamic acid. *Am. J. Med.* 84:1016–1022, 1988.

30. Jain, R. K. Determinants of tumor blood flow: A review. *Cancer Res.* 48:2641–2658, 1988.

31. Johnson, D. H., et al. A randomized comparison of high-dose versus conventional-dose cyclophosphamide, doxorubicin and vincristine for extensive-stage small-cell lung cancer: A phase III study of the Southeast Cancer Study Group. *J. Clin. Oncol.* 5:1731–1738, 1987.

32. Karnofsky, D. A., et al. The use of nitrogen mustards in the palliative treatment of carcinoma. *Cancer* 1:634–656, 1948.

33. Kies, M. S., et al. Multimodality therapy for limited small-cell lung cancer: A randomized study of induction combination chemotherapy with or without radiation in complete responders; and with wide-field versus reduced-field radiation in partial responders. *J. Clin. Oncol.* 5:592–600, 1987.

34. Lad, T., et al. The benefit of adjuvant treatment for resected, locally advanced non-small-cell lung cancer. *J. Clin. Oncol.* 6:9–17, 1988.

35. Le Chevalier, T., et al. Radiotherapy alone versus combined chemotherapy and radiotherapy in nonresectable non-small-cell lung cancer: First analysis of a randomized trial in 353 patients. *J. Natl. Cancer Inst.* 83:417–423, 1991.

36. Lee, J. S., et al. Edatrexate improves the antitumor effects of cyclophosphamide and cisplatin against non-small cell lung cancer. *Cancer* 68:959–964, 1991.

37. Lird, A. K. The dynamics of tumor growth. *Br. J. Cancer.* 28:490–502, 1966.

38. Lowenbraun, S., et al. The superiority of combination chemotherapy over single agent chemotherapy in small cell lung carcinoma. *Cancer* 44:406–413, 1979.

39. Lowenbraun, S., et al. Combination chemotherapy in small cell lung carcinoma: A randomized study of two intensive regimens. *Cancer* 54:2344–2350, 1984.

40. The Lung Cancer Study Group: Effects of postoperative mediastinal radiation on completely resected stage II and stage III epidermoid cancer of the lung. *N. Engl. J. Med.* 315:1377–1381, 1986.

41. McCracken, J. D., et al. Concurrent chemotherapy/radiotherapy for limited small-cell lung carcinoma: A Southwest Oncology Group Study. *J. Clin. Oncol.* 8:892–898, 1990.

42. Mattison, K., et al. Inoperable non-small cell lung cancer: Radiation with or without chemotherapy. *Eur. J. Cancer. Clin. Oncol.* 24:477–482, 1988.

43. Mosteller, R. D. Simplified calculation of body surface area. *N. Engl. J. Med.* 317:1098, 1987.

44. Rosen, S. T., et al. Role of prophylactic cranial irradiation in prevention of central nervous system metastases in small cell lung cancer. *Am. J. Med.* 74:615–624, 1983.

45. Roth, B. J., et al. Randomized study of cyclophosphamide, doxorubicin, and vincristine versus etoposide and cisplatinum versus alternation of these two regimens in extensive small-cell lung cancer: A phase III trial of the Southeastern Cancer Study Group. *J. Clin. Oncol.* 10:282–291, 1992.

46. Ruckdeschel, J. C., et al. A randomized trial of the four most active regimens for metastatic non-small-cell lung cancer. *J. Clin. Oncol.* 4:14–22, 1986.

47. Samson, M. K., et al. Mitomycin C in advanced adenocarcinoma and large cell carcinoma of the lung. *Cancer Treat. Rep.* 62:163–165, 1978.

48. Shackney, S. E., et al. Growth patterns of solid tumors and their

relation to responsiveness to therapy: An analytical review. *Ann. Intern. Med* 89:107–121, 1978.

49. Soresi, E., et al. A randomized clinical trial comparing radiation therapy v radiation therapy plus cis-dichlorodiammine platinum (II) in the treatment of locally advanced non-small cell lung cancer. *Semin. Oncol.* 15:20–25, 1988.
50. Spiro, S. G., et al. Duration of chemotherapy in small cell lung cancer: A cancer research campaign trial. *Br. J. Cancer.* 59:578–583, 1989.
51. Stanley, K. E. Prognostic factors for survival in patients with inoperable lung cancer. *J. Natl. Cancer Inst.* 65:25–32, 1980.
52. Van Echo, D. A., et al. The pharmacology of carboplatin. *Semin. Oncol.* 16 (Suppl. 5):1–6, 1992.
53. Vichi, P., and Tritton, T. R. Adriamycin: Protection from cell death by removal of extracellular drug. *Cancer Res.* 52:4135–4138, 1992.
54. Vincent, R. G., et al. Evaluation of methotrexate in the treatment of bronchogenic carcinoma. *Cancer* 36:873–880, 1975.
55. Vokes, E. E., et al. Role of systemic therapy in advanced non-small-cell lung cancer. *Am. J. Med.* 89:777–786, 1990.

11

Kaposi's Sarcoma

John F. Wiley
Samuel V. Spagnolo

First described in 1872, Kaposi's sarcoma was a rare disease in the United States and was seen only occasionally in patients of Eastern European, Italian, or Russian descent. However, during the 1980s, with the onset of acquired immunodeficiency syndrome (AIDS) epidemic, the incidence of Kaposi's sarcoma greatly increased. By 1993, more than 24,000 cases of AIDS-associated Kaposi's sarcoma were reported to the Centers for Disease Control [2,16]. Over 95% of AIDS-associated Kaposi's sarcoma are seen in homosexual or bisexual men.

Clinically, there are four categories of Kaposi's sarcoma: classic, endemic African, iatrogenic (seen in transplant recipients on immunosuppressive therapy), and AIDS associated. The last group is by far the most common type seen in the United States. The AIDS-associated Kaposi's sarcoma is also more widespread in the body than the other forms, and it can involve the skin and mucous membranes, lymph nodes, and various organ systems such as the GI tract and the lung.

Kaposi's sarcoma lesions appear as blue to reddish nodules, macules, or plaques. Histopathologically, these lesions consist of pleomorphic perivascular spindle cells and vascular structures. There is an inflammatory picture in early lesions; however, this usually subsides as the lesion develops. The origin of the spindle cell remains controversial, but recent data suggest that is is derived from a mesenchymal precursor for smooth muscle [23,24].

Pulmonary Involvement

Lung involvement in patients with AIDS-associated Kaposi's sarcoma is common; many cases remain undiagnosed until autopsy.

The incidence of lung involvement is estimated to be between 18 and 40% [16,19,21,27]. Several studies suggest that the pulmonary involvement with Kaposi's sarcoma carries a worse prognosis [10,16]. Almost all patients with lung involvement from Kaposi's sarcoma will have preexisting cutaneous involvement, but there are reported cases of isolated pulmonary involvement [18].

The clinical presentation of pulmonary Kaposi's sarcoma is similar to that of an opportunistic pneumonia [1,4] and can present with a variety of respiratory complaints, such as dry cough, dyspnea, chest pain, and hemoptysis [4,7].

Diagnosis of lung involvement with Kaposi's sarcoma is determined by visualization of the characteristic endobronchial lesion during fiberoptic bronchoscopy. The finding of such a lesion is diagnostic in the setting of clinical AIDS [3,4]. In a recent study, 19 of 20 patients with pulmonary Kaposi's sarcoma had endobronchial lesions [7]. The chest roentgenograms are also abnormal in these patients. In this same report, 80% of patients demonstrated interstitial infiltrates, and 50% had hilar adenopathy by chest roentgenogram. The interstitial infiltrates were somewhat more nodular and progressed more slowly than those seen as a result of *Pneumocystis carinii* pneumonia [27].

Treatment

Pre-AIDS, the treatment of Kaposi's sarcoma usually involved local therapy due to the nonaggressive nature of tumor [2]. For this reason, little information was available regarding the systemic therapy of the more aggressive Kaposi's sarcoma that is seen in AIDS patients. Currently, two types of systemic therapy are commonly used (in addition to antiretroviral therapy): (1) treatment with chemotherapy agents such as adriamycin, bleomycin, and vincristine and (2) the use of the immune modulator alpha-interferon.

Response rates following treatment now range from 26% to 88% [6,8,15,25]. Since there is currently no uniform staging system for the treatment of Kaposi's sarcoma, comparisons among studies are difficult [2]. Furthermore, the treatments may actually decrease survival by increasing the rate of opportunistic infections since no control groups have been used. A recent study compared treatment with adriamycin alone versus adriamycin plus bleomycin and vincristine (ABV) [8]. The authors found a significantly higher response rate with ABV (88%) than with adriamycin alone (48%). There were similar toxicities in both groups. In the same study, only a small percentage of patients developed opportunistic infections during treatment. Despite treatment, the duration of the response and survival were both poor.

Alpha-interferon has activity against AIDS-associated Kaposi's sarcoma used alone or in combination with zidovudine. Using high dosages, response rates of up to 50% have been seen, with longer durations of response than seen in the chemotherapy group [9,22,26]. Alpha-interferon has been used for maintenance therapy following treatment with combination chemotherapy using ABV [5].

The following guidelines suggested by Kahn et al. are based on the patient's immune status [11]:

1. Patients with CD_4 counts greater than 500/mm^3 should be treated with local therapy.
2. Patients with CD_4 counts of 200–500/mm^3 should receive alpha-interferon in combination with zidovudine. If this treatment is ineffective, systemic chemotherapy should be tried.
3. CD_4 counts below 200/mm^3 will need systemic chemotherapy.

These authors also point out that this treatment is palliative and not curative.

Bleomycin

PHARMACOKINETICS AND CLINICAL INDICATIONS

Bleomycin (Blenoxane), a water-soluble toxic antimicrobial isolated from *Streptomyces verticillus,* probably works by inhibiting DNA synthesis. It has activity against AIDS-associated Kaposi's sarcoma as a single agent [14] or in combination with adriamycin and vinblastine [15], viscristine [6], or adriamycin and vincristine [8]. The drug must be given parenterally. Bleomycin is mainly eliminated through the kidney, and its half-life is approximately 2 hours in a patient with a normal creatinine clearance.

DOSAGE AND ADMINISTRATION

Following a test dose, bleomycin is given in dosages of 5–10 mg/m^2 in cycles of 2–4 weeks [6,8,14,15].

ADVERSE EFFECTS

The most serious side effect of bleomycin is a pneumonitis (occurring in about 10% of patients on bleomycin), which can progress to pulmonary fibrosis. Approximately 1% of patients treated with bleomycin die of pulmonary fibrosis. Patients with bleomycin-induced pulmonary fibrosis are at a much higher risk of oxygen toxicity; this can occur at oxygen levels that are usually considered safe. The most common side effects from bleomycin are skin and mucous membrane abnormalities, seen in 50% of patients.

Doxorubicin

PHARMACOKINETICS

Doxorubicin (Adriamycin), a cytoxic anthracycline antimicrobial isolated from strains of *Streptomyces peucetius,* works by binding to DNA and inhibiting nucleic acid synthesis. Doxorubicin is given intravenously, and its major excretory route is through the bile. After intravenous infusion, doxorubicin is cleared rapidly from the plasma and undergoes significant tissue binding.

Caution: Extravasation of doxorubicin during administration can cause severe cellulitis and even tissue necrosis.

CLINICAL INDICATIONS

Doxorubicin is effective in treating AIDS-associated Kaposi's sarcoma in combination with bleomycin and vincristine [8]. It can also be used with bleomycin and vinblastine [15] or as a single agent [8].

DOSAGE AND ADMINISTRATION

The dosage of doxorubicin used is 20–40 mg/m^2 as a single IV injection [18,11,19]. (See Chap. 10.)

ADVERSE EFFECTS

The major side effects of doxorubicin are myelosuppression and cardiotoxicity; the latter occurs as total dosages approach 550 mg/m^2. Other systemic side effects are reversible alopecia, nausea and vomiting, and occasional hypersensitivity reactions. Cumulative cardiac toxicity occurs regularly as cumulative dosages exceed 500 mg/m^2. Elderly patients may develop cardiac toxicity at lower dosages. A decrease in cardiac ejection fraction is an early sign of doxorubicin toxicity.

Etoposide

PHARMACOKINETICS

Etoposide, or VP-16 (Vepesid) is a semisynthetic derivative of podophyllotoxin, which works by inhibiting DNA synthesis. It can be given N or PO. Its terminal elimination half-life is 4–11 hours. Etoposide is excreted mainly through the kidney (although some is excreted in the bile, and some is metabolized).

CLINICAL INDICATIONS

Etoposide has activity against AIDS-associated Kaposi's sarcoma as a single agent [15]. In that study, patients were treated with 150 mg/m^2 IV daily for 3 days, with the dosages repeated every 28 days. Infusion should be given over at least 30 minutes.

ADVERSE EFFECTS (See also Chap. 10.)

The most common adverse effects of etoposide are nausea and vomiting, alopecia, anorexia, diarrhea, and myelosuppression. Bone marrow recovery occurs by day 20 with no cumulative effect. Rapid IV infusion may cause acute hypotension and bronchospasm.

Alpha-Interferon

PHARMACOKINETICS AND CLINICAL USE

Recombinant alpha-interferon (Roferon-A, INTRON) is a water-soluble protein that has anti-HIV activity and is effective in treating AIDS-associated Kaposi's sarcoma. It can be given by intralesional, IM, or SC injection [11]. The peak serum dose occurs 3–12 hours following injection, and its half-life is 2–3 hours.

DOSAGE AND ADMINISTRATION

Alpha-interferon's effectiveness and toxicities are both dosage related; the best response is seen with dosages of 30–36 million units/day IM [22]. The best-tolerated doses are 5 million units/day IM [12]. The effect of alpha-interferon at low dosages can be enhanced by combining it with zidovudine therapy [12].

ADVERSE EFFECTS

The major side effect of alpha-interferon is a combination of flulike symptoms (including fever) seen commonly at high dosages. Fatigue, headache, anorexia, confusion, dyspnea, and GI disturbances are also seen.

Vinblastine

PHARMACOKINETICS

Vinblastine (Velban) an alkaloid extract from the periwinkle, works by interfering with microtubule formation in the mitotic spindle, thus arresting cell division in metaphase.

CLINICAL INDICATIONS

Vinblastine was one of the first chemotherapeutic drugs used in the treatment of AIDS-associated Kaposi's sarcoma [11] and can be used both as a single agent [25] or in combination with adriamycin and bleomycin [15]. Vinblastine must be given transvenously, as extravasation can cause cellulitis; its major route of elimination is probably through the bile.

DOSAGE AND ADMINISTRATION

The dosage of vinblastine is dependent on the amount of leukopenia that it causes. In one study, a starting dosage of 4 mg IV weekly was given; this was increased weekly until the leukocyte count dropped, that dosage being titrated to maintain a total leukocyte count of greater than 2500 cells/mm^3 [25]. (The median dosage is usually 6 mg.)

ADVERSE EFFECTS

The most common adverse reaction of vinblastine is leukopenia; in addition, alopecia, constipation, hypertension, paresthesis, headaches, convulsions, malaise, and bone pain may be seen.

Vincristine

PHARMACOKINETICS

Vincristine (Oncovin), also an alkaloid obtained from the periwinkle plant, works by inhibiting microtubule formation in the mitotic spindle, thus arresting cell division in metaphase. Vincristine also must be given IV since extravasation can cause irritation; the major route of elimination is through the bile. It should never be given intrathecally, as this can cause death. Vincristine has great affinity for blood elements, especially platelets. Vincristine does not cross blood-brain barrier and dosage adjustments are needed for hepatic dysfunction.

CLINICAL INDICATIONS

Vincristine can be used as a single agent in the treatment of AIDS-associated Kaposi's sarcoma [17] or in combination with bleomycin [6] or with adriamycin and bleomycin [8].

DOSAGE AND ADMINISTRATION

The usual dosage is 1.4 mg/m^2 given IV every 2 to 3 weeks, with 2 mg the maximum dosage [6,18].

ADVERSE EFFECTS (See also Chap. 10.)

The side effects of vincristine are usually dosage-related and reversible. The most common side effect is alopecia; the most serious are neuromuscular, such as paresthesia, difficulty walking, loss of deep tendon reflexes, and muscle wasting. Also seen are leukopenia, constipation, anorexia, and hypersensitivity reactions. Severe shortness of breath and bronchospasm have been reported after administration of the drug, usually in combination with mitimycin-C.

References

1. Baum, G. L., and Wolinsky, E. *Textbook of Pulmonary Diseases* (4th ed.). Boston: Little, Brown, 1989.
2. DeVita, V. T., et al. *AIDS: Etiology, Diagnosis, Treatment and Prevention* (3d ed.) Philadelphia: JB Lippincott, 1992.
3. Fouret, P. J., et al. Pulmonary Kaposi's sarcoma in patients with acquired immunodeficiency syndrome: A clinicopathologic study. *Thorax* 42:262–268, 1987.
4. Garay, S. M., et al. Pulmonary manifestations of Kaposi's sarcoma. *Chest* 91:39–43, 1987.
5. Gill, P. A. Phase I/II trials of alpha-interferon alone or in combination with zidovudine as maintenance therapy following induction chemotherapy in the treatment of acquired immunodeficiency syndrome-related Kaposi's sarcoma. *Semin. Oncol.* 18 (Suppl. 7):53–57, 1991.
6. Gill, P., et al. Treatment of advanced Kaposi's sarcoma using a combination of bleomycin and vincristine. *Am. J. Clin. Oncol.* 13:315–319, 1990.
7. Gill, P. S., et al. Pulmonary Kaposi's sarcoma: Clinical findings and results of therapy. *Am. J. Med.* 87:57–61, 1989.
8. Gill, P. S., et al. Systemic treatment of AIDS-related Kaposi's sarcoma: Results of a randomized trial. *Am. J. Med.* 90:427–433, 1991.
9. Groopman, J. E., et al. Recombinant alpha-2 interferon therapy for Kaposi's sarcoma associated with acquired immunodeficiency syndrome. *Ann. Intern. Med.* 100:671–676, 1984.
10. Hamm, P. G., et al. Diagnosis of pulmonary Kaposi's sarcoma with

fiberoptic bronchoscopy and endobronchial biopsy. *Cancer* 59:807–810, 1987.

11. Kahn, J. D., et al. AIDS-associated Kaposi's sarcoma. *AIDS Clin. Rev.* New York: Marcel Dekker. Pp. 261–280, 1992.
12. Kovacs, J. A., et al. Combined zidovudine and interferon-alpha in patients with Kaposi's sarcoma and the acquired immunodeficiency syndrome (AIDS). *Ann. Intern. Med.* 111:280–287, 1989.
13. Krigel, R., et al. Kaposi's sarcoma: A new staging classification. *Cancer Treat. Rep.* 67:531–534, 1983.
14. Lassoued, K., et al. Treatment of the acquired immune deficiency syndrome–related Kaposi's sarcoma with bleomycin as a single agent. *Cancer* 66:1869, 1990.
15. Laubenstein, L. J., et al. Treatment of epidemic Kaposi's sarcoma with etoposide or a combination of doxorubicin, bleomycin, and vincristine. *J. Clin. Oncol.* 2:1115–1120, 1984.
16. Meduri, G. U., et al. Pulmonary Kaposi's sarcoma in the acquired immunodeficiency syndrome. *Am. J. Med.* 81:11–18, 1986.
17. Mintzer, D. M., et al. Treatment of Kaposi's sarcoma and thrombocytopenia with vincristine in patients with the acquired immunodeficiency syndrome. *Ann. Intern. Med.* 102:200–202, 1985.
18. Nash, G., and Fligiel, S. Kaposi's sarcoma presenting as pulmonary disease in the acquired immunodeficiency syndrome: Diagnosis by lung biopsy. *Hum. Pathol.* 15:999–1001, 1984.
19. Ognibene, F. P., and Shelhamer, J. Kaposi's sarcoma. *Clin. Chest Med.* 9:459–465, 1988.
20. *Physician's Desk Reference* (47th ed.). Oradell, NJ: Medical Economics Co., 1993.
21. Pitchnik, A. E., et al. Kaposi's sarcoma of the tracheobronchial tree. *Chest* 87:122–124, 1985.
22. Real, F. X., et al. Kaposi's sarcoma and the acquired immunodeficiency syndrome: Treatment with high and low doses of recombinant leukocyte A interferon. *J. Clin. Oncol.* 4:544–551, 1986.
23. Salahuddin, S. Z., et al. Angiogenic properties of Kaposi's sarcoma–derived cells after long-term culture in vitro. *Science* 242:430–433, 1988.
24. Thompson, E. W., et al. Supernatants of acquired immunodeficiency syndrome–related Kaposi's sarcoma cells induce endothelial cell chemotaxis and invasiveness. *Cancer Res.* 51:2670–2676, 1991.
25. Volberding, P. A., et al. Vinblastine therapy for Kaposi's sarcoma in the acquired immunodeficiency syndrome. *Ann. Intern. Med.* 103:335–338, 1985.
26. Volberding, P. A., et al. Treatment of Kaposi's sarcoma with interferon alpha-2b (Intron A). *Cancer* 59:620–625, 1987.
27. Zibrak, J. D., et al. Bronchoscopic and radiologic features of Kaposi's sarcoma involving the respiratory system. *Chest* 90:476–479, 1986.

12

Asthma During Pregnancy

Samuel V. Spagnolo
Richard A. Nicklas

Although there was concern in the past about an association between increased perinatal mortality and morbidity and maternal asthma, recent information suggests that optimal control of asthma during pregnancy actually reduces this risk [3,11]. In addition, emerging data show that the currently accepted goals of asthma therapy are beneficial for the fetus, as well as for the mother.

Asthma severity may increase, decrease, or remain unchanged during pregnancy. Some studies suggest that women with more severe asthma are more prone to face increased asthma severity during pregnancy. The course of asthma during a previous pregnancy may not be helpful in predicting the patient's course, since only about 60% of patients react in a similar way in regard to the course of asthma with successive pregnancies [7].

Treatment

The avoidance of known asthmatic triggers is particularly important during pregnancy. An asthmatic patient should discontinue smoking since smoking not only aggravates asthma but has a direct adverse effect on the fetus and the course of pregnancy [1,2,9].

The choice of medications for use during pregnancy is based on available information about their gestational use and their efficacy in asthma, as well as the knowledge that their use during pregnancy is less than the risk of the uncontrolled asthma that could result if they were not used [5]. When treating the pregnant asthmatic patient, it is important to discuss with the patient the risks of uncontrolled asthma in the mother and the fetus, the alternative asthma medications available, and the rationale for choosing among those alternatives. For example, based mainly on animal data, cromolyn and terbutaline have a better risk factor rating than beclomethasone [4,6].

Recommendations for the stepwise pharmacologic management of chronic asthma during pregnancy (with no demonstrable evidence of a concurrent infection or self-limited triggering factor) in the generally recommended order of trial according to increasing severity of asthma is as follows:

Terbutaline (beta agonist)
Cromolyn
Theophylline
Prednisone

Based on animal studies, terbutaline has a safer teratogenic profile, but there are no human data that indicate that one beta agonist is safer than another. For inhalation use two metered-dose inhalations (MDI) q4h as needed up to 8 MDI per day are recommended.

Patients requiring regular inhaled beta agonist medication should initially receive inhaled cromolyn. If a 1-month trial of cromolyn is ineffective, beclomethasone should be substituted or added, and if this is not adequate, regular oral theophylline should be added. Oral prednisone should be used in short courses or chronically at the lowest effective dosage if asthma is not controlled with beta agonists, cromolyn, and theophylline. The use of prednisone will ultimately depend on factors such as the severity of the asthma-triggering events and the clinical course and response of previous acute asthma episodes for each patient.

Patients adequately controlled on theophylline prior to pregnancy and who have not previously received cromolyn or beclomethasone might warrant trials on those medications during pregnancy. Such an approach should also be considered if (1) the patient has nausea, gastroesophageal reflux, or gestational hypertension, which might be exacerbated by theophylline; (2) the patient is experiencing other theophylline side effects; (3) there is concern about the compliance of the patient; and (4) subjective and objective indexes of severity dictate the need for additional therapy.

Antimicrobials

Antimicrobials are used only when there is evidence of infection. Tetracyclines are **contraindicated** during pregnancy. Sinusitis-induced exacerbations of asthma may represent a particular indication for use of antimicrobials since (1) sinusitis has been reported to be six times more common during pregnancy than in nonpregnant patients [10] and (2) the classic signs of sinusitis may be absent in approximately half of the women with documented sinusitis during pregnancy.

Severe Intractable Asthma

We currently define severe intractable asthma as persistent asthma that fails to improve or continues to worsen while the patient is receiving optimal initial dosages of inhaled or injected sympathomimetics (and possible IV aninophylline). Severe asthma may develop quite rapidly and occasionally move from a mild attack to a fatal outcome in a matter of minutes. Refractory asthma requires prompt recognition and an understanding of the physiologic abnormalities occurring as a consequence of increasing airflow resistance. Early in an asthmatic exacerbation, ventilation/perfusion mismatches are the predominant physiologic abnormality, and the arterial pO_2 will decrease. Therefore, oxygen administration is indicated in patients with intractable asthma. Early in the treatment of intractable asthma, parenteral and inhaled sympathomimetic agents are equally effective in most patients. However, parenteral sympathomimetic agents are indicated for patients who are not ventilating well enough to deliver adequate amounts of nebulized drug to the lower respiratory tract.

Nearly all patients with intractable asthma will require corticosteroid administration (see Chapter 1). Severe intractable asthma occurring during pregnancy that results in respiratory failure should probably be treated in an intensive care unit setting. Specific management will depend on the severity of the respiratory impairment, but careful and frequent monitoring of the patient is essential. The pharmacologic agents used in the treatment of severe intractable asthma during pregnancy have been previously described in Chapter 1.

Summary

1. During a normal pregnancy, a compensated respiratory alkolosis (normal pH) will develop, and patients will have a slightly higher pO_2 and a slightly lower pCO_2 than in the nonpregnant state.
2. The finding of a pCO_2 greater than 35 or a pO_2 less than 70 associated with acute asthma may represent a more severe respiratory compromise during pregnancy than would similar arterial blood gases in the nonpregnant state.
3. In patients with intractable severe asthma, use parenteral sympathomimetic agents when patients are not ventilating well enough to deliver adequate amounts of inhaled drug to the lower respiratory tract.
4. A lag time of several hours may occur before any clinical effect is noted after parenteral corticosteroid administration.
5. Large negative peak intrapleural pressures and overhydration increase the possibility of pulmonary interstitial edema and alveolar edema occurring during the treatment of severe intractable asthma.

References

1. Brooke, O. G., et al. Effects on birth weight of smoking, alcohol, caffeine, socioeconomic factors, and psychosocial stress. *Br. Med. J.* 298:795–801, 1989.
2. Cnattinquis, S., et al. Cigarette smoking as risk factor for late fetal and early neonatal deaths. *Br. Med. J.* 297:258–261, 1988.
3. Fitzsimmons, R., et al. Outcome of pregnancy in women requiring corticosteroids for severe asthma. *J. Allergy Clin. Immunol.* 78:349–353, 1986.
4. Greenberger, P. A., and Patterson, R. Beclomethasone dipropriate for severe asthma during pregnancy. *Ann. Intern. Med.* 98:478, 1983.
5. Mawhinney, H., and Spector, S. L. Optimum management of asthma in pregnancy. *Drugs* 32:1786–1787, 1986.
6. Schatz, M. Asthma during pregnancy: Interrelationships and management. *Ann. Allergy* 68:123–133, 1992.

7. Schatz, M., et al. The course of asthma during pregnancy, postpartum, and with successive pregnancies; a prospective analysis. *J. Allergy Clin. Immunol.* 81:509–517, 1988.

8. Schatz, M., et al. The Course and Management of Asthma and Allergic Diseases during Pregnancy. In E. Middleton, Jr., et al. (eds.), *Allergy Principles and Practice* (3d ed.). St. Louis: C. V. Mosby, 1988.

9. Shiono, P. H., et al. Smoking and drinking during pregnancy: Their effects on pre-term birth. *JAMA* 255:8284, 1986.

10. Sorri, M., et al. Rhinitis during pregnancy. *Rhinology* 18:83, 1980.

11. Stenius-Aarnicala, B., et al. Asthma in pregnancy: A prospective study of 198 pregnancies. *Thorax* 43:12–18, 1988.

Index

UNIVERSITY OF IOWA
3 1858 052 030 149